OPPORTUNISTIC INFECTIONS IN PATIENTS WITH THE ACQUIRED IMMUNODEFICIENCY SYNDROME

INFECTIOUS DISEASE AND THERAPY

Series Editors

Brian E. Scully, M.B., B.Ch.

College of Physicians
and Surgeons
Columbia University
New York, New York

Harold C. Neu, M.D.

College of Physicians
and Surgeons
Columbia University
New York, New York

Additional Volumes in Preparation

OPPORTUNISTIC INFECTIONS IN PATIENTS WITH THE ACQUIRED IMMUNODEFICIENCY SYNDROME

edited by

GIFFORD LEOUNG
University of California, San Francisco
San Francisco, California

JOHN MILLS
University of California, San Francisco
and
San Francisco General Hospital
San Francisco, California

MARCEL DEKKER   New York and Basel

Library of Congress Cataloging-in-Publication Data

Opportunistic infections in patients with the acquired immunodeficiency
    syndrome / edited by Gifford Leoung and John Mills.
        p. cm. — — (Infectious disease and therapy ; v. 3)
    Includes index.
    ISBN 0-8247-8080-9 (alk. paper)
        1. AIDS (Disease) 2. Opportunistic infections. I. Leoung
Gifford. II. Mills, John. III. Series.
        [DNLM: 1. Acquired Immunodeficiency Syndrome——complications.
2. Infection——complications.   W1 IN406HMN v. 3 / WD 308 062]
RC607.A26067 1989
616.97'92——dc20
DNLM/DLC
for Library of Congress   89-7793
                                                                            CIP

This book is printed on acid-free paper.

MARCEL DEKKER, INC.
270 Madison Avenue, New York, New York 10016

Current printing (last digit):
10 9 8 7 6 5 4 3 2 1

PRINTED IN THE UNITED STATES OF AMERICA

Series Introduction

Marcel Dekker, Inc., has for many years specialized in the publication of high-quality monographs in tightly focused areas in a variety of medical disciplines. These have been of great value to both the practicing physician and the research scientist as sources of detailed and up-to-date information presented in an attractive format. During the last decade, there has been a veritable explosion in knowledge in the various fields related to infectious diseases and clinical microbiology. Antimicrobial resistance, antibacterial and antiviral agents, AIDS, Lyme disease, infections in immunocompromised patients, and parasitic diseases are but a few of the areas in which an enormous amount of significant work has been published. This new Infectious Disease and Therapy series will cover carefully chosen topics which should be of interest and value to the practicing physician, the clinical microbiologist, and the research scientist.

Brian E. Scully, M.B., B.Ch.
Harold C. Neu, M.D.

Foreword

The epidemic of HIV infection poses challenges to the medical system that we are still just beginning to appreciate. We find ourselves asked to respond to an ever-growing number of patients infected with the virus for which we have no uniformly effective therapy—a virus which in the absence of this treatment may kill most of those affected. Moreover, many of these patients will experience numerous episodes of opportunistic infections and malignancies that are either difficult or impossible to eradicate.

The remarkably complex set of medical problems seen in AIDS has been accompanied by rapid changes in diagnostic and therapeutic options and strategies, often employing drugs that are either newly approved or still investigational. Adding yet more to the challenge is the high frequency and unique nature of the toxic drug reactions so common in the setting of the HIV infection.

For these and other reasons, many physicians in some hospitals have been reluctant to become involved in the care of patients with AIDS or other manifestations of HIV infection. This reluctance is understandable, given the many complexities in the field of AIDS and the small number of physicians who feel competent in dealing with these issues. Thus, it is critical for the medical system to make it as easy as possible for the practicing physician to care for the AIDS patient.

Certainly, one of the areas that we can best control is the dissemination of accurate and up-to-the-minute information to help in the clinical management of AIDS-associated problems. Considering the high frequency of serious opportunistic infections in the setting of HIV and the enormous complexity in diagnosing and managing these patients, *Opportunistic Infections in Patients with the Acquired Immunodeficiency Syndrome* should find a place in many physicians' offices. It summarizes many of the latest developments in the diagnosis and management of AIDS-related opportunistic infections, with contributions by leaders in each specific area. Furthermore, the book is organized to provide ready access to this information.

The first part provides clinically relevant overviews of essential background information on the epidemiology, biology, and pathophysiology of HIV infection.

In Part II, the spectrum of HIV disease from acute infection to specific syndromes is presented along with details of management schemes. A framework is offered for managing patients who present with common symptom complexes such as neurologic or cutaneous disease, and a separate chapter discusses the unique features of HIV infection in pediatric populations.

The final parts of the book review the management of specific opportunistic infections and offer guidelines for the use of laboratory diagnostic tests. Information in this is again practical in content while also pointing out the context of these infections in the AIDS epidemic, i.e., the often unique presentations and toxicities in the HIV-infected population.

Taken as a whole, this book is a substantial and welcome addition to the information available to the physician community. It is hoped that this type of resource will enable additional practicing physicians to offer expert care for the AIDS patients that the epidemic seems destined to give us.

Paul Volberding, M.D.
Associate Professor of Medicine
Chief, AIDS Activities Division
San Francisco General Hospital

Preface

In the decade since it was recognized as a distinct clinical entity, AIDS has become an enormous international health problem. The total number of persons with AIDS in the United States will probably exceed 100,000 this year, and the worldwide total may be several times that number. Millions of persons are already infected with the human immunodeficiency virus (HIV), and most of those infected will eventually develop AIDS.

Opportunistic infections are the paramount clinical problem confronting physicians caring for AIDS patients. *Pneumocystis carinii* pneumonia alone accounts for 65% of index AIDS diagnoses, and over 80% of patients will have at least one episode. Opportunistic infections will dominate the clinical picture of HIV infection until highly effective and nontoxic antiretroviral drugs, or a vaccine against HIV, can be developed.

Some physicians feel that aggressive treatment of opportunistic infections in the HIV-infected subject is unnecessary, given the inexorable progression of the underlying viral infection and its fatal outcome. However, all clinicians who have cared for patients infected with this retrovirus are aware that treatment of opportunistic infections decreases suffering and prolongs life, and that successful prevention of these infections has an even more dramatic effect on length of survival and quality of life. As there are currently available numerous nontoxic and inexpensive drugs that are active against most opportunistic pathogens, the likelihood is high that chemotherapy will be successful.

For these reasons, we felt that there was a clear need for a book that focused on the unique problems of managing opportunistic infections in HIV-infected patients. Our main intention was to provide a practical approach to patient management, although basic science and pathophysiologic issues have been discussed where relevant. Hence, full details of diagnostic testing, drug dosing, and laboratory monitoring have been supplied. The authors, who are all authorities in their respective areas, bring experience in direct patient care to their writing.

This book is divided into four parts. The first, a general introduction, reviews the epidemiology, virology, and immunology of HIV infection, with specific reference to opportunistic infections. Part II provides a systematic approach to the evaluation of HIV-infected patients who present with clinical syndromes such as fever, cough, or diarrhea. The next part discusses all of the major infections, grouped by etiologic agent, known to occur in HIV-infected patients and offers specific advice regarding diagnostic techniques and therapy. Finally, there is a part on the optimal usage of laboratory services.

We would like to thank the many individuals who helped to make this book possible. The work of the contributing authors is especially appreciated, particularly in light of their heavy workloads. Thanks go to Rosie Enesi, Debbie Gillespie and Colleen Chafian for their secretarial and word processing efforts. Burroughs Wellcome Company and Upjohn Company are thanked for their generous contributions toward the color reproductions that illustrate this book. Finally, we would like to express our gratitude to the faculty physicians, nurses, residents and students who helped us care for these patients, and to the patients themselves for teaching us about this disease.

Gifford Leoung
John Mills

Contents

Part VII: Ancillary Services

Contributors

Dale E. Bredesen, M.D. Assistant Adjunct Professor, Department of Neurology, University of California, San Francisco, California

Michel Carael Institute of Sociology, Free University of Brussels, Brussels, Belgium

Richard E. Chaisson, M.D.* Assistant Clinical Professor of Medicine, Department of Medicine, University of California, San Francisco, California

Michael Clement, M.D. Medical Director, Department of Inpatient AIDS Services, Assistant Clinical Professor of Medicine, Division of AIDS/Oncology, San Francisco General Hospital, San Francisco, California

Clay J. Cockerell, M.D.† Assistant Professor, Department of Dermatology, New York University Medical Center, New York, New York

Nathan Clumeck, M.D. Associate Professor and Chief of Infectious Diseases, Department of Internal Medicine, Free University of Brussels, Brussels, Belgium

Suzanne Crowe, M.D. San Francisco General Hospital, San Francisco, California

William E. Dismukes, M.D. Professor and Vice-Chairman for Education, Department of Medicine, School of Medicine, University of Alabama at Birmingham, Birmingham, Alabama

---

Present affiliations:
*Assistant Professor of Medicine and Epidemiology, Department of Medicine, The Johns Hopkins University School of Medicine, Baltimore, Maryland
†Assistant Professor, Departments of Dermatology and Pathology, University of Texas Southwestern Medical Center, Dallas, Texas

Kim S. Erlich, M.D.* Post-Doctoral Fellow, Division of Infectious Diseases, University of California, San Francisco, California

Alvin E. Friedman-Kien, M.D. Professor of Dermatology and Microbiology, Department of Dermatology, New York University Medical Center, New York, New York

Deborah Greenspan, B.D.S. Associate Clinical Professor, Division of Oral Medicine, Department of Stomatology, School of Dentistry, University of California, San Francisco, California

John S. Greenspan, B.D.S., Ph.D., F.R.C.Path. Professor of Oral Biology and Pathology, Chair, Division of Oral Biology, and Director, Oral AIDS Center, Department of Stomatology, School of Dentistry, and Professor of Pathology, School of Medicine, University of California, San Francisco, California

W. Keith Hadley, M.D., Ph.D. Professor of Clinical Laboratory Medicine, University of California, San Francisco, California, and Chief, Division of Microbiology, Department of Laboratory Medicine, San Francisco General Hospital, San Francisco, California

Mark A. Jacobson, M.D. Assistant Professor in Residence, Department of Medicine, University of California, and San Francisco General Hospital, San Francisco, California

Jane E. Koehler, M.D. Fellow, Infectious Diseases, Division of Infectious Diseases, Department of Medicine, University of California, San Francisco, California

Joseph A. Kovacs, M.D. Senior Investigator, Critical Care Medicine Department, National Institutes of Health, Bethesda, Maryland

Robert M. Levy, M.D., Ph.D. Assistant Professor, Departments of Surgery (Neurosurgery) and Physiology, Northwestern University Medical School, Chicago, Illinois

Pearl Ma, Ph.D. Chief of Microbiology, Department of Laboratories, St. Vincent's Hospital and Medical Center of New York, New York, New York

Valerie L. Ng, Ph.D., M.D. Assistant Professor in Residence, Department of Laboratory Medicine and Medicine, University of California, San Fran-

* *Present affiliation*: Consultant, Division of Infectious Disease, Seton Medical Center, Daly City, California

cisco, California, and Assistant Chief, Division of Microbiology, Department of Laboratory Medicine, San Francisco General Hospital, San Francisco, California

Carolyn Petersen, M.D. Adjunct Assistant Professor of Medicine, Division of Infectious Diseases, Department of Medicine, University of California, and San Francisco General Hospital, San Francisco, California

John P. Phair, M.D. Professor of Medicine, Chief of Infectious Disease, Department of Medicine, Northwestern University Medical School, Chicago, Illinois

Mark L. Rosenblum, M.D. Professor, Department of Neurosurgery, University of California, San Francisco, California

George W. Rutherford, M.D. Medical Director, AIDS Office, San Francisco Department of Public Health, San Francisco, California

Gisela F. Schecter, M.D., M.P.H.* Tuberculosis Controller, Bureau of Communicable Disease Control, Department of Public Health, San Francisco, California

Gwendolyn B. Scott, M.D. Associate Professor of Pediatrics, Department of Pediatrics, University of Miami School of Medicine, Miami, Florida

Michael S. Simberkoff, M.D. Chief, Infectious Diseases Section, New York Veterans Administration Medical Center, and Associate Professor of Medicine, New York University School of Medicine, New York, New York

James P. Steinberg, M.D. Associate of Clinical Medicine, Section of Infectious Diseases, Department of Medicine, Northwestern University Medical School, Chicago, Illinois

Michael G. Threlkeld, M.D. Fellow, Division of Infectious Diseases, Department of Medicine, University of Alabama at Birmingham School of Medicine, Birmingham, Alabama

Philippe Van de Perre, M.D. Reference Laboratory for HIV Infections, National AIDS Control Programme and Rwandese-Belgian Medical Cooperation, Kigali, Rwanda

Peggy S. Weintrub, M.D. Assistant Clinical Professor, Department of Pediatric Infectious Diseases and Immunology, University of California, San Francisco, California

---

* *Present affiliation*: Assistant Clinical Professor of Medicine, Infectious Diseases Division, Department of Medicine, University of California, San Francisco, California

Constance B. Wofsy, M.D. Associate Clinical Professor of Medicine, University of California; Co-Director, AIDS Activities Division; and Assistant Chief, Department of Infectious Diseases, San Francisco General Hospital, San Francisco, California

Abigail Zuger, M.D. Assistant Professor of Medicine, Albert Einstein College of Medicine, Bronx, New York

OPPORTUNISTIC INFECTIONS IN PATIENTS WITH THE ACQUIRED IMMUNODEFICIENCY SYNDROME

Part I
Introduction

1
The Epidemiology of Human Immunodeficiency Virus and the Acquired Immunodeficiency Syndrome

George W. Rutherford   *San Francisco Department of Public Health, San Francisco, California*

INTRODUCTION

The epidemiology of acquired immunodeficiency syndrome (AIDS) and of its causative agent, human immunodeficiency virus (HIV), have been well described in the 6 years since AIDS was first reported. During this period, over 60,000 cases have been reported worldwide, and it is likely that several million people have been infected with HIV and are at risk of developing AIDS. This chapter reviews the epidemiology of AIDS and HIV infection and examines possible future trends of this pandemic.

Historical Background

In June 1981, the Centers for Disease Control (CDC) reported a cluster of five previously healthy homosexual men from Los Angeles with *Pneumocystis càrinii* pneumonia and candidiasis (1). Three of these patients had in vitro abnormalities of cell-mediated immunity, and the reported concluded that the cluster suggested "the possibility of a cellular immune dysfunction related to a common exposure that predisposes individuals to opportunistic infections such as pneumocystosis and candidiasis (1)."

By August 1981, 111 cases of *P. carinii* pneumonia and Kaposi's sarcoma had been reported to the CDC, and national surveillance and a national case-control study had been organized (2). The epidemiology of this new disorder was striking—99% of the patients were male, 95% were 25 to 49 years old,

94% were homosexual or bisexual, 77% were white, and, most importantly, 40% were dead (2).

These and other earlier reports (3-8) heralded the beginning of the AIDS epidemic. Subsequently, AIDS has been described in intravenous drug users (5,9), Haitians (10), hemophiliacs (11,12), blood transfusion recipients (13), infants of mothers at increased risk for AIDS (14), female sexual partners of men with AIDS (15,16), and health care workers (17), groups all now recognized to be at increased risk for HIV infection.

Definitions

Definition of AIDS

AIDS is a clinical syndrome characterized by diseases that are at least moderately predictive of abnormal cell-mediated immunity in a person with no known underlying cause for cellular immunodeficiency (18). For purposes of AIDS reporting and surveillance, a case definition of AIDS was first published in 1982 (18) and successively modified to increase its specificity and sensitivity (19-24). The current national surveillance definition of AIDS is shown in Table 1 (24).

Because of a slightly different clinical spectrum of AIDS and a variety of congenital immunodeficiency syndromes that must be excluded before a diagnosis is established, the CDC established a separate definition for surveillance of AIDS in children under 13 years of age in 1984 (21). The current surveillance definition of pediatric AIDS is also shown in Table 1 (24).

Definition of HIV Infection

The other clinical manifestations of HIV infection, including AIDS-related complex (ARC) and progressive generalized lymphadenopathy, have until recently, been less rigidly defined. Three classification systems for HIV infection in adult patients have been published (25-27), each describing a spectrum of clinical disease ranging from asymptomatic infection to clinically evident AIDS. The current CDC definition for clinical HIV infection is shown in Table 2 (27). A somewhat similar classification scheme for HIV infection in children has also been described (28).

NATURAL HISTORY OF HIV INFECTION

Transmission of HIV Infection

Detailed epidemiologic studies have demonstrated that HIV is transmitted in three ways: sexually, parenterally, and perinatally. The classic AIDS transmission categories reflect these routes of transmission with homosexual and bisexual men and heterosexual patients having been infected sexually; heterosexual

TABLE 1 CDC Surveillance Case Definition of AIDS

I. WITHOUT LABORATORY EVIDENCE REGARDING HIV INFECTION

If laboratory tests for HIV were not performed or gave inconclusive results and the patient had no other cause of immunodeficiency listed in Section I.A below, then any disease listed in Section I.B indicates AIDS, if it was diagnosed by a definitive method.

    A. Causes of Immunodeficiency that Disqualify Diseases as Indicators of AIDS in the Absence of Laboratory Evidence for HIV Infection

        1. High-dose or long-term systemic corticosteroid therapy or other immunosuppressive/cytotoxic therapy $\leq$ 3 months before the onset of the indicator diseases

        2. Any of the following diseases diagnosed $\leq$ 3 months after diagnosis of the indicator disease: Hodgkin's disease, non-Hodgkin's lymphoma (other than primary brain lymphoma), lymphocytic leukemia, multiple myeloma, any other cancer of lymphoreticular or histiocytic tissue, or angioimmunoblastic lymphadenopathy

        3. A genetic (congenital) immunodeficiency syndrome or an acquired immunodeficiency syndrome atypical of HIV infection, such as one involving hypogammaglobulinemia

    B. Indicator Diseases Diagnosed Definitively

        1. Candidiasis of the esophagus, trachea, bronchi, or lungs

        2. Cryptococcosis, extrapulmonary

        3. Cryptosporidiosis with diarrhea persisting > 1 month

        4. Cytomegalovirus disease of an organ other than liver, spleen, or lymph nodes in a patient > 1 month of age

        5. Herpes simplex virus infection causing a mucocutaneous ulcer that persists longer than 1 month; or bronchitis, pneumonitis, or esophagitis for any duration affecting a patient > 1 month of age

        6. Kaposi's sarcoma affecting a patient < 60 years of age

        7. Lymphoma of the brain (primary) affecting a patient < 60 years of age

        8. Lymphoid interstitial pneumonia and/or pulmonary lymphoid hyperplasia (LIP/PLH complex) affecting a child < 12 years of age

        9. *Mycobacterium avium* complex or *M. kansasii* disease, disseminated (at a site other than or in addition to lungs, skin, or cervical or hilar lymph nodes)

       10. *Pneumocystis carinii* pneumonia

       11. Progressive multifocal leukoencephalopathy

       12. Toxoplasmosis of the brain affecting a patient > 1 month of age

II. WITH LABORATORY EVIDENCE FOR HIV INFECTION

Regardless of the presence of other causes of immunodeficiency (I.A), in the presence of laboratory evidence of HIV infection, any disease listed above (I.B) or below (II.A or II.B) indicates a diagnosis of AIDS.

Table 1 (continues)

TABLE 1 Continued

A. Indicator Diseases Diagnosed Definitively

  1. Bacterial infections, multiple or recurrent (any combination of at least two within a 2-year period), of the following types affecting a child < 13 years of age:

     septicemia, pneumonia, meningitis, bone or joint infection, or abscess of an internal organ or body cavity (excluding otitis media or superficial skin or mucosal abscesses), caused by *Haemophilus*, *Streptococcus* (including pneumococcus), or other pyogenic bacteria

  2. Coccidioidomycosis, disseminated (at a site other than or in addition to lungs or cervical or hilar lymph nodes)

  3. HIV encephalopathy (also called "HIV dementia," "AIDS dementia," or "subacute encephalitis due to HIV")

  4. Histoplasmosis, disseminated (at a site other than or in addition to lungs or cervical or hilar lymph nodes)

  5. Isosporiasis with diarrhea persisting > 1 month

  6. Kaposi's sarcoma at any age

  7. Lymphoma of the brain (primary) at any age

  8. Other non-Hodgkin's lymphoma of B-cell or unknown immunologic phenotype and the following histologic types:

     a. Small noncleaved lymphoma (either Burkitt or non-Burkitt type)

     b. Immunoblastic sarcoma (equivalent to any of the following, although not necessarily all in combination: immunoblastic lymphoma, large-cell lymphoma, diffuse histiocytic lymphoma, diffuse undifferentiated lymphoma, or high-grade lymphoma)

     Note: Lymphomas are not included here if they are of T-cell immunologic phenotype or their histologic type is not described or is described as "lymphocytic," "lymphoblastic," "small cleaved," or "plasmacytoid lymphocytic."

  9. Any mycobacterial disease caused by mycobacteria other than *M. tuberculosis*, disseminated (at a site other than or in addition to lungs, skin, or cervical or hilar lymph nodes)

  10. Diseases caused by *M. tuberculosis*, extrapulmonary (involving at least one site outside the lungs, regardless of whether there is concurrent pulmonary involvement)

  11. *Salmonella* (nontyphoid) septicemia, recurrent

  12. HIV wasting syndrome (emaciation, "slim disease")

B. Indicator Diseases Diagnosed Presumptively

  Note: Given the seriousness of diseases indicative of AIDS, it is generally important to diagnose them definitively, especially when therapy that would be used may have serious side effects or when definitive diagnosis is needed for eligibility for antiretroviral therapy. Nonetheless, in some situations, a patient's condition will not permit the performance of definitive tests. In

Table 1 (continues)

TABLE 1 Continued

other situations, accepted clinical practice may be to diagnose presumptively based on the presence of characteristic clinical and laboratory abnormalities.

  1. Candidiasis of the esophagus
  2. Cytomegalovirus retinitis with loss of vision
  3. Kaposi's sarcoma
  4. Lymphoid interstitial pneumonia and/or pulmonary lymphoid hyperplasia (LIP/PLH complex) affecting a child < 13 years of age
  5. Mycobacterial disease (acid-fast bacilli with species not identified by culture), disseminated (involving at least one site other than or in addition to lungs, skin, or cervical or hilar lymph nodes)
  6. *Pneumocystis carinii* pneumonia
  7. Toxoplasmosis of the brain affecting a patient > 1 month of age

III. WITH LABORATORY EVIDENCE AGAINST HIV INFECTION

With laboratory test results negative for HIV infection, a diagnosis of AIDS for surveillance purposes is ruled out *unless*:

  A. All the other causes of immunodeficiency listed above in Section I.A are excluded; **AND**
  B. The patient has had either:
    1. *Pneumocystis carinii* pneumonia diagnosed by a definitive method; *OR*
    2. a. Any of the other diseases indicative of AIDS listed above in Section I.B diagnosed by a definitive method; **AND**
       b. A T-helper/inducer (CD4) lymphocyte count < 400/mm^3.

Source: Ref. 24.

TABLE 2 Summary of Classification System for Human Immunodeficiency Virus

Group I. Acute infection
Group II. Asymptomatic infection[a]
Group III. Persistent generalized lymphadenopathy[a]
Group IV. Other disease
      subgroup A. Constitutional disease
      subgroup B. Neurologic disease
      subgroup C. Secondary infectious diseases
            category C-1. Specified secondary infectious diseases listed in the CDC surveillance definition for AIDS[b]
            category C-2. Other specified secondary infectious diseases
      subgroup D. Secondary cancers[b]
      subgroup E. Other conditions

[a]Patients in Groups II and III may be subclassified on the bases of a laboratory evaluation.
[b]Includes those patients whose clinical presentation fulfills the definition of AIDS used by CDC for national reporting.
Source: Ref. 27.

TABLE 3   AIDS Cases by Transmission Category and Sex, United States[a]

Category	Males Number	(%)	Females Number	(%)	Total Number	(%)
Adults/Adolescents[b]						
homosexual/bisexual male	33,369	(70)			33,369	(65)
intravenous (IV) drug abuser	6,961	(15)	1,916	(51)	8,877	(17)
homosexual/bisexual male and IV drug abuser	3,858	(8)			3,858	(7)
hemophilia/coagulation disorder	499	(1)	20	(1)	519	(1)
heterosexual cases[c]	948	(2)	1,110	(29)	2,058	(4)
transfusion, blood/ components	793	(2)	413	(11)	1,206	(2)
undetermined[d]	1,248	(3)	332	(9)	1,580	(3)
Subtotal [% of all cases]	47,676	[93]	3,791	[7]	51,467	[100]
Children[e]						
hemophilia/coagulation disorder	40	(9)	3	(1)	43	(5)
parent at risk of AIDS[f]	305	(72)	298	(82)	603	(76)
transfusion, blood/ components	63	(15)	45	(12)	108	(14)
undetermined[d]	18	(4)	17	(5)	35	(4)
Subtotal [% of all cases]	426	[54]	363	[46]	789	[100]
Total [% of all cases]	48,102	[92]	4,154	[8]	52,256[g]	[100]

[a]These data are provisional to February 1, 1988.

[b]Cases with more than one risk factor other than the combinations listed in the tables or footnotes are tabulated only in the category listed first.

[c]Includes 1174 persons (260 men 914 women) who have had heterosexual contact with a person with AIDS or at risk for AIDS and 884 persons (688 men, 196 women) without other identified risks who were born in countries in which heterosexual transmission is believed to play a major role, although precise means of transmission have not yet been defined.

[d]Includes patients on whom risk information is incomplete (due to death, refusal to be interviewed, or loss to follow-up), patients still under investigation, men reported only to have had heterosexual contact with a prostitute, and interviewed patients for whom no specific risk was identified.

[e]Includes all patients under 13 years of age at time of diagnosis.

[f]Epidemiologic data suggests transmission from an infected mother to her fetus or infant during the perinatal period.

[g]Includes 3400 patients who meet only the 1987 revised surveillance definition for AIDS.

intravenous drug users, hemophiliacs, transfusion recipients, and health care workers having been infected parenterally; and children of parents with or at risk for AIDS having been infected perinatally. Homosexual and bisexual men with histories of intravenous drug use have been infected either sexually or parenterally. In the United States, sexual transmission is the most common route of HIV infection among reported AIDS patients and parenteral transmission the second most common route (Table 3).

Sexual Transmission

Sixty-nine percent of adult and adolescent AIDS patients in the United States acquired HIV infection sexually. This route of transmission was the first one recognized, with early case-control studies of AIDS in homosexual and bisexual men demonstrating a correlation between sexual activity, as measured by numbers of sexual partners and histories of certain sexually transmitted diseases, and the development of AIDS (29-31). The risk of sexually acquiring HIV infection depends on two variables: the probability of exposure to an infected partner and the probability of transmission from an infected partner (32). As the prevalence of HIV infection increases in a population, the probability of a randomly chosen sexual partner being infected increases so that, for instance, the risk of exposure per contact now is substantially higher for a homosexual man than it was in 1980. The second variable, the risk of actual transmission, depends on the probability of an infectious inoculum of HIV infecting the T4 (CD4)-helper cells of a previously uninfected host (32). More recent studies of HIV seroconversion among homosexual men have demonstrated that sexual activities in which the rectal mucosa of the uninfected partner is traumatized, such as receptive anal intercourse, douching, and fisting, and sexually transmitted diseases in which the genital epithelium is disrupted by ulcers, such as syphilis, herpes simplex, and chancroid (35-37), are correlated with infection. They have also suggested that the risk of infection per partner with whom receptive anal intercourse is practiced (as a marker of risk per episode of intercourse) is 9% (38). Further studies are under way to delineate the relative risk of other sexual activities such as insertive anal intercourse and oral intercourse and the protective effect of condoms.

Among women, the number of sexual contacts with an HIV-infected man has been associated with seroconversion (39-40). The prevalence of HIV infection among steady female sex partners of infected men has ranged from 9.5% to 71% (41-45). Additionally, receptive anal intercourse has also been associated with increased risk of transmission from men to women (45), but both male-to-female transmission and female-to-male transmission have occurred in the absence of anal intercourse (41-48).

Parenteral Transmission

Currently, 28% of adult and adolescent AIDS patients and 19% of pediatric AIDS patients acquired HIV infection parenterally, that is, from blood contact. This number includes 17% of the adult and adolescent patients who are heterosexual intravenous drug users, 8% who are homosexual or bisexual male intravenous drug users, 1% who are hemophiliacs or have coagulation disorders, and 2% who are blood or blood component transfusion recipients, 5% of the pediatric patients who are hemophiliacs, and 13% who are blood transfusion recipients.

As with sexual transmission, the risk of parenteral transmission is determined by the risk of exposure and the probability of transmission occurring during that exposure. Because the body fluid in parenteral transmission is by definition blood, the probability of transmission is presumably dependent on the volume of blood, that is, there is a minimal infecting dose. For instance, a patient who received multiple infected units of blood has a higher probability of acquiring HIV infection than a health care worker who sustained a single needle-stick injury from an infected patients (49,50). Among intravenous drug users, the risk of transmission appears to be related to the frequency of needle sharing (51-53), presumably reflecting both an increased risk of exposure (53,54) and the relative efficiency of HIV transmission through drug paraphernalia. Transmission is likely facilitated by the practice of "booting" or aspirating blood into the syringe, thus leaving larger amounts of residual blood in the syringe and needle together than, for instance, that in a needle in a needle-stick injury. Among hemophiliacs, HIV transmission was clearly related to factor VIII use before factor VIII became routinely heat treated to inactivate HIV (55-57), and patients with greater factor VIII dependency have higher rates of infection than those with less severe disease (58).

Perinatal Transmission

Perinatally transmitted cases currently comprise 77% of all pediatric AIDS cases. Perinatal transmission can occur from mother to child in the prepartum, intrapartum, or immediate postpartum periods (59). Although transmission presumably occurs transplacentally or as the placenta separates from the uterine wall at birth, a single case of postnatal transmission presumably through breast milk has been described (60), and HIV has been isolated from milk (61). The risk of transmission from an infected mother varies between 20% and 65% in various series (62-64), but it is generally believed to be around 50%. Because of passively transfused maternal antibody, all infants will be seropositive for several months after birth (59), except for a small number who exhibit immunotolerance and are viremic and seronegative (D. Wara, personal communication).

Other Routes of Transmission

Currently, no clear route of transmission has been determined for 3% of adolescent and adult AIDS patients and for 4% of pediatric AIDS patients. Patients in this "undetermined" category include those for whom risk information is incomplete because of death, who refused to be interviewed, or who were lost to follow-up; those still under investigation; men reported to have had sexual contact with female prostitutes; and those who were interviewed and for whom no specific risk could be determined (65). Approximately one-half of this heterogeneous group include people on whom risk information is incomplete and also some proportion probably represents non-AIDS-related cases of Kaposi's sarcoma (65). Although 64% of these patients are nonwhite, the proportion of the total cases falling into this category has remained stable over time (39).

None of the identified cases of HIV infection in the United States is known to have been transmitted in school, day-care, or foster care settings or through casual person-to-person contact (66). Other than sexual partners of HIV-infected patients, infants born to infected mothers, or two cases involving apparent percutaneous transmission of HIV to persons providing extended nursing care (67,68), none of the family members of AIDS patients reported to CDC have developed AIDS or HIV infection (66). Studies from the United States (41,67-76) and Africa (77) have failed to demonstrate HIV transmission to adults who were not sexual contacts of the infected patients or to children who were not already infected perinatally. In addition to evidence against casual household transmission, case-control studies of the prevalence of antibodies to a variety of arboviruses in HIV-infected persons and controls have failed to demonstrate evidence of vector-borne transmission (78).

Prevalence of HIV Infection

The current prevalence of HIV infection in the United States is not known. Among blood donors and military recruits, groups that have been widely used as surrogates for the population at large, the prevalence has ranged from 0.04% among blood donors (79) to 0.15% among military recruits (80). In both these groups the prevalence among men (0.07% in blood donors and 0.16% in military recruits) has been greater than among women (0.006% and 0.06% respectively). Additionally, prevalence has varied by race among military recruits with 0.09% of whites, 0.39% of blacks, and 0.26% of others (Hispanics, Asians, and American Indians) being infected (80).

The prevalence of HIV infection among selected risk groups can be somewhat more easily estimated. Studies of homosexual and bisexual men living in large cities in the United States and Europe have found seroprevalences of 32% to 42% in Seattle (81), 42% in Los Angeles (82), 21% to 51% in

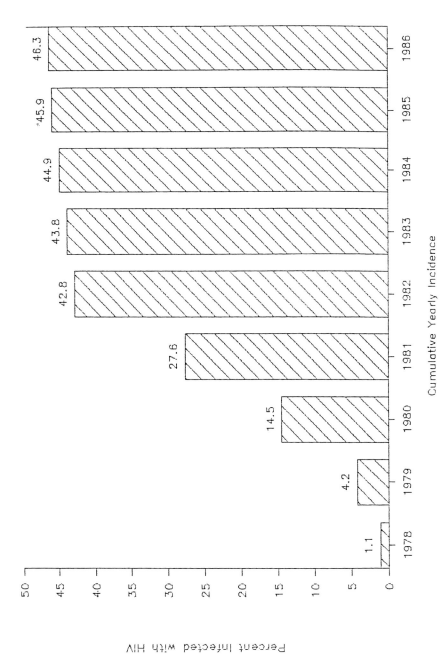

FIGURE 1 Prevalence of HIV infection by year; San Francisco City Clinic Cohort Study, 1978-1986 (from Ref. 43).

Manhattan (83-87), 33% to 73% in San Francisco (88-95), 48% in Vancouver (96), 17% in London (97), 34% in Paris (98), 31% in Amsterdam (99), 10% in Zurich (100), and 8% in Denmark (84). From these studies it can be shown that the first cases of HIV infection in this population occurred in the late 1970s and that new cases are continuing to occur, although at a much slower rate (93-95; Fig. 1).

Among intravenous drug users, the prevalence of HIV infection has been reported to range between 2% in California (101), 50% in New Jersey (102), and 72% in New York City (54,102). In Europe, the prevalence among intravenous drug users has been reported to be as high as 51%, 52% to 60%, 51%, and 50%, in Edinburgh, Italy, southern France, and Spain, respectively (103-107). Among hemophiliacs in the United States, between 40% and 88% are now estimated to be infected (108-110).

Incidence of HIV Infection

Data on the annual incidence, that is, new cases per year, of HIV infection are limited. In three cohorts of homosexual and bisexual men from San Francisco, the annual incidence between 1985 and 1986, was 3% to 5% (92-95). However, when compared with previous years, this incidence was quite low, paralleling a similar decline in the incidence of gonococcal proctitis among men in San Francisco (94; Fig. 2). Similar trends have been observed in Stockholm (111), Melbourne (112), and New York (86,87,113). Nonetheless, homosexual and bisexual men are continuing to seroconvert, albeit in low numbers (82,83,91,93,114). One report suggests that black homosexual and bisexual men are seroconverting at a higher rate than white men (115), and another that the sexually disinhibiting effects of drugs and alcohol may be correlated with more recent seroconversion (116).

The annual incidence of HIV infection among intravenous drug users has been estimated from serial seroprevalence surveys of methadone and detoxification clients. In a 1-year period between 1985 and 1986, the prevalence of infection in a San Francisco methadone clinic rose from 10% to 14% (117; R.E. Chaison, personal communication), whereas during a 2-year period, 1984-1986, the prevalence rose from 5% to 20% to 64% among treatment populations in Edinburgh (103). These and similar data from New York, New Jersey, and Italy demonstrate the potential for rapid spread of HIV infection among intravenous drug users.

Persistence of HIV Infection

As with other mammalian retroviral diseases, HIV infection possibly persists for the life of the host (49). Persistent viremia for up to 69 months has

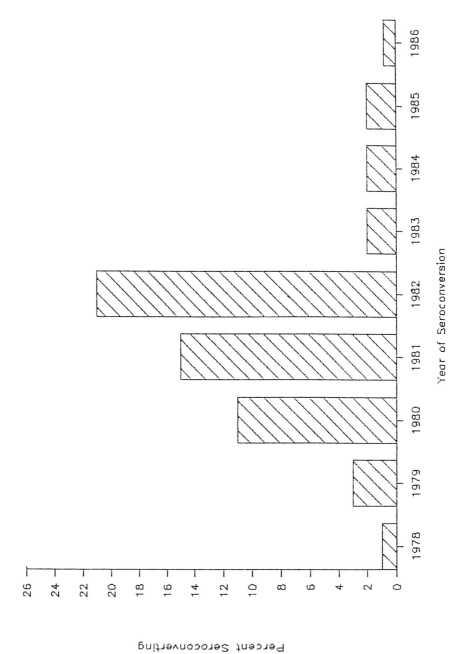

FIGURE 2 Incidence of HIV infection by year, San Francisco City Clinic Cohort Study, 1978-1986 (from Ref. 43).

been documented in homosexual men (118), and seropositivity has been clearly correlated with viremia in between 67% and 85% of symptomatic and asymptomatic individuals (118-123). Because of this close association between seropositivity and viremia, seropositivity should be considered presumptive evidence of HIV infection and transmissability (49).

Outcome of HIV Infection

Natural History of HIV Infection

Human immunodeficiency virus can cause a broad spectrum of clinically apparent diseases ranging from an acute mononucleosislike syndrome (124, 125) to clinically evident AIDS (25-27). Cohort studies of homosexual men (95,96,126-146), intravenous drug users (147,148), and hemophiliacs (149-150), using survival analysis, have predicted that between 6% and 40% of infected patients will develop AIDS over periods ranging from 36 to 88 months.

In a study of 63 homosexual and bisexual men whose dates of seroconversion were known, 30% had developed AIDS, 21% had developed other clinically significant HIV-related symptoms (including persistent fever, diarrhea, weight loss, candidiasis, or hairy leukoplakia), 27% had developed generalized lymphadenopathy, and 22% had remained asymptomatic over an average follow-up of 76 months after infection (135; Table 4). Additionally, by use of survival analysis, it could be estimated that 36% (95% confidence interval, 26%-46%), of these men and 92 hepatitis B vaccine trial participants would develop AIDS within 88 months of infection (135; Fig. 3). In this cohort, the mean incubation period between infection and diagnosis of AIDS was 55 months (135).

Among transfusion recipients with AIDS, patients whose date of infection is known, the mean incubation period observed, to date, is 29 months for

TABLE 4   Clinical Outcomes of 63 Men with Long-Term HIV Infection, San Francisco City Clinic Cohort Study[a]

	Cases	Percentage	95% Confidence interval
AIDS	19	30	19-41
AIDS-related conditions[b]	13	21	11-31
Generalized lymphadenopathy	17	27	16-38
Asymptomatic	14	22	12-32

[a]Mean follow-up, 76 months (date of seroconversion to AIDS or last examination).
[b]Oral candidiasis, weight loss, or persistent idiopathic fever or diarrhea. Nine participants had coincident generalized lymphadenopathy.
Source: Ref. 135.

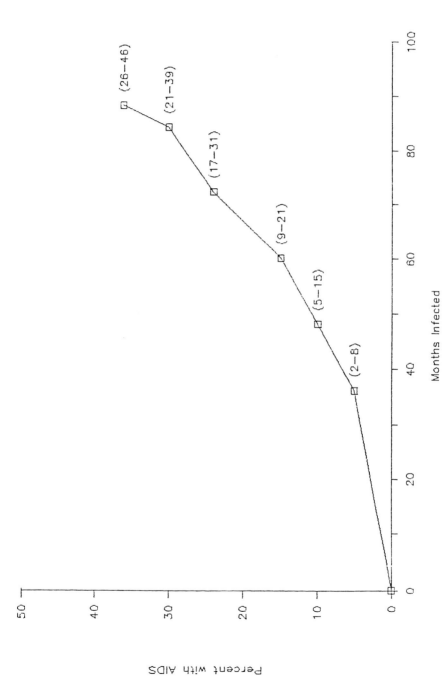

FIGURE 3   Predicted AIDS-free interval by duration of HIV infection, San Francisco City Clinic Cohort Study, 1986; 95% confidence interval in parenthesis (from Ref. 69).

adults and 14 months for infants (151,152). Among infants with perinatally transmitted HIV infection, the mean age at diagnosis of AIDS is 12 months, which represents the minimal incubation period for perinatally acquired AIDS (59). However, these estimates are likely underestimates of the true incubation period because cases with a longer incubation period may not yet have been diagnosed (153).

Risk Factors for the Development of Clinical Disease

With the development of an effective HIV antibody test, cofactors for the development of clinical disease, as opposed to those associated with sero-conversion, could be studied separately. Preliminary data from case-control studies suggested that volatile alkyl nitrites, substances known to be in vitro immunosuppressants and widely used by homosexual men (154), were possibly a cofactor in the development of Kaposi's sarcoma (155-160). Other studies, however, have not confirmed this finding (128,161-165). The most consistent cofactors that have been demonstrated, to date, are duration of infection (131,135,161) and older age (143,166), neither of which can be effectively modified at the present time.

Immunologic and Virologic Correlates of Clinical Disease

Immunologic, virologic, and other laboratory parameters that have been correlated with progression to AIDS include a progressive decline in T4 (CD4)-helper cell numbers (96,128,129,137,141-143,145,146,167-171), the presence of HIV antigenemia (127,143,171-174), a high T8 (CD8)-suppressor cell number (127,146), hyperimmunoglobulinemia A (96,143,168) and G (96), falling levels of HIV antibody (143,166,175), low HIV-neutralizing antibody titers (175-177), low lymphocyte 5'-nucleotidase (169), decreased reactions to intradermal antigens (169), decreased lymphocyte response to pokeweed mitogen (171), low levels of antibody to Epstein-Barr virus nuclear antigens (169) and high levels of antibody to cytomegalovirus (143), low serum albumin levels (169), low hemoglobin levels (96,141,143,168,169), thrombocytopenia (168), viramia (178), and absence of hepatitis B antigenemia (179). Immuno-genetic factors that have been associated with progression to AIDS are histocompatibility (HLA) antigens DR1 and DR2 (180) and the cell membrane receptor protein Gc (181).

AIDS IN THE UNITED STATES

Descriptive Epidemiology

As of February 1, 1988, 52,256 cases of AIDS and 29,206 (56%) deaths from AIDS had been reported in the United States. The incidence of AIDS is currently 227 cases per million population. Of these 52,256 patients, 47,676

TABLE 5 AIDS Cases and Incidence by Standard Metropolitan Statistical Areas, United States[a]

	Cases	Population[b]	Incidence[b]
New York, NY	12,225	9.12	1,340.5
San Francisco, CA	4,783	3.25	1,471.7
Los Angeles, CA	4,219	7.48	564.0
Houston, TX	1,760	2.91	604.8
Washington, DC	1,618	3.06	528.8
Newark, NJ	1,416	1.97	718.8
Miami, FL	1,387	1.63	850.9
Chicago, IL	1,303	7.10	183.5
Dallas, TX	1,127	2.97	379.5
Philadelphia, PA	1,034	4.72	219.1
Atlanta, GA	828	2.03	407.9
Boston, MA	790	2.76	286.2
San Diego, CA	700	1.86	376.3
Fort Lauderdale, FL	665	1.02	652.0
Jersey City, NJ	617	0.56	1,101.8
Nassau-Suffolk, NY	567	2.61	217.2

[a]Provisional data to February 1, 1988.
[b]Incidence, cases per million population.
Source: Centers for Disease Control.

(91%) were adult and adolescent men, 3791 (7%) were adult and adolescent women, and 789 (2%) were children (see Table 3). Sixty percent of patients were white, 25% black, 14% Latino, 1% Asian and Pacific islanders, and less than 1% were American Indians or Alaskan Natives. Cases have now been reported from all 50 states, the District of Columbia, Puerto Rico, the Virgin Islands, Guam, and the Trust Territory of the Pacific, but they tend to be clustered in major metropolitan areas (Table 5).

Sixty-five percent of adult and adolescent patients were homosexual or bisexual men; 17% heterosexual intravenous drug users; 7% homosexual or bisexual men with histories of intravenous drug use; 4% heterosexual partners of persons with AIDS, at risk for AIDS, or heterosexuals from tropical countries where heterosexual transmission is the predominate mode of transmission; 2% blood transfusion recipients; 1% hemophiliacs; and 3% persons with undetermined risk (see Table 3). Among children under 13 years old, 76% were born to parents with or at risk for AIDS, 14% were blood transfusion recipients, 5% were hemophiliacs, and 4% were persons with undetermined risk (see Table 3). Blacks and Latinos comprise 79% of heterosexual intravenous drug users with AIDS, 83% of heterosexually transmitted cases, and 86% of infants with perinatally transmitted infection.

Homosexual and Bisexual Men

Sixty-five percent of adult and adolescent AIDS patients were homosexual and bisexual men who acquired HIV infection sexually. AIDS was first described in this population, and AIDS is the leading cause of death among homosexual and bisexual men. In some cohort studies of homosexual and bisexual men, the overall AIDS-specific morbidity exceeds 7% and the AIDS-specific mortality 4% (135). Homosexual and bisexual men with AIDS are predominantly white, 30 to 49 years old, and from major urban areas including New York City, San Francisco, Los Angeles, and Houston. This disease is expected to continue to be principally a disease of homosexual and bisexual men, with 62% of patients with this diagnosis in 1991 being homosexual and bisexual men and 8% gay men with histories of intravenous drug use (182).

Homosexual and Bisexual Male Intravenous Drug Users

Seven percent of adult and adolescent AIDS patients were homosexual or bisexual men with histories of intravenous drug use. These men may have been infected sexually or parenterally by sharing needles contaminated with infected blood. In addition to possible needle exposure, behavioral studies have demonstrated a correlation between alcohol and drug use and high-risk sexual activities, suggesting also an indirect disinhibitory role for alcohol and drugs in HIV transmission (116).

Heterosexuals

Four percent of adult and adolescent AIDS cases involve persons who acquired HIV infection through heterosexual contact. Of these 2058 patients, 1174 (57%), including 260 men and 914 women, were sexual contacts of a person with AIDS or at risk for AIDS; and 884 (43%), including 688 men and 196 women, were born in Haiti or Central Africa and had no other identifiable risk factors. Patients who were sexual contacts of persons with or at risk for AIDS were primarily contacts of intravenous drug users, black and Latino, and from the urban Northeast. It is expected that in 1991, 5.0% of all AIDS cases will be in this category (182). Given the high incidence of sexually transmitted diseases in these populations and potential bidirectional transmission, the possibility for multiple generation transmission from intravenous drug users to their communities certainly exists.

Haitian immigrants in southern Florida and New York City comprise the large majority of patients from tropical countries with endemic sexually transmitted HIV infection. Many of these patients acquired HIV infection early in the epidemic, either sexually or through infected transfusions or needles in Haiti before immigrating to the United States (183); therefore, cases among Haitians are expected to decrease to 0.3% of the total in 1991 (182).

In addition, transmission has also been described as the result of infected semen during artificial insemination (62). Although the method of inoculation of semen may influence infectivity, universal screening of sperm donors for HIV antibody has been recommended (184).

Intravenous Drug Users

Heterosexual intravenous drug users currently account for 17% of all adolescent and adult AIDS cases. Among these 8877 patients are 1916 (22%) women and 7104 (80%) nonwhites. Fifty-one percent of all women with AIDS and 35% of all adult and adolescent nonwhites with AIDS are heterosexual intravenous drug users. They tend to cluster predominantly in the large urban centers of the Northeast with relatively few cases, as yet, in California. However, cases in San Francisco have recently doubled over one 6-month period suggesting that the exponential phase of the epidemic in this group is now beginning in the West (185). Nationally, in 1991, heterosexual intravenous drug users are expected to comprise 16.4% of adult cases (182).

Heterosexual intravenous drug users also are the major source of secondary spread of HIV infection, both sexually and perinatally. Currently, over two-thirds of the female heterosexual contact cases and one-half of the perinatally transmitted cases can be attributed to secondary or tertiary intravenous drug users (186-188). Additionally, the disinhibitory influences of drugs may contribute to sexual transmission of HIV among intravenous drug users in high-prevalence areas, much as has been described for homosexual and bisexual men (116).

Transfusion Recipients

Recipients of infected blood or blood products currently account for 2% of all adult and adolescent AIDS cases, 14% of all pediatric AIDS cases, and 3% of overall AIDS cases. When compared with other AIDS patients, patients with transfusion-associated AIDS tend to be older with a median age range of 50 to 59 years (192). Among adult and adolescent patients, 76% are white, but among pediatric patients, 55% are white; the reason for this disparity is unknown. The HIV virus has been transmitted in whole blood, red cells, plasma, and platelets (13,151,152,189), and also in transplanted kidneys (190). There is no laboratory or epidemiologic evidence of HIV in immune serum globulin (191) or hepatitis B vaccine (192). National screening of all donated blood, plasma, and organs, was initiated in April 1985, to prevent further transfusion-associated transmission (184), but because of the long incubation period of AIDS, cases will continue to occur over the next several years. In 1991, 2.5% of all adolescent and adult AIDS cases are expected to be transfusion-associated (182).

Hemophiliacs

Currently, 1% of all adolescent and adult AIDS patients, 5% of all pediatric AIDS patients, and 1% of overall AIDS patients are hemophiliacs. Because hemophilia A, the major coagulation disorder requiring pooled plasma products for treatment, is a sex-linked disease, 96% of these cases are in males. Clotting factor concentrates and cryoprecipitate have been implicated in HIV transmission (11,55,149,150,193,194). Heat treatment of factor VIII and other clotting factor concentrates to inactivate HIV was begun in 1985 (57,195); but again, because of the long incubation period, cases are expected to continue to occur with 1.4% of cases in 1991 involving hemophiliacs (182).

Health Care Workers

The transmission of HIV from infected patients to health care workers following needle-stick injury has been reported (17,196,197). However, the risk of HIV transmission following needle-stick injury from a known infected patient is believed to be very low, probably less than 0.5% (50), and it is certainly many times lower than the risk of hepatitis B transmission (198). Additionally, there are case reports of a mother providing extended nursing care for her child with transfusion-associated AIDS who seroconverted after prolonged and repeated mucous membrane exposure to AIDS blood (67) and of a nurse with severe dermatitis providing home care for an AIDS patient who seroconverted and developed AIDS after prolonged and repeated percutaneous exposure to blood (68). Prevention of transmission to health care workers has focused on minimizing needle sticks and percutaneous and mucous membrane exposure to blood (150,199-203).

Children of Parents at Risk for AIDS

Seventy percent of perinatally transmitted AIDS cases have been in children born to a parent with a history of intravenous drug use, 17% have been in children born to Haitian parents, and 13% have been in children born to parents with other risk factors for AIDS (182). The median age for diagnosis of AIDS in these patients is 12 months (59), and the male/female ratio is approximately 1:1. Eighty-seven percent of these children are nonwhite, and 88% of all pediatric AIDS cases among blacks and 81% of cases among Latinos are perinatallly transmitted. Because of the correlations between intravenous drug use and Haitian ancestry and perinatal transmission, these cases cluster in New York, New Jersey, and southern Florida (59). However, as the geographic distribution of intravenous drug-use-associated HIV infection changes, the distribution of perinatally transmitted cases will change as well.

TABLE 6 Opportunistic Diseases Reported in ≥ 0.1% of AIDS Patients in the United States, Ranked in Descending Order of Frequency

Disease	Percentage of AIDS patients
1. *Pneumocystis carinii* pneumonia	63.6
2. Oral/pharyngeal candidiasis (thrush)	44.8[a,b]
3. Kaposi's sarcoma	20.8
4. Esophageal candidiasis	10.6
5. Extrapulmonary cryptococcosis	6.8
6. Cytomegalovirus disease (internal organ infection)	5.0
7. Herpes zoster	4.8[a,b]
8. Disseminated infection with *Mycobacterium avium* complex	4.2
9. Chronic mucocutaneous herpes simplex	3.6
10. Chronic enteric cryptosporidiosis	3.1
11. Toxoplasmosis of the brain	2.5
12. Tuberculosis (at any site)	1.9[b]
13. Immunoblastic sarcoma (other than primary of the brain)	1.0
14. Primary lymphoma of the brain	0.7
15. Disseminated histoplasmosis	0.6
16. Progressive multifocal leukoencephalopathy	0.6
17. Bronchopulmonary candidiasis	0.5
18. Small noncleaved (Burkitt's) lymphoma	0.3
19. Disseminated mycobacteriosis of undetermined species	0.3[b]
20. Chronic enteric isosporiasis	0.2
21. Disseminated *Mycobacterium kansasii* infection	0.2
22. *Salmonella* septicemia	0.2[b]
23. *Legionella* pneumonia	0.1[b]
24. Aspergillosis	0.1[b]
25. Herpes simplex virus pneumonia	0.1
26. Coccidioidomycosis	0.1[b]
27. Nocardiosis	0.1[b]

[a]Provisional data as of February 9, 1987 (*n* = 30,632). The data for thrush and herpes zoster used a smaller denominator than was used for the other diseases: 6545 AIDS cases reported during June 1983-March 1985.
[b]These diseases were not used as an indicator of AIDS in the case definition.
Source: Ref. 204.

Opportunistic Infections and Malignancies

The most common opportunistic infection or malignancy reported among AIDS patients in the United States is *Pneumocystis carinii* pneumonia (63.6%), followed by oral and pharyngeal candidiasis (44%), Kaposi's sarcoma (20.8%), esophageal candidiasis (10.8%), extrapulmonary cryptococcosis (6.8%), and cytomegalovirus disease (5.0%; 204). The other opportunistic infections and malignancies that occur in AIDS patients are reported in fewer than 5% of patients (204; Table 6). Additionally, lymphoid interstitial pneumonitis is reported in 44.3% of pediatric AIDS patients and histologically confirmed in 19.7% (204).

Kaposi's sarcoma tends to be a disease predominantly of homosexual and bisexual men (204,205), although it also occurs significantly more frequently in Haitians than in other heterosexuals with AIDS and in children born to Haitian mothers than other children with AIDS (204; Table 7). Cryptococcosis occurs more commonly in heterosexual intravenous drug users and Haitians; cytomegalovirus occurs more commonly in children; toxoplasmosis, tuberculosis, and isosporiasis occur more commonly in Haitians; and chronic herpes simplex occurs more commonly in female intravenous drug users (204; see Table 7).

TABLE 7 Percentage of AIDS Patients with Particular Diseases by Patient Characteristics, United States[a]

Characteristics	n	P. carinii pneumonia	Kaposi's sarcoma	Eosphageal candidiasis	Cryptococcosis (extrapulmonary)	Cytomegalovirus (internal organ histopathology)
Homosexual/bisexual male	19,795	62.8[c]	27.7[b]	8.5[c]	5.2[c]	5.5[b]
Homosexual/bisexual male and intravenous (IV) drug abuser	2,332	61.6	24.6	10.0	8.0	4.9
IV drug abuser	5,128	67.1[b]	2.9[c]	15.4[b]	11.5[b]	2.1[c]
Hemophilia/coagulation disorder	276	68.5	1.1[c]	15.6	8.3	3.6
Persons born in Haiti (HIV presumed infected by heterosexual transmission)	601	49.2[c]	8.8[c]	16.8[b]	11.2[c]	4.5
Heterosexual sex partners of persons in any of the above groups	544	77.4[b]	2.2[c]	14.9	5.2	3.7
Children (age < 13) with mother infected or in one of the above groups	350	49.7[c]	3.4[c]	15.4	0.6[c]	14.9[b]
Transfusion, blood/ components	622	70.6[b]	3.0[c]	19.0[b]	6.8	6.6
Undetermined	984	67.4	8.6[c]	14.5[b]	10.1[b]	7.0
Total	30,632	63.6	20.8	10.6	6.8	5.0

Table 7 (continues)

TABLE 7 Continued

Characteristics	M. avium complex (disseminated)	Chronic herpes simplex	Chronic cryptosporidiosis	Toxoplasmosis (internal organ histopathology)	Tuberculosis (at any site)
Homosexual/bisexual male	4.2	3.7	3.5[b]	2.0[c]	1.0[c]
Homosexual/bisexual male and intravenous (IV) drug abuser	4.2	4.0	3.7	2.7	2.1
IV drug abuser	4.2	2.9	1.7[c]	3.1	3.4[b]
Hemophilia/coagulation disorder	4.4	2.9	4.7	2.9	1.1
Persons born in Haiti (HIV presumed infected by heterosexual transmission	2.5	5.0	4.0	13.3[b]	21.1[b]
Heterosexual sex partners of persons in any of the above groups	5.0	3.3	2.8	2.9	1.8
Children (age < 13) with mother infected or in one of the above groups	5.1	3.4	3.4	0.3	0.0
Transfusion, blood/ components	3.9	3.0	1.8	2.9	1.6
Undetermined	3.7	4.6	2.4	4.5[b]	2.0
Total	4.2	3.6	3.1	2.5	1.9

[a]Provisional data as of February 9, 1987, for AIDS-indicative diseases reported in more than 1% of AIDS cases and tuberculosis.
[b]The percentage with this disease for patients in this group is significantly greater than that for all other AIDS patients combined ($p < 0.001$, Fisher's exact test).
[c]The percentage with this disease for patients in this group is significantly less than that for all other AIDS patients combined ($p < 0.001$, Fisher's exact test).
Source: Ref. 204.

The geographic location of patients in the United States also is associated with specific opportunistic infections. Histoplasmosis occurs 10 times more frequently in AIDS patients residing in states in the Mississippi Valley, and coccidioidomycosis occurs 100 times more frequently in residents of Arizona than in residents in other states (204).

The percentages of AIDS patients presenting with various opportunistic infections and malignancies have changed over time, with the most pronounced changes being an increase in P. carinii pneumonia and a decrease in Kaposi's sarcoma (204; Fig. 4). Smaller changes have occurred in patients presenting

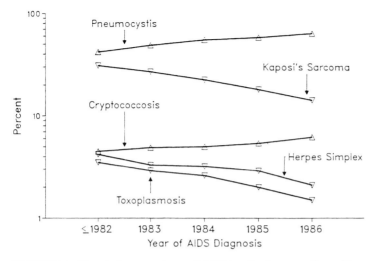

FIGURE 4 Trends in percentage of AIDS patients presenting with specific opportunistic diseases (from Ref. 204).

with extrapulmonary cryptococcosis, chronic herpes simplex, and cerebral
toxoplasmosis (204; see Fig. 4). The reasons for the declining incidence of
Kaposi's sarcoma are unclear, although the decline is independent of the increase in *P. carinii* pneumonia (204) and not an artifact of reporting or diagnostic practices (205). Possible explanations include the parallel declining
incidence of postulated cofactors for Kaposi's sarcoma, including amyl nitrite inhalants (154-160) and cytomegalovirus infection (206-209), or a shorter
incubation period of Kaposi's sarcoma (210). None of these, however, have
been proved (143,161,167,210).

Survival

Survival of patients after an AIDS diagnosis has been reported to be 347
days in New York City (211) and 12.1 months in San Francisco (212). Longer
survival times in both studies were associated with Kaposi's sarcoma and
younger age (211,212), and in the New York study with race (white) and sex
(male; 211). Both studies also found that survival following diagnosis of *P.
carinii* pneumonia was increased over time, gradually from 1981 to 1985 in
the New York study (211), and abruptly from 1985 to 1986 in the San Francisco study (212).

Trends

The number of cases of AIDS diagnosed in the United States will continue to increase over the next several years, arising primarily from individuals already infected with HIV (182). Projections of the number of cases in the United States have been made by fitting quadratic equations to the present epidemic curve (182). This model predicts that there will be 270,000 cases reported by the end of 1991 and that there will be 74,000 cases diagnosed in 1991 alone (182). By using a 1985 estimate of the overall prevalence of HIV infection in the United States of between 500,000 and 1 million people (46) and assuming that no further transmission occurs, this model predicts that 27% to 54% of people infected with HIV will eventually develop AIDS. This estimate is consistent with observed AIDS morbidity from cohort studies (131,135).

Quadratic modeling also has been used to predict changes in transmission category, geographic distribution, age, race, and sex. Major trends that have been predicted included increasing numbers of transfusion-associated and heterosexual contact cases to 2.5% and 5.0% of the 1991 cases, respectively, and a redistribution of cases away from New York City, San Francisco, and Florida, with 76.9% of cases in 1991 diagnosed outside of these areas, as opposed to 52.6% in 1986 (182). Emergence of new transmission patterns, such as bidirectional heterosexual transmission among adolescents or low-income populations, effective measures to prevent infection, such as vaccination, or therapeutic interventions to limit the progression of clinical disease among persons with asymptomatic or mildly symptomatic HIV infection, may markedly change both the overall projections and projections by age, sex, race, geographic distribution, and transmission category.

CONCLUSIONS

Both AIDS and HIV have spread rapidly throughout the world since the initial description of AIDS in 1981 and are now, with over 60,000 cases reported, considered pandemics. In the absence of effective antiviral therapy, cases of AIDS should be expected to continue to increase well into the future, even if HIV transmission could be interrupted today. Certain types of HIV transmission, such as transfusion- or hemophilia-associated transmission, can be interrupted with careful screening of donated blood and heat treatment of clotting factors, but the other modes of transmission will require unprecedented health education efforts even to be slowed (213-216). It is likely that definitive prevention will be dependent on the development of a safe, effective, and inexpensive vaccine. However, given the magnitude of the AIDS pandemic, it is unacceptable to wait for a vaccine. The medical profession, community groups, educational institutions, churches, and industry need to reach out and frankly educate the public about sexuality, drug use, and other factors involved in the prevention of AIDS.

REFERENCES

1. CDC (1981). *Pneumocystis* pneumonia—Los Angeles. *MMWR 30*:250-252.
2. CDC (1981). Follow-up on Kaposi's sarcoma and *Pneumocystis* pneumonia. *MMWR 30*:409-410.
3. CDC (1981). Kaposi's sarcoma and *Pneumocystis* pneumonia among homosexual men—New York City and California. *MMWR 30*:305-308.
4. Hymes, K. B., Cheung, T., Greene, J. B. et al. (1981). Kaposi's sarcoma in homosexual men—a report of eight cases. *Lancet 2*:598-600.
5. Gottlieb, M., Schroff, R., Schauber, H. et al. (1981). *Pneumocystis carinii* pneumonia and mucosal candidiasis in previously healthy homosexual men. *N. Engl. J. Med. 305*:1425-1431.
6. Masur, H., Michelis, M. A., Greene, J. B. et al. (1981). An outbreak of community-acquired *Pneumocystis carinii* pneumonia: Initial manifestation of cellular immune dysfunction. *N. Engl. J. Med. 305*:1431-1438.
7. Siegal, F. P., Lopez, C., Hammer, G. S., et al. (1981). Severe acquired immunodeficiency in male homosexuals, manifested by chronic perianal ulcerative Herpes simplex lesions. *N. Engl. J. Med. 305*:1439-1444.
8. Durack, D. T. (1981). Opportunistic infections and Kaposi's sarcoma in homosexual men [Editorial]. *N. Engl. J. Med. 305*:1465-1467.
9. CDC (1982). Update on Kaposi's sarcoma and opportunsitic infections in previously healthy persons—United States. *MMWR 31*:294, 300-301.
10. CDC (1982). Opportunistic infections and Kaposi's sarcoma among Haitians in the United States. *MMWR 31*:353-354, 360-361.
11. CDC (1982). *Pneumocystis carinii* pneumonia among persons with hemophilia A. *MMWR 31*:365-367.
12. CDC (1982). Update on acquired immunodeficiency syndrome (AIDS) among patients with hemophilia A. *MMWR 31*:644-646, 652.
13. CDC (1982). Possible transfusion-associated acquired immune deficiency syndrome (AIDS)—California. *MMWR 31*:652-654.
14. CDC (1982). Unexplained immunodeficiency and opportunistic infections in infants—New York, New Jersey, California. *MMWR 31*:665-667.
15. Masur, H., Michelis, M. A., Wormser, G. P. et al. (1982). Opportunistic infection in previously healthy women: Initial manifestations of a community-acquired cellular immunodeficiency. *Ann. Intern. Med. 97*:533-539.
16. CDC (1983). Immunodeficiency among female sexual partners of males with acquired immunodeficiency syndrome. *MMWR 31*:697-698.
17. CDC (1985). Update: Evaluation of human T-lymphotropic virus type III/lymphadenopathy-associated virus infection in health-care personnel—United States. *MMWR 34*:575-578.

18. CDC (1982). Update on acquired immune deficiency syndrome (AIDS)—United States. *MMWR 31*:507-508, 513-514.

19. Jaffe, H. W., Bregman, D. J., and Selik, R. M. (1983). Acquired immune deficiency syndrome in the United States: The first 1,000 cases. *J. Infect. Dis. 148*: 339-345.

20. Jaffe, H. W., and Selik, R. M. (1984). Acquired immune deficiency syndrome: Is disseminated aspergillosis predictive of underlying cellular deficiency? [Letter]. *J. Infect. Dis. 149*:829.

21. Selik, R. M., Haverkos, H. W., and Curran, J. W. (1984). Acquired immune deficiency syndrome (AIDS) trends in the United States, 1979-1982. *Am. J. Med. 76*:493-500.

22. CDC (1984). Update: Acquired immunodeficiency syndrome (AIDS)—United States. *MMWR 32*:688-691.

23. CDC (1985). Revision of the case definition of acquired immunodeficiency syndrome for national reporting—United States. *MMWR 43*:373-375.

24. CDC (1987). Revision of the case definition for acquired immunodeficiency syndrome. *MMWR 36*(suppl. 2S):1S-15S.

25. Haverkos, H. W., Gottlieb, M. S., Killen, J. Y., and Edelman, R. (1985). Classification of HTLV-III/LAV-related diseases [Letter]. *J. Infect. Dis. 152*:1095.

26. Redfield, R. R., Wright, D. C., and Tramont, E. C. (1986). The Walter Reed staging classification for HTLV-III/LAV infection. *N. Engl. J. Med. 314*:131-132.

27. CDC (1986). Classification system for human T-lymphotropic virus type-III/lymphadenopathy-associated virus infections. *MMWR 35*:334-339.

28. CDC (1987). Classification system for human immunodeficiency virus (HIV) infection in children under 13 years of age. *MMWR 36*:225-230, 235-236.

29. Jaffe, H. W., Choy, K., Thomas, P. A. et al. (1983). National case-control study of Kaposi's sarcoma and *Pneumocystis carinii* pneumonia in homosexual men: Part I. Epidemiologic results. *Ann. Intern. Med. 99*:145-151.

30. Goedert, J. J., Sarngahdaran, M. G., Biggar, R. J. et al. (1984). Determinants of retrovirus (HTLV-III) antibody and immunodeficiency conditions in homosexual men. *Lancet 2*:711-716.

31. Marmor, M., Friedman-Klein, A. E., Zolla-Pazner, S. et al. (1984). Kaposi's sarcoma in homosexual men: A seroepidemiologic case-control study. *Ann. Intern. Med. 100*:809-815.

32. Peterman, T. A., and Curran, J. W. (1986). Sexual transmission of human immunodeficiency virus. *JAMA 256*:2222-2226.

33. Darrow, W. W., Echenberg, D. F., Jaffe, H. W. et al. (1987). Risk factors for human immunodeficiency virus (HIV) infection in homosexual men. *Am. J. Public Health 77*:479-483.

34. Winkelstein, W. Jr., Lyman, D. M., Padian, N. et al. (1987). Sexual practices and risk of infection by the human immunodeficiency virus: The San Francisco Men's Health Study. *JAMA 257*:321-325.

35. Handsfield, H. H., Ashley, R. L., Rompalo, A. M., Stamm, W. E., Wood, R. W., and Corey, L. (1987). Association of anogenital ulcer diseases with human

immunodeficiency virus infection in homosexual men. III International Conference on AIDS, Washington, D.C., June 1987.

36. Holmberg, S. D., Steward, J. A., Gerber, A. R. et al. (1988). Prior herpes simplex virus type 2 (HSV-2) infection as a risk factor for human immunodeficiency virus (HIV) infection. *JAMA* (in press).

37. Katzenstein, D. A., Latif, A., Bassett, M. T., and Emmanuel, J. C. (1987). Risks for heterosexual transmission in Zimbabwe. III International Conference on AIDS, Washington, D.C., June 1987.

38. Winkelstein, W., Wiley, J., Lang, W., Grant, R., Samuel, M., and Levy, J. A. (1986). Reduction in AIDS virus transmission: Seroconversion in San Francisco 1982-1985. International Conference on AIDS, Paris, France, June 1986.

39. CDC (1984). Update: Acquired immunodeficiency syndrome (AIDS)—United States. *MMWR 33*:661-664.

40. Padian, N. S. (1987). Heterosexual transmission of acquired immunodeficiency syndrome: International perspectives and national projections. *Rev. Infect. Dis. 9*:947-960.

41. Peterman, T. A., Stoneburner, R. L., and Allen, J. R. (1986). Risk of HTLV-III/LAV transmission to household contacts of persons with transfusion-associated AIDS. International Conference on AIDS, Paris, France, June 1986.

42. Kreiss, J. K., Kitchen, L. W., Prince, H. E. et al. (1985). Antibody to human T-lymphotropic virus type III in wives of hemophiliacs: Evidence for heterosexual transmission. *Ann. Intern. Med. 102*:623-626.

43. Jason, J., McDougal, J. S., Dixon, G. et al. (1986). HTLV-III/LAV antibody and immune status of household contacts and sexual partners of persons with hemophilia. *JAMA 255*:212-215.

44. Redfield, R. R., Markham, P. D., Salahuddin, S. Z. et al. (1985). Frequent transmission of HTLV-III among spouses of patients with AIDS-related complex and AIDS. *JAMA 253*:1571-1573.

45. Padian, N., Marquis, L., Francis, D. P. et al. (1987). Male-to-female transmission of human immunodeficiency virus. *JAMA 258*:788-790.

46. Kreiss, J. K., Koech, D., Plummer, F. A. et al. (1986). AIDS virus infection in Nairobi prostitutes. *N. Engl. J. Med. 31*:414-418.

47. Hira, S. K., Perine, P. L., Redfield, R. R. et al. (1986). The epidemiology and clinical manifestations of the acquired immune deficiency syndrome (AIDS) and its related complex (ARC) in Zambia. International Conference on AIDS, Paris, France, June 1986.

48. Mann, J. M., Quinn, T., Francis, H. et al. (1986). Sexual practices associated with LAV/HTLV-III seropositivity among female prostitutes in Kinshasa, Zaire. International Conference on AIDS, Paris, France, June 1986.

49. Curran, J. W., Morgan, W. M., Hardy, A. M., Jaffe, H. W., Darrow, W. W., and Dowdle, W. R. (1985). The epidemiology of AIDS: Current status and future prospects. *Science 229*:1352-1357.

50. Sande, M. A. (1986). Transmission of AIDS: The case against casual contagion [Editorial]. *N. Engl. J. Med. 314*:380-382.

51. Robertson, J. R., Bucknall, A. B. V., Welsby, P. D. et al. (1986). Epidemic of AIDS-related virus (HTLV-III/LAV) infection among intravenous drug abusers. *Br. Med. J. 292*:527-529.
52. Weiss, S. H., Ginzburg, H. V., Goedert, J. J., Biggar, R. J., Mohica, B. A., and Blattner, W. A. (1985). Risk for HTLV-III exposure and AIDS among parenteral drug abusers in New Jersey. International Conference on Acquired Immunodeficiency Syndrome (AIDS), Atlanta, Georgia, April 1985.
53. Cohen, H., Marmor, M., DesJarlais, D., Spira, T., Friedman, S., and Yancovitz, S. (1985). Behavioral risk factors for HTLV-III/LAV seropositivity among intravenous drug abusers. International Conference on Acquired Immunodeficiency Syndrome (AIDS), Atlanta, Georgia, April 1985.
54. Spira, T. J., Des Jarlais, D. C., Bokos, D. et al. (1985). HTLV-III/LAV antibodies in intravenous (IV) drug abusers—comparison of high and low risk areas for AIDS. International Conference on Acquired Immunodeficiency Syndrome (AIDS), Atlanta, Georgia, April 1985.
55. Evatt, B. L., Gomperts, E. D., McDougal, J. S. et al. (1985). Coincidental appearance of LAV/HTLV-III in hemophiliacs and the onset of the AIDS epidemic. *N. Engl. J. Med. 312*:483-486.
56. Evatt, B. L., Ramsey, R. B., Lawrence, D. N. et al. (1984). The acquired immunodeficiency syndrome in patients with hemophilia. *Ann. Intern. Med. 100*:499-504.
57. CDC (1984). Update: Acquired immunodeficiency syndrome in persons with hemophilia. *MMWR 33*:589-591.
58. Ramsey, R. B., Palmer, E. L., McDougal, J. S. et al. (1984). Antibody to lymphadenopathy-associated virus in hemophiliacs with and without AIDS [Letter]. *Lancet 2*:397-398.
59. Rogers, M. F. (1985). AIDS in children: A review of the clinical, epidemiologic and public health aspects. *Pediatr. Infect. Dis. 4*:230-236.
60. Ziegler, J. B., Cooper, D. A., Johnson, R. O., and Gold, J. (1985). Postnatal transmission of AIDS-associated retrovirus from mother to infant. *Lancet 1*:896-898.
61. Thiry, L., Sprecher-Goldberger, S., Jonckheer, T. et al. (1985). Isolation of AIDS virus from cell-free breast milk of three healthy virus carriers [Letter]. *Lancet 2*:891-892.
62. Stewart, G. J., Tyler, J. P. P., Cunningham, A. L. et al. (1985). Transmission of human lymphotropic virus type III (HTLV-III) by artificial insemination by donor. *Lancet 2*:581-585.
63. Scott, G. B., Fischl, M. A., Klimas, N. et al. (1985). Mothers of infants with the acquired immunodeficiency syndrome: Evidence for both symptomatic and asymptomatic carriers. *JAMA 235*:363-366.
64. Scott, G. B., Fischl, M. A., Klimas, N., Fletcher, M., Dickinson, G., and Parks, W. (1985). Mothers of infants with the acquired immunodeficiency syndrome: Outcome of subsequent pregnancies. International Conference on Acquired Immunodeficiency Syndrome (AIDS), Atlanta, Georgia, April 1985.

65. CDC (1985). Heterosexual transmission of human T-lymphotropic virus type III/lymphadenopathy-associated virus. *MMWR 34*:561-563.
66. CDC (1985). Education and foster care of children infected with human T-lymphotropic virus type III/lymphadenopathy-associated virus. *MMWR 34*:517-521.
67. Fishl, M. A., Dickinson, G. M., Scott, G. B., Klimas, N., Fletcher, M. A., and Parks, W. (1986). Heterosexual and household transmission of the human T-lymphotropic virus type III. International Conference on AIDS, Paris, France, June 1986.
68. Grint, P. and McEvoy, M. (1985). Two associated cases of the acquired immune deficiency syndrome (AIDS). *Commun. Dis. Rep. 42*:4.
69. Jason, J. M., McDougal, J. S., Lawrence, D. N., Kennedy, D. S., Hilgartner, M., and Evatt, B. L. (1986). Lymphadenopathy-associated virus (LAV) antibody and immune status of household contacts and sexual partners of persons with hemophilia. *JAMA 255*:212-215.
70. Kaplan, J. E., Oleske, J. M., Getchell, J. P. et al. (1985). Evidence against transmission of HTLV-III/LAV in families of children with AIDS. *Pediatr. Infect. Dis. 4*:468-471.
71. Lawrence, D. N., Jason, J. M., Bouhasin, J. D. et al. (1985). HTLV-III/LAV antibody status of spouses and household contacts assisting in home infusion of hemophilia patients. *Blood 66*:703.
72. Lewin, E. B., Zack, R., and Ayodele, A. (1985). Communicability of AIDS in a foster care setting. International Conference on Acquired Immunodeficiency Syndrome (AIDS), Atlanta, Georgia, April 1985.
73. Redfield, R. R., Markham, P. D., Salahuddin, S. Z. et al. (1985). Frequent transmission of HTLV-III among spouses of patients with acquired immunodeficiency syndrome (AIDS) or AIDS-related complex: A family study. *JAMA 253*:1571-1573.
74. Rogers, M. F., White, C. R., Sanders, R. et al. (1986). Can children transmit human T-lymphotropic virus type III/lymphadenopathy-associated virus (HTLV-III/LAV)? International Conference on AIDS, Paris, France, June 1986.
75. Saltzman, B. R., Freidland, G. H., Rogers, M. F. et al. (1986). Lack of household transmission of HTLV-III/LAV infection. International Conference on AIDS, Paris, France, June 1986.
76. Thomas, P. A., Lubia, K., Enlow, R. W. et al. (1985). Comparison of HTLV-III serology, T-cell levels, and general health status of children whose mothers have AIDS with children of healthy inner city mothers in New York. International Conference on Acquired Immunodeficiency Syndrome (AIDS), Atlanta, Georgia, April 1985.
77. Mann, J. M., Quinn, T., Francis, H. et al. (1986). Prevalence of HTLV-III/LAV in household contacts of patients with controls in Kinshasa, Zaire. *JAMA 256*:721-724.
78. CDC (1986). Update: AIDS—Palm Beach County, Florida. *MMWR 35*:609-612.
79. Schorr, J. B., Berkowitz, A., Cumming, P. D., Katz, A. J., and Sandler, S. G. (1985). Prevalence of HTLV-III antibody in American blood donors [Letter]. *N. Engl. J. Med. 313*:384-385.

80. CDC (1986). Human T-lymphotropic virus type III/lymphadenopathy-associated virus antibody prevalence in U.S. Military recruit applicants. *MMWR* *35*:421-424.

81. Collier, A. C., Barnes, R. C., and Handsfield, H. H. (1986). Prevalence of antibody to LAV/HTLV-III among homosexual men in Seattle. *Am. J. Public Health* *76*:564-565.

82. Schwartz, K., Vischer, B. R., Detels, R., Taylor, J., Nishanian, P., and Fahey, J. L. (1985). Immunological changes in lymphadenopathy virus positive and negative symptomiess male homosexuals: Two years of observation [Letter]. *Lancet 2*:831-832.

83. Safai, B., Sarngadharan, M. G., Groopman, J. E. et al. (1984). Seroepidemiological studies of human T-lymphotropic retrovirus type III in acquired immunodeficiency syndrome. *Lancet 1*:1438-1440.

84. Blattner, W. A., Biggar, R. J., Weiss, S. H. et al. (1986). 3-year AIDS incidence after HTLV-III: 5 cohorts and cofactor analysis. International Conference on AIDS, Paris, France, June 1986.

85. Stevens, C. E., Taylor, P. E., Rodriquez de Cordoba, S., and Rubinstein, P. (1986). AIDS virus infection in homosexual men and volunteer blood donors in New York City. International Conference on AIDS, Paris, France, June 1986.

86. Stevens, C. E., Taylor, P. E., Zang, E. A., Rodriquez de Cordoba, S., and Rubenstein, P. (1987). Incidence of HIV infection in homosexual men in a high risk area: Implications for vaccine trials design. III International Conference on AIDS, Washington, D.C., June 1987.

87. Marmor, M., Zelenrich-Jacquette, A., Zolla-Pazner, S., El-Sadr, W., Thomas, P., and Spira, T. J. (1987). Cohort study of New York City male homosexuals, 1981-86. III International Conference on AIDS, Washington, DC, June 1987.

88. Anderson, R. E. and Levy, J. A. (1985). Prevalence of antibody to AIDS-associated retrovirus in single men in San Francisco [Letter]. *Lancet 1*:250.

89. Osmond, D., Moss, A. R., Bachetti, P., Volberding, P., Barre-Sinoussi, F., and Cherman, J.-C. (1985). A case-control study of risk factors for AIDS in San Francisco. International Conference on Acquired Immunodeficiency Syndrome (AIDS), Atlanta, Georgia, April 1985.

90. Jaffe, H. W., Darrow, W. W., Echenberg, D. F. et al. (1985). The acquired immunodeficiency syndrome in a cohort of homosexual males: A 6-year follow-up study. *Ann. Intern. Med. 103*:210-214.

91. CDC (1985). Update: Acquired immunodeficiency syndrome in the San Francisco Cohort Study. *MMWR 34*:573-575.

92. Moss, A. R., Osmond, D., Bachetti, P., Cherman, J.-C., Carlson, J., and Casavant, C. (1986). Progression to AIDS in men seropositive for LAV/HTLV-III— 1-year follow-up of the San Francisco General Hospital Study [Poster]. International Conference on AIDS, Paris, France, June 1986.

93. Winkelstein, W., Wiley, J., Lang, W., Grant, R., Samuel, M., and Levy, J. A. (1986). Reduction in AIDS virus transmission: Seroconversion in San Francisco, 1982-1985. International Conference on AIDS, Paris, France, June 1986.

94. Echenberg, D. F., Rutherford, G. W., Darrow, W. W., O'Malley, P. M., Bodecker, T., and Jaffe, H. W. (1986). The incidence and prevalence of LAV/

HTLV-III infection in the San Francisco City Clinic Cohort Study, 1985 [Poster]. International Conference on AIDS, Paris, France, June 1986.

95. Hessol, N. A., O'Malley, P. M., Rutherford, G. W. et al. (1987). Sexual transmission of human immunodeficiency virus infection in homosexual and bisexual men who participated in hepatitis B vaccine trials. 20th Annual Meeting of the Society for Epidemiologic Research, Amherst, Massachusetts, June 1987.

96. Schecter, M. T., Boyko, W. J., Weaver, M. S., Douglas, B., Willoughby, B., and McLeod, A. W. (1987). Progression to AIDS, predictors of AIDS, and seroconversion in a cohort of homosexual and bisexual men: Results of a four year prospective study. III International Conference on AIDS, Washington, DC, June 1987.

97. Cheingsong-Popov, R., Weiss, R. A., Dalgleish, A. et al. (1984). Prevalence of antibody to human T-lymphotropic virus type III in AIDS and AIDS-risk patients in Britain. *Lancet 2*:477-480.

98. Rouzioux, C., Bucquet, D., Mettetal, J. F., Delaqueau, J. F., and Messiah, A. (1987). HIV-1 and HIV-2 infection in a French cohort of homosexual and bisexual men in Paris. III International Conference on AIDS, Washington, DC, June 1987.

99. VanGriensven, G. J. P., Tielman, R. A. P., Goudsmit, J., Van der Noordaa, J., DeWolf, F., and deContingho, R. A. (1986). Prevalence of LAV/HTLV-III antibodies in relation to lifestyle characteristics in homosexual men in the Netherlands. International Conference on AIDS, Paris, France, June 1986.

100. Schupback, J., Haller, O., Vogt, M. et al. (1985). Antibodies to HTLV-III in Swiss patients with AIDS and pre-AIDS and in groups at risk for AIDS. *N. Engl. J. Med. 312*:265-270.

101. Levy, N., Carlson, C. R., Hinrichs, S., Lerche, N., Schenker, M., and Gardner, M. B. (1986). The prevalence of HTLV-III/LAV antibodies among intravenous drug users attending treatment programs in California: A preliminary report [Letter]. *N. Engl. J. Med. 314*:446.

102. Weiss, S. H., Ginzburg, H. M., Goeddert, J. J. et al. (1985). Risk for HTLV-III exposure and AIDS among parenteral drug abusers in New Jersey. International Conference on Acquired immunodeficiency Syndrome (AIDS), Atlanta, Georgia, April 1985.

103. Robertson, J. R., Bucknall, A. B. V., and Wiggins, P. (1986). Regional variations in HIV antibody seropositivity in British intravenous drug users [Letter]. *Lancet 1*:1435-1436.

104. Angarano, G., Pastore, G., Monno, L., Santantonio, T., Luchena, N., and Schiraldi, O. (1985). Rapid spread of HTLV-III infection among drug addicts in Italy [Letter]. *Lancet 2*:1302.

105. Lazzarin, A., Crocchiolo, P., Galli, M., Uberti Foppa, C., Re, T., and Moroni, M. (1986). Milan as a possible starting point of LAV/HTLV-III infection among Italian drug addicts. International Conference on AIDS, Paris, France, June 1986.

106. Federlin, M., Smilovici, W., Montalegre, A., Watrigant, M. P., Ducos, J., and Armengaud, M. (1986). LAV/HTLV-III virus endemic among a popula-

tion of 431 former drug users. International Conference on AIDS, Paris, France, June 1986.

107. Rodrigo, J. M., Serra, M. A., Aguilar, E., Del Olmo, J. A., Gimeno, V., and Aparisi, L. (1985). HTLV-III antibodies in drug addicts in Spain [Letter]. *Lancet 2*:156-157.

108. Ragni, M. V., Tegtmeier, G. E., Handwerk-Leber, C., Lewis, J. H., Mayer, W. L., and Spero, J. A. (1985). Prevalence and seroconversion of human T-lymphotropic retrovirus (HTLV-III) antibody in patients with hemophilia. International Conference on Acquired Immunodeficiency Syndrome (AIDS), Atlanta, Georgia, April 1985.

109. Jason, J., McDougal, J. S., Holman, R. C. et al. (1985). Human T-lymphotropic retrovirus type III/lymphadenopathy-associated virus antibody. Association with hemophiliacs' immune status and blood component usage. *JAMA 253*:3409-3415.

110. Goedert, J. J., Sarngadharan, M. G., Eyster, M. E. et al. (1985). Antibodies reactive with human T-cell leukemia viruses in the serum of hemophiliacs receiving factor VIII concentrate. *Blood 65*:492-495.

111. Bratt, G., Karlsson, A., von Krogh, G., Mobeig, L., Biberfeld, G., and Sandstrom E. (1987). HIV-seroconversion in a cohort of homosexual men in Stockholm between 1983 and 1986 [Poster]. III International Conference on AIDS, Washington, D.C., June 1987.

112. Mulhall, B. P., Crapper, R. M., Frazer, I. H., and McKay, I. R. (1987). The Melbourne Cohort after 3 years: half of sero-conversion to HIV and predictors of immune-deficiency. III International Conference on AIDS, Washington, D.C., June 1987.

113. Martin, J. L. (1987). Prevalence and incidence of AIDS, ARC and HIV infection in a gay NYC cohort. III International Conference on AIDS, Washington, DC, June 1987.

114. Winkelstein, W., Jr., Samuel, M., Padian, N. S. et al. (1987). The San Francisco Men's Health Study: III. Reduction in human immunodeficiency virus transmission among homosexual/bisexual men, 1982-1986. *Am. J. Public Health 76*:685-689.

115. Samuel, M. C., and Winkelstein, W., Jr. (1987). Prevalence of human immunodeficiency virus (HIV) infection in ethnic minority homosexual/bisexual men [Poster]. III International Conference on AIDS, Washington, D.C., June 1987.

116. Stall, R., McKusick, L., Wiley, J., Coates, T. J., and Ostrow, D. G. (1986). Alcohol and drug use during sexual activity and compliance with safe sex guidelines for AIDS: The AIDS Behavioral Research Project. *Health Educ. Q. 13*:359-371.

117. Chaisson, R. E., Moss, A. R., Onishi, R., Osmond, D., and Carlson, J. R. (1987). Human immunodeficiency virus infection in heterosexual intravenous drug users in San Francisco. *Am. J. Public Health 77*:169-172.

118. Jaffe, H. W., Feorino, P. M., Darrow, W. W. et al. (1985). Isolation of a T-lymphotropic virus type III/lymphadenopathy-associated virus in apparently healthy homosexual men. *Ann. Intern. Med. 102*:627-628.

119. Barre-Sinoussi, F., Cherman, J.-C., Rey, F. et al. (1983). Isolation of a T-lymphotropic retrovirus from a patient at risk for acquired immune deficiency syndrome (AIDS). *Science 220*:868-871.
120. Gallo, R. C., Salahuddin, S. Z., Popovic, M. et al. (1984). Frequent detection and isolation of cytopathic retroviruses (HTLV-III) from patients with AIDS and at risk for AIDS. *Science 224*:500-503.
121. Levy, J. A., Hoffman, A. D., Kramer, A. D. et al. (1984). Isolation of lymphocytopathic retrovirus from San Francisco patients with AIDS. *Science 225*: 840-842.
122. Feorino, P. M., Jaffe, H. W., Palmer, E. et al. (1985). Transfusion-associated acquired immunodeficiency syndrome: Evidence for persistent infection in blood donors. *N. Engl. J. Med. 312*:1293-1296.
123. McCormick, J. B., Krebs, J. W., Mitchell, S. W. et al. (1987). Isolation of human immunodeficiency virus from African AIDS patients and persons without AIDS or IgG antibody to human immune deficiency virus. *Am. J. Trop. Med. Hyg. 36*:102-106.
124. Cooper, D. A., Gold, J., Maclean, P. et al. (1985). Acute AIDS retrovirus infection: Definition of a clinical illness associated with seroconversion. *Lancet 1*:537-540.
125. McLeod, A. W., Schecter, M. T., Boyko, W. J., Craib, K. J. P., Willoughby, B., and Douglas, B. (1987). Primary infection with human immunodeficiency virus: Clinical and laboratory features of 73 cases. III International Conference on AIDS, Washington, DC, June 1987.
126. Abrams, D. I., Feigal, D. W., and Levy, J. A. (1987). AIDS-related immune thrombocytopenia: HIV expression and progression to AIDS [Poster]. III International Conference on AIDS, Washington, D.C., June 1987.
127. Abrams, D. I., Kirn, D. H., Feigal, D. W., Volberding, P. A. (1987). Persistent generalized lymphadenopathy: Update of a 60-month prospective study [Poster]. III International Conference on AIDS, Washington, D.C., June 1987.
128. Biggar, J. R., Melbye, M., Ebbesen, P. et al. (1984). T-lymphocyte ratios in homosexual men: Epidemiologic evidence for a transmissable agent. *JAMA 251*:1441-1446.
129. Collier, A. C., Murphy, V. L., Roberts, P. L., and Handsfield, H. H. (1987). Clinical course of HIV-seropositive homosexual men [Poster]. III International Conference on AIDS, Washington, D.C., June 1987.
130. De Wolf, F., Goudsmit, J., Paul, D. A., Lange, J. M. A., Hooykaas, C., and Continho, R. A. (1987). HIV antigenemia: Association with decreased numbers of T4-cells and increased risk for AIDS [Poster]. III International Conference on AIDS, Washington, D.C., June 1987.
131. Goedert, J. J., Biggar, R. J., Ebbesen, P. et al. (1986). Three-year incidence of AIDS in five cohorts of HTLV-III-infected risk group members. *Science 231*:992-995.
132. Goedert, J. J., Biggar, R. J., Winn, D. M. et al. (1985). Decreased helper T-lymphocytes in homosexual men: I. Sexual contact in high-incidence areas for the acquired immunodeficiency syndrome. *Am. J. Epidemiol. 121*:629-636.

133. Goedert, J. J., Biggar, R. J., Winn, D. M. et al. (1985). Decreased helper T-lymphocytes in homosexual men: II. Sexual practices. *Am. J. Epidemiol. 121*: 637-644.

134. Goedert, J. J., Sarngadharan, J. G., Biggar, R. J. et al. (1984). Determinants of retrovirus (HTLV-III) antibody and immunodeficiency conditions in homosexual men. *Lancet 2*:711-716.

135. Hessol, N. A., Rutherford, G. W., O'Malley, P. M. et al. (1987). The natural history of human immunodeficiency virus (HIV) infection in a cohort of homosexual and bisexual men: A 7-year follow-up study. III International Conference on AIDS, Washington, D.C., June 1987.

136. Karlsson, A., Morfeldt-Mansson, Ø., Buttinger, B., von Krogh, G., Moberg, L., and Sandstrom, E. (1987). A three-year prospective study of initially asymptomatic HIV positive gay men in Stockholm, Sweden [Poster]. III International Converence on AIDS, Washington, D.C., June 1987.

137. Lang, W., Anderson, R., Winkelstein, W., Jr., Royce, R., Perkins, H. (1987). In a cohort of HIV seropositive men followed for 30 months, initial low 3a T-lymphocyte counts predict subsequent declines in T-cell counts, clinical findings and AIDS. III International Conference on AIDS, Washington, D.C., June 1987.

138. Mayer, K., McCusher, J., Stoddard, A. M., Saltzman, S. P., Moon, M. W., and Groopman, J. E. (1987). Clinical and behavioral predictors of developing AIDS and related outcomes among asymptomatic HIV seropositive homosexual men in Boston [Poster]. III International Conference on AIDS, Washington, D.C., June 1987.

139. Melbye, M. (1986). The natural history of human T-lymphotropic virus-III infection: The cause of AIDS. *Br. Med. J. 292*:5-12.

140. Melbye, M., Biggar, R. J., Ebbesen, P. et al. (1984). Seroepidemiology of HTLV-III antibody in Danish homosexual men: Prevalence, transmission, and disease outcome. *Br. Med. J. 289*:573-575.

141. Moss, A. R., Osmond, D., Bacchetti, P., Casavant, C., Cherman, J.-C., and Carlson, J. (1987). Three-year progression to clinical AIDS in seropositive men: San Francisco General Hospital Study [Poster]. III International Conference on AIDS, Washington, D.C., June 1987.

142. Nicholson, J. K. A., Spira, T. J., Jones, B. M., and McDougal, J. S. (1987). Serial T-cell phenotypes in homosexual men who did or did not progress to AIDS [Poster]. III International Conference on AIDS, Washington, D.C., June 1987.

143. Polk, B. F., Fox, R., Brookmeyer, R. et al. (1987). Predictors of the acquired immunodeficiency syndrome developing in a cohort of seropositive homosexual men. *N. Engl. J. Med. 316*:61-66.

144. Stevens, C. E., Taylor, P. E., Zang, E. A. et al. (1986). Human T-cell lymphotropic virus type III infection in a cohort of homosexual men in New York City. *JAMA 255*:2167-2172.

145. Taylor, J. M. G., Schwartz, K., and Detels, R. (1986). The time from infection with human immunodeficiency virus (HIV) to the onset of AIDS. *J. Infect. Dis. 154*:694-697.

146. Tindall, B., Cooper, D. A., Bureham, J., Donovan, B., Barns, T., and Penny, S. (1987). The Sydney AIDS Project: Factors associated with progression to AIDS [Poster]. III International Conference on AIDS, Washington, D.C., June 1987.

147. Orangio, G. R., Pitlick, S. D., della Latta, P. et al. (1984). Soft tissue infections in parenteral drug abusers. *Ann. Surg. 199*:97-100.

148. Orangio, G. R., della Latta, P., Mario, C. et al. (1983). Infections in parenteral drug abusers: Further immunologic studies. *Am. J. Surg. 146*:738-741.

149. Eyster, E., Goedert, J. J., Sarngadhavan, M. G. et al. (1985). Development and early natural history of HTLV-III antibodies in persons with hemophilia. *JAMA 253*:2219-2223.

150. Goedert, J. J., Sarngadhavan, M. G., Eyster, M. E. et al. (1985). Antibodies reactive with human T-cell leukemia virus (HTLV-III) in the sera of hemophiliacs receiving factor VIII concentrate. *Blood 65*:492-495.

151. Curran, J. W., Lawrence, D. N., Jaffe, H. W. et al. (1984). Acquired immunodeficiency syndrome (AIDS) associated with transfusion. *N. Engl. J. Med. 310*:69-75.

152. Peterman, T. A., Jagge, H. W., Feorino, P. M. et al. (1985). Transfusion-associated AIDS in the United States. International Conference on Acquired Immunodeficiency Syndrome (AIDS). Atlanta, Georgia, April 1985.

153. Peterman, T. A., Drotman, D. P., and Curran, J. W. (1985). Epidemiology of the acquired immunodeficiency syndrome (AIDS). *Epidemiol. Rev. 7*:1-21.

154. Newell, G. R., Adams, S. C., Mansell, P. W. A., and Hersh, E. M. (1984). Toxicity, immunosuppressive effects and carcinogenic potential of volatile nitrites: Possible relationship to Kaposi's sarcoma. *Pharmacotherapy 4*:284-291.

155. Marmor, M., Friedman-Klein, A. E., Laubenstein, L. et al. (1982). Risk factors for Kaposi's sarcoma in homosexual men. *Lancet 1*:1083-1087.

156. Haverkos, H. W., Pinsky, P. F., Drotman, D. P. et al. (1985). Disease manifestations among homosexual men with acquired immunodeficiency syndrome (AIDS): A possible role of nitrites in Kaposi's sarcoma. *Sex. Trans. Dis. 12*: 203-208.

157. Goedert, J. J., Newland, C. Y., Wallen, W. C. et al. (1982). Amyl nitrite may alter T-lymphocytes in homosexual men. *Lancet 1*:412-416.

158. Mathur-Wagh, U., Enlow, R. W., Spigland, I. et al. (1984). Longitudinal study of persistent generalized lymphadenopathy in homosexual men: Relation to acquired immunodeficiency syndrome. *Lancet 1*:1033-1038.

159. Mathur-Wagh, U., Mildvan, D., and Senie, R. T. (1985). Follow-up at 4-1/2 years on homosexual men with generalized lymphadenopathy [Letter]. *N. Engl. J. Med. 313*:1541-1543.

160. Osmond, D., Moss, A. R., Bachetti, P., Volberding, P., Barre-Sinoussi, F., and Chermann, J.-C. (1985). A case-control study of risk factors for AIDS in San Francisco. International Conference on Acquired Immunodeficiency Syndrome (AIDS), Atlanta, Georgia, April 1985.

161. Darrow, W. W., Byers, R. H., Jaffe, H. W., O'Malley, P., Rutherford, G. W., and Echenberg, D. F. (1986). Cofactors in the development of AIDS and AIDS-related conditions. International Conference on AIDS, Paris, France, June 1986.

162. CDC Task Force on Kaposi's Sarcoma and Opportunistic Infections (1982). Epidemiologic aspects of the current outbreak of Kaposi's sarcoma and opportunistic infections. *N. Engl. J. Med. 306*:248-252.

163. Marmor, M., Friedman-Klein, A. E., Zolla-Pazner, S. et al. (1984). Kaposi's sarcoma in homosexual men: A seroepidemiologic case-control study. *Ann. Intern. Med. 100*:809-815.

164. Roland, A., Feigal, D. W., Abrams, D., Volberding, P. A., Hollander, H., and Connant, M. A. (1987). Recreational drug use does not cause AIDS progression [Poster]. III International Conference on AIDS, Washington, D.C., June 1987.

165. Stevens, C. E., Taylor, P. E., Rodriquez, S., and Robinstein, P. (1987). Recreational drugs and HIV infection: Relationship to risk of infection and immune deficiency [Poster]. III International Conference on AIDS, Washington, D.C., June 1987.

166. Wiley, J. A., Rutherford, G. W., Moss, A. R., Winkelstein, W., Jr. (1987). Age and cumulative incidence of AIDS among seropositive homosexual men in high incidence areas of San Francisco. III International Conference on AIDS, Washington, D.C., June 1987.

167. Goedert, J. J., Biggar, R. J., Melbye, M. et al. (1987). Effect of T4 count and co-factors on the incidence of AIDS in homosexual men infected with human immunodeficiency virus. *JAMA 257*:331-334.

168. Munoz, A., Carey, V., Polk, B. F., Saah, A., Phair, J., Kingsley, L., and Fahey, J. (1987). Relationships between decline in CD4 lymphocytes and other variables among 1,828 seropositive gay men [Poster]. III International Conference on AIDS, Washington, D.C., June 1987.

169. McCutchan, J. A., Jacobson, D., Kennedy, C., Spector, S., Klauber, M., and Richman, D. (1987). Risk factors for infection by HIV and development of AIDS in a cohort of gay men [Poster]. III International Conference on AIDS, Washington, D.C., June 1987.

170. Fahey, J., Detels, R., Visscher, B., Munzo, A., Saah, A., and Clark, V. (1987). Maintaining a stable level of CD-4 cells is a favorable prognostic sign among HIV positive men [Poster]. III International Conference on AIDS, Washington, D.C., June 1987.

171. Lindhart, B., Hoffman, B., and Ulrich, K. (1987). Correlation between number of T-helper (Th) cells, lymphocyte response to pokeweed mitogin (PWM) and HIV antigenemia in seropositive homosexual men [Poster]. III International Conference on AIDS, Washington, D.C., June 1987.

172. Osmond, D., Chaisson, R., Leuther, M., Allain, J. P., and Moss, A. R. (1987). Serum HIV antigen (HIV-Ag) as a predictor of progression to AIDS and ARC in homosexual men [Poster]. III International Conference on AIDS, Washington, D.C., June 1987.

173. Pedersen, C. and Neilsen, J. O. (1987). HIV antigenemia precedes the development of AIDS or ARC in patients with HIV infection. III International Conference on AIDS, Washington, D.C., June 1987.

174. Phair, J. P., Chmiel, J., Wallemark, C.-B., Wu, W., and Huprikar, J. (1987). HIV antigenemia and AIDS. III International Conference on AIDS, Washington, D.C., June 1987.

175. Ong, K. R., Klein, E. B., Shriver, K., Goldstein, L., and Cooper, L. Z. (1987). Are absence or progressive loss of antibody to individual viral proteins of HIV predicator for development of AIDS? [Poster]. III International Conference on AIDS, Washington, D.C., June 1987.

176. Robert-Guroff, M., Goeddert, J. J., Jennings, A., Blattner, W. A., and Gallo, R. C. (1987). High HTLB-III/LAV neutralizing antibody titers correlate with better clinical outcome. III International Conference on AIDS, Washington, D.C., June 1987.

177. Weber, J., Clapham, P., Weiss, R., Parker, D., and Cheinsong-Popov, R. (1987). Anti-gag antibodies to HIV: Association with neutralization and clinical outcome in cohorts of homosexual men. III International Conference on AIDS, Washington, D.C., June 1987.

178. Spira, T. J., Kaplan, J. E., Feorino, P. M., Warfield, D. T., Fishbein, D. B., and Bozeman, L. H. (1987). Human immujnodeficiency virus viremia as a prognostic indicator in homosexual men with lymphadenopathy syndrome [Letter]. *N. Engl. J. Med.* *317*:1093-1094.

179. Osmond, D., Chaisson, R., Beasley, P., Bacchetti, P., and Moss, A. (1987). Hepatitis B virus coinfection in homosexual men seropositive for human immunodeficiency virus antibody. III International Conference on AIDS, Washington, D.C., June 1987.

180. Mann, D. L., Murray, C., Goedert, J. J., Blattner, W. A., and Robert-Guroff, M. (1987). HLA phenotypes are possible risk factors for development of AIDS. III International Conference on AIDS, Washington, D.C., June 1987.

181. Eales, L. J., Hye, K. E., Parkin, J. M. et al. (1987). Association of different allelic forms of group specific component with susceptibility to and clinical manifestation of human immunodeficiency virus infection. *Lancet* *1*:999-1002.

182. Morgan, W. M. and Curran, J. W. (1986). Acquired immunodeficiency syndrome: Current and future trends. *Public Health Rep.* *101*:459-465.

183. Pitchenik, A. E., Fishl, M. A., Dickinson, Ø. et al. (1983). Opportunistic infection and Kaposi's sarcoma among Haitians: Evidence of a new acquired immunodeficiency state. *Ann. Intern. Med.* *98*:277-284.

184. CDC (1985). Provisional Public Health Service inter-agency recommendations for screening donated blood and plasma for antibody to the virus causing acquired immunodeficiency syndrome. *MMWR 34*:1-5.

185. San Francisco Department of Public Health (1986). AIDS among intravenous drug users—San Francisco. *San Francisco Epidemiol. Bull.* *2*(6):1-3.

186. CDC (1985). Heterosexual transmission of human T-lymphotropic virus type III/lymphadenopathy-associated virus. *MMWR 34*:561-563.

187. Guinan, M. E. and Hardy, A. (1987). Epidemiology of AIDS in women in the United States. *JAMA 257*:2039-2042.

188. Schwarcz, S. K. and Rutherford, G. W. (in press). Acquired immunodeficiency syndrome in infants, children, and adolescents. *J. Drug. Issues.*

189. Curran, J. W., Lawrence, D. L., Jaffe, H. et al. (1984). Acquired immunodeficiency syndrome (AIDS) associated with transfusions. *N. Engl. J. Med.* *310*:69-75.

190. Prompt, C. A., Reis, M. M., Grillo, F. M. et al. (1985). Transmission of AIDS virus at renal transplantation. *Lancet 2*:672.

191. Food and Drug Association (1986). Safety of immune globulins in relation to HTLV-III. *FDA Drug Bull. 16*:3.

192. CDC (1984). Hepatitis B vaccine: Evidence confirming lack of AIDS transmission. *MMWR 33*:685-687.

193. CDC (1985). Changing patterns of acquired immunodeficiency syndrome in hemophilia patients—United States. *MMWR 34*:241-243.

194. McGrady, G., Gjerset, G., and Kennedy, S. (1985). Risk of exposure to HTLV-III/LAV and type of clotting factor used in hemophilia. International Conference on AIDS, Atlanta, Georgia, April 1985.

195. CDC (1987). Survey of non-U.S. hemophilia treatment centers for HIV seroconversions following therapy with heat-treated factor concentrates. *MMWR 36*:121-124.

196. *Lancet* (1984). Needlestick transmission of HTLV-III from a patient infected in Africa. *2*:1376-1377.

197. Stricoff, R. L. and Morse, D. L. (1986). HTLV-III seroconversion in a health care worker following an occupational needlestick injury. 114th Annual Meeting of the American Public Health Association, Las Vegas, Nevada, September 1986.

198. Gerberding, J. L., Hopewell, P. C., Kamingley, L. S., and Sande, M. A. (1985). Transmission of hepatitis B without transmission of AIDS by accidental needlestick [Letter]. *N. Engl. J. Med. 312*:56.

199. CDC (1982). Acquired immunodeficiency syndrome (AIDS): Precautions for clinical and laboratory staffs. *MMWR 31*:577-580.

200. CDC (1983). Acquired immunodeficiency syndrome (AIDS): Precautions for health-care workers and allied professionals. *MMWR 32*:450-451.

201. CDC (1985). Recommendations for preventing transmission of infection with human T-lymphotropic virus type III/lymphadenopathy-associated virus in the workplace. *MMWR 34*:682-686, 691-695.

202. CDC (1986). Recommendations for preventing transmission of infection with human T-lymphotropic virus type III/lymphadenopathy-associated virus during invasive procedures. *MMWR 35*:221-223.

203. CDC (1986). Human T-lymphotropic virus type III/lymphadenopathy-associated virus: Agent summary statement. *MMWR 35*:540-542.

204. Selik, R. M., Starcher, E. T., and Curran, J. W. (1987). Opportunistic infections reported in AIDS patients: Frequencies, associations, and trends. *AIDS 1*:175-182.

205. Rutherford, G. W., Echenberg, D. F., Rauch, K. J. et al. (1986). The epidemiology of AIDS-related Kaposi's sarcoma in San Francisco: Evidence for decreasing incidence. International Conference on AIDS, Paris, France, June 1986.

206. Giraldo, G., Beth, E., and Huang, E. S. (1980). Kaposi's sarcoma and its relationship to cytomegalovirus (CMV). III. CMV DNA and CMV early antigens in Kaposi's sarcoma. *Int. J. Cancer 26*:23-29.

207. Drew, W. L., Conant, M. A., Miner, R. C. et al. (1982). Cytomegalovirus and Kaposi's sarcoma in young homosexual men. *Lancet 2*:125-127.
208. Drew, W. L., Mint, L., Miner, R. C., Sands, M., and Ketterer, B. (1981). Prevalence of cytomegalovirus infection in homosexual men. *J. Infect. Dis. 143*: 188-192.
209. Drew, W. L., Mills, J., Hauer, L., Gottlieb, A., and Miner, R. (1986). Declining prevalence of Kaposi's sarcoma in homosexual AIDS patients is paralleled by declining incidence of CMV infection. International Conference on AIDS, Paris, France, June 1986.
210. Lifson, A. R., Bodecker, T. W., Barnhart, J. L. et al. (1987). AIDS in the San Francisco City Clinic Study. 27th Interscience Conference on Antimicrobial Agents and Chemotherapy, New York, New York, October 1987.
211. Rothenberg, R., Woelfel, M., Stonburner, R., Milberg, J., Parker, R., and Truman, B. (1987). Survival with the acquired immunodeficiency syndrome: Experience with 5833 cases in New York City. *N. Engl. J. Med. 317*:1297-1302.
212. Lemp, G. F., Barnhart, J. L., Rutherford, G. W., Temelso, T., and Werdegar, D. (1987). Predictors of survival for AIDS cases in San Francisco. 115th Annual American Public Health Association Meeting, New Orleans, Louisiana, October 1987.
213. Office of the Assistant Secretary for Health (1986). Surgeon General's Report on Acquired Immunodeficiency Syndrome. Washington, D.C.: Public Health Service.
214. MacDonald, D. I. (1986). Coolfont report: A PHS plan for prevention and control of AIDS and the AIDS virus. *Public Health Rep. 101*:341-348.
215. Acheson, E. D. (1986). AIDS: A challenge for the public health. *Lancet 1*: 662-666.
216. Francis, D. P. and Chin, J. (1987). The prevention of AIDS in the United States: An objective strategy for medicine, public health, business, and the community. *JAMA 257*:1357-1366.

2

The African AIDS Experience in Contrast with the Rest of the World

Nathan Clumeck and **Nathan Carael** *Free University of Brussels, Brussels, Belgium*

Philippe Van de Perre *National AIDS Control Programme and Rwandese-Belgian Medical Cooperation, Kigali, Rwanda*

Human immunodeficiency virus (HIV) infection is now endemic in most sub-Saharan African countries. By April 1987, 3538 cases from 36 countries have been reported to the World Health Organization. However, this is undoubtedly a large underestimate of the reality, as it is thought that 50,000 to 100,000 people, so far, have suffered or died from acquired immunodeficiency syndrome (AIDS) in that continent. Seroprevalence rates of 1% to 20% are found in the general population, and 27% to 88% of certain groups, such as female prostitutes and their clients, may be infected; thus, it is evident that, at present, several million HIV-infected individuals must exist in Africa. The HIV infection is creating a major public health problem in Africa, on the same scale as parasitic, diarrheal, and respiratory diseases. In that continent, more than anywhere else in the world, health care costs for HIV-infected patients are putting a tremendous burden on budgets already limited by sparce resources. In addition, in some parts of Africa, most AIDS patients are found predominantly in high socioeconomic classes and in the most productive stage of their lives. Thus, the years of potential active life lost because of AIDS will have dramatic and far-reaching consequences on socioeconomic development. From the beginning of the epidemic, with the recognition of the first cases among African residents in Europe (1,2) and, subsequently, in Rwanda and Zaire (3,4), some striking epidemiological and clinical differences from cases from Western countries were noted. From a historical viewpoint, it is interesting that evidence of heterosexual transmission of AIDS virus has been questioned vigorously (5,6), and hypotheses very distant from the African reality have been elaborated in an attempt to explain the characteristics of the African epidemic.

So far, AIDS cases in Africa have had a male/female ratio of about 1, in contrast with the 19:1 male/female ratio in the United States, and a peak age-specific AIDS case incidence and HIV seroprevalence between 20 to 49 years of age. In contrast with Western countries, male homosexuality, intravenous drug use, and hemophilia are not found among African AIDS patients. Risk factors for HIV infection in Africa include heterosexual contacts, blood transfusions, parenteral administration of unsterile material, and mother-to-infant transmission before, during, or shortly after birth. From the clinical point of view, the natural history of HIV infection in Africa is very similar to that described among homosexuals in the United States, Europe, and Australia (7,8). However, differences exist in clinical presentation and type of opportunistic infections, which undoubtedly reflect exposure of the host to local pathogens.

This chapter discusses differences between HIV infection in Africa and in Western countries.

WHICH VIRUSES ARE INVOLVED IN AFRICAN AIDS?

From the beginning of the epidemic, it was apparent that HIV isolates from central African patients were similar to American or European isolates in their biologic and serologic properties. However, a larger polymorphism was noted, indicating that they may have been evolving over a longer period (9). In 1985, retroviruses different from HIV-1 were isolated from individuals residing in West Africa, an area of the continent where the reported incidence of AIDS is lower than in Central Africa. Kanki and colleagues isolated a retrovirus in subhuman primates that they called simian T-lymphotropic virus type III (STLV-III, now known as SIV; 10). Seropositivity against SIV-like virus was further found among healthy prostitutes from Senegal (11). The virus isolated was termed human T-lymphotropic virus type IV (HTLV-IV) and demonstrated 50% to 60% genetic homology to HIV-1 (12). The HTLV-IV now named HIV-2 is widespread among healthy heterosexually active adults in West African countries (mostly Guinea Bissau, Burkina Fasso, Senegal, and Ivory Coast; 13). By the end of 1985 Clavel and collaborators identified, among several West African patients with AIDS or AIDS-related complex (ARC), a virus that was named lymphadenopathy virus type 2 (LAV-2; 14). This virus also shows envelope and genomic similarity with SIV and seems more closely related to the monkey virus than to HIV-1. In vitro LAV-2, also called HIV-2, has cytopathogenicity similar to that of HIV-1 in contrast with HIV-2/HTLV-IV which appears to have limited cytopathogenicity and, so far, has not been found to be associated with clinical immunodeficiency. Thus, the designation HIV-2 refers to at least two related retroviruses predominant in West Africa: HIV-2/HTLV-IV and HIV-2/LAV-2. These viruses are serologically indistinguishable because they have homologous antigens that crossreact immunologically. Epidemiologic surveys have shown that HIV-2 is almost absent in central African countries (13,15).

HETEROSEXUAL TRANSMISSION: RISK FACTORS AND COFACTORS

The epidemiologic pattern of the African AIDS epidemic strongly favors bidirectional heterosexual transmission as the primary mode by which HIV is spread within this continent. Because HIV is a sexually transmitted disease, prostitutes are at great risk of exposure, and contact with prostitutes has been identified as an important risk factor for men in some areas. A case-control study of heterosexual African men with AIDS showed a strong association between HIV infection and a history of contact with prostitutes (81% versus 34%) and an increased number of female partners per year (32% versus 3%) (16).

Two studies, one from Butare, Rwanda (17) and the other from Nairobi, Kenya (18), provide further evidence that female prostitutes are playing a central role in the spread of HIV in African cities. In the Rwandese study, the risk of seropositivity in the male customers of prostitutes increased significantly with the annual number of female sexual partners, most of whom are prostitutes. Interviews of the prostitutes enrolled in these studies, showed that most of them were reluctant to practice oral or anal intercourse, and also to use condoms (17,18; M. Carael, personal observation). Subsequent studies from various African countries confirmed that female prostitute populations who do not use drugs have high rates of HIV infection (19). However, some regional variations exist. As shown in Table 1, the prevalence of HIV among selected groups of prostitutes is higher in eastern and central African countries (27% to 88%) than in West and North Africa (1% to 20%). These very high prevalence rates indicate that central Africa is currently the most heavily infected area, suggesting that the epidemic would have started earlier there than in areas of East or West Africa. Indeed, longitudinal studies performed in Nairobi, Kenya, showed a rising prevalence of HIV infection among prostitutes, from 4% in 1981 to 59% in 1985 and to 90% in 1987 (P. Piot, personal communication).

An analysis of risk factors in various subsets of urban adults from Zaire, Kenya (19,21), and Rwanda showed that an increasing number of sexual

TABLE 1 Prevalence of HIV Antibodies[a] Among African Prostitutes, by Countries

Country (Ref.)	Year of sampling	No. tested	Percentage with antibody
Central and East Africa			
Rwanda (17)	1983	51	74.5
	1984	33	88
Kenya (18,19)	1980-1981	116	4
	1983-1984	130	51
	1985-1986	215	59
Zaire (urban) (54)	1985	377	27
Zaire (rural) (55)	1986	283	11
Western Africa			
Ivory Coast (56)	1986	232	20
Ghana (57)	1986	98	1
Cameroon (58)	1985	358	3
Northern Africa			
Tunisia (59)	1985	108	2
Horn of Africa			
Ethiopia (20)	1986-1987	60	7

[a]Enzyme-linked immunoassay confirmed by Western blot (reactive to > two bands).

encounters, a history of sexually transmitted diseases, and sexual contacts with prostitutes were the major factors predicting HIV infection. It has been hypothesized that these associations could reflect only the exposure to unsterile needles used for parenteral treatments of sexually transmitted infections (22). The fact that the association between HIV infection and history of sexually transmitted infections is stronger than the one between HIV infection and parenteral treatment of sexually transmitted infections in Rwandese men is not in favor of this assertion. Moreover, the disclosure of the same aforementioned associations in Europeans infected with HIV in Africa and who received injections with only disposable materials (23), together with the description of clusters of HIV infection in subjects linked by only sexual contacts (4,24) confirms that the heterosexual route is directly involved in most of the cases of HIV transmission among African adults.

Why is the pattern of transmission of HIV so different in Africa compared with the Western world? Female infibulation (circumcision), which likely increases mucosal trauma during intercourse, may play a role by facilitating contact between blood and sperm and, thus, male-to-female transmission of HIV (25). However, this female circumcision ritual is practiced exclusively in rural areas of northern eastern Africa, where HIV seroprevalence is low compared with central and East Africa (26). More convincing is the association noted between HIV seropositivity and an history of past or present sexually transmitted infections (18,27). This association is stronger in those with a history of genital ulcers than with nonulcerative sexually transmitted infections (28,29), suggesting that ulcerated skin or mucosa could facilitate transmission of the virus during intercourse. In a study of 603 central African people, antibodies to herpes simplex virus type 2 were found in 86% of the patients with HIV infection in comparison with only 39% and 37% of matched control groups consisting, respectively, of healthy Africans living in Brussels and blood donors from Rwanda (30). Moreover, among the controls, infection with HIV and HSV-2 tended to coexist. As a marker of an active sexual life, HSV-2 is associated with HIV infection in central Africa, where it could be an important cofactor among promiscuous heterosexual people. Human immunodeficiency virus has also been successfully isolated from vaginal secretions (31,32) and has been shown to be mainly cell-associated (32). Very recently, indirect immunofluorescence with monoclonal antibody, has shown the presence of HIV p17 antigen in lymphocytes but not in cervicovaginal epithelial cells of African women with both HIV infection and a concurrent sexually transmitted infection (P. Van de Perre, personal observation). Thus, lymphocytes in the female genital tract may serve as target cells and reservoir of HIV. It is then likely that times during which the female genital tract is enriched in lymphocytes—e.g., sexually transmitted infections, menstruation, chronic cervicitis—may facilitate the acquisition and transmission of HIV through heterosexual contact, even in the absence of disruption of the genital skin or mucosa.

For obvious financial reasons, many African prostitutes do not interrupt their sexual activity during menstruation (M. Carael, personal observation). In addition, sexually transmitted infections, including genital ulcers (33), are one of the major public health problems in many African countries (34), being responsible for secondary infertility (35,36), ectopic pregnancies, and pelvic inflammatory disease (37). Sexually transmitted diseases are most prevalent in urban centers, where rupture of traditional social structures, an excess of young recent emigres who are single wage earners, and unawareness of the danger of sexually transmitted infections, are factors facilitating access of men to female prostitutes and exposure to sexually transmitted infections (34). In some large African cities as many as 75% of single men admit to at least one sexual contact with a prostitute each year. This could explain the rapid spread of HIV infection in central and East African cities. Female prostitutes who do not use condoms, and the high prevalence of classic sexually transmitted infections, are the crucial factors responsible for the AIDS epidemic in African cities. Only public health strategies aimed at fighting the spread of HIV, combined with more general measures to prevent sexually transmitted infections, for instance, promotion of condom and spermicide use (38-40), and promotion of social alternatives to prostitutes, will slow the AIDS epidemic in Africa.

CLINICAL ASPECTS OF HIV INFECTION IN AFRICA

The natural history of HIV infection among African patients is similar to that observed among Western patients (7,8). Primary infection may present with a mononucleosislike syndrome or unexplained lymphocytic meningitis (41). The HIV-infected patients can be classified as asymptomatic, lymphadenopathic, AIDS-related complex, and AIDS. Studies of a cohort of 170 African patients seen in Brussels have demonstrated that these different stages reflect different levels of host immune impairment (42). Several studies have shown striking differences in the type and frequency of various opportunistic infections between African and American AIDS patients (Table 2). Similar clinical discrepancies have also been noted among Haitian patients with AIDS, when compared with Americans (43). They reflect the different spectrum of latent infections in developed versus developing countries, and in the future we can expect to find infections with other pathogens more common in the tropical setting. Table 3 summarizes the clinical manifestations seen in African patients in Brussels. *Pneumocystis carinii* was isolated from only 22% of these patients, despite extensive diagnostic procedures such as bronchoalveolar lavage. In contrast, esophageal candidiasis, cerebral toxoplasmosis, cryptococcal infection, and mucocutaneous herpes simplex infection are the most frequent manifestations of immunodeficiency among African patients. Associated infections were diagnosed in 10% to 25% of the patients and included non-typhi salmonellae, tuberculosis (pulmonary and extrapulmonary), and severe extensive varicella-zoster. These

TABLE 2 Comparison Between African and American AIDS Patients

	Percentage of group with indicated infection	
Disease	African[a] $n = 313$	American[b] $n = 12,000$
PCP and/or interstitial pneumonitis	25	50-63
Cryptococcal meningitis	13	7
Toxoplasma gondii encephalitis	21	4

[a]Total patients obtained from Ref. 1,2,3,4,42,51.
[b]Ref. 60.

TABLE 3 Clinical Infections of 59 African Patients with AIDS St. Pierre Hospital, Brussels—1982-1987[a]

Type of infection	Percentage with finding
Opportunistic infections	
esophageal candidiasis	37
cerebral toxoplasmosis	24
mucocutaneous herpes simplex infection	17
cryptococcal meningitis	17
pneumocystis carinii pneumonitis	22
Disseminated cytomegalovirus infection	7
cryptosporidiosis	2
Other associated infections	
septicemia caused by	
non-typhi salmonella	7
pyogenic bacteria	20
(*Escherichia coli*, pneumococcus,	
Staphylococcus aureus)	
tuberculosis (pulmonary and extrapulmonary)	24
varicella-zoster	8

[a]N. Clumeck et al., unpublished data.

latter clinical manifestations, occurring among young sexually active adults, are to be considered as at least indicative of a possible HIV infection in developing countries (44,53). So far, the most typical manifestation of HIV infection in Africa is a diarrhea-wasting syndrome, called "slim disease," characterized by severe weight loss, chronic diarrhea, itchy papular rash, prolonged fever, and oral candidiasis (45). Occasionally, cytomegalovirus inclusions, *Cryptosporidium* parasites, and *Isospora belli* may be found during intestinal biopsies, but in many patients, no specific cause for the diarrhea is apparent. This enteropathic form of AIDS seems to be predominant in some parts of Africa (Zaire, Uganda), but we did not find it to be so among our patients seen in Brussels (42). It is possible that the African patients seen in Europe are less prone to enteropathogen infections because of a high level of hygiene related to their better social status and environment.

African patients also seem to be more prone to mucocutaneous lesions than patients in developed countries (Table 4). These lesions are fairly specific for HIV infection and may lead to an early diagnosis of ARC or AIDS. A generalized papular pruritic eruption (prurigo) is found in approximately 20% of the patients and could be the major complaint in an early stage of the infection. In Kinshasa, Zaire, 87% of consecutive adult outpatients with prurigo were HIV antibody-positive (44). The lesions, which consist of papules,

TABLE 4 Mucocutaneous Lesions Among African Patients with HIV Infection

---

Frequent (10% to 30%)
  generalized papular pruritic eruption (prurigo)
  varicella-zoster
  herpes genitalis
  oral candidiasis
Less frequent (1% to 10%)
  Kaposi's sarcoma
  seborrheic dermatitis
  molluscum contagiosum
  oral hairy leukoplakia
  thrombocytopenic purpura

---

scratch lesions, and hyperpigmented macules, are most frequently found on the extremities and are symmetrically distributed over the body. Histologic features are nonspecific and the etiology is unknown.

The unique and troublesome existence of Kaposi's sarcoma (KS) in central Africa has led some to claim that endemic Kaposi's sarcoma was an evidence against the concept of AIDS as a new disease in Africa (46). The patterns of the two forms of KS that coexist in central Africa (classic and HIV-associated) are summarized in Table 5. In equatorial Africa, KS is an extremely common tumor, and accounts for 12.8% of all malignant tumors in Zaire, 4.5% in Tanzania, 4.2% in Uganda, and 2.9% in Kenya (47). In adults, the disease,

TABLE 5 Differences Between Classic and AIDS-Associated Kaposi's Sarcoma in Central Africa

Characteristic	Classic form	Associated with HIV infection and AIDS
Sex ratio, M/F	15:1	2:1
Geographic distribution	East Zaire, Rwanda, and Uganda only	All area with HIV infection
Clinical form	Cutaneous localized, mostly lower extremities	Cutaneous localized, deep organ involvement is common
Evolution	Chronic, indolent	Rapidly fatal
Cellular immunity	Grossly normal	Severely impaired
Evidence of HIV infection	No	Yes

as defined prior to 1975 (48), was mainly cutaneous, nodular, located predominantly on feet or hands, and with a benign clinical course. Some patients had more aggressive illness, usually developing after several years of indolent disease, with extensive cutaneous lesions on one or more extremities and generally associated with involvement of adjacent bone. Cutaneous lesions in the florid, classic group are exophytic tumors, whereas in Kaposi's sarcoma related to HIV infection, deep lesions associated with dense fibrosis predominate. Over 90% of classic KS patients responded promptly to actinomycin D and vincristine (50). Among these patients, prospective studies performed in the endemic areas (East Zaire or Zambia) failed to demonstrate any significant impairment of cellular immunity, and the patients uniformly lacked antibodies to HIV (49).

The changing pattern of KS was first noted in 1983, in Lusaka, Zambia (50). The "new" pattern of KS among African patients consists of generalized lymphadenopathy, oral, gastrointestinal, or bronchial lesions, together with cutaneous infiltrative plaques on the trunk, the genital organs, the face, or more rarely, the limbs. When associated with opportunistic infection, the disease is rapidly fatal. These patients respond about as well to therapy with high doses of recombinant α-interferon or vinblastine/vincristine (i.e., response rates < 50%) as American or European homosexual patients (N. Clumeck, unpublished data). The 6% to 15% prevalence of aggressive KS among African heterosexual patients seems to be lower than the 25% to 30% prevalence noted among homosexuals or bisexuals from Western countries (2-4,51). A similar lower rate of KS has been noted among IV-drug users in the United States (52). This finding suggests that homosexuals or bisexuals, in contrast with heterosexuals (whether African or IV-drug user), are more susceptible to KS because of cofactors in them that have not yet been identified.

CONCLUSIONS

Human immunodeficiency virus infection in Africa is characterized by heterosexual transmission of the virus in the general population, especially in urban areas. As a consequence of the high seroprevalence rate among young women in their childbearing years, HIV infection is also affecting children, and one can expect major demographic consequences in the forthcoming decades in that continent. Social, economic, and cultural backgrounds and the high prevalence of other sexually transmitted infections have favored the explosive spread of HIV among heterosexuals. In Africa, as well as in Western countries, measures aimed at avoiding any further spread of the epidemic among heterosexuals should focus on prevention, detection, and treatment of sexually transmitted infections in general. A community-based approach to sexually transmitted infection control, focused on prostitutes and other women with multiple sexual partners, patients with sexually transmitted infections, and adolescents, should be implemented, together with control of blood donation, and health education programs should be instituted to inform the population about the risk of HIV transmission through contaminated needles, skin piercing instruments, and sexual contact.

Major impediments to such programs in Africa are cost, logistic problems, and misinformation.

ACKNOWLEDGMENT

This study has been supported by a grant from the European Community, TSD-M-422-B (TT).

REFERENCES

1. Clumeck, N., Sonnet, J., Taelman, H., Mascart-Lemone, F., De Bruyere, M., Van de Perre, P., Dasnoy, J., Marcelis, L., Lamy, M., Jonas, C., Eyckmans, L., Noel, H., Vanhaeverebeek, M., and Butzler, J. P. (1984). Acquired immune deficiency syndrome in African patients. *N. Engl. J. Med. 310*:492-497.
2. Clumeck, N., Sonnet, J., Taelman, H., Cran, S., and Henrivaux, P. (1984). Acquired immune deficiency syndrome in Belgium and its relation to Central Africa. *Ann. N.Y. Acad. Sci. 437*:264-269.
3. Van de Perre, P., Rouvroy, D., Lepage, P., Bogaerts, J., Kestelyn, P., Kayhigi, J., Hekker, A. C., Butzler, J. P., and Clumeck, N. (1984). Acquired immunodeficiency syndrome in Rwanda. *Lancet 2*:62-65.
4. Piot, P., Taelman, H., Minlangu, K. B., Mbendi, N., Ndangi, K., Kalambayi, K., Bridts, C., Quinn, T. C., Feinsod, F. M., Odio, W., Mazebo, P., Stevens, W., Mitchell, S., and McCormick, J. B. (1984). Acquired immunodeficiency syndrome in an heterosexual population in Zaire. *Lancet 2*:65-69.
5. Padian, N. and Pickering, J. (1986). Female-to-male transmission of AIDS: A reexamination of the African sex ratio of cases. *JAMA 256*:590.
6. Pearce, R. B. (1986). Heterosexual transmission of AIDS. *JAMA 256*:590-591.
7. Mann, J. M., Colebunders, R. L. Khonde, N., Nzilambi, N., Jansegers, L., McCormick, J. B., Quinn, T. C., Kalemba, K., Bosenge, N., Malonga, M., Francis, H., Piot, P., and Curran, J. W. (1986). Natural history of human immunodeficiency virus infection in Zaire. *Lancet 2*:707-709.
8. Clumeck, N., Hermans, P., and De Wit, S. (1986). Disease outcome among heterosexual Africans with HTLV-III/LAV infection. *Abstr. 26th Intersci. Conf. Antimicrob. Agents Chemother.*, September 1986, New Orleans, p. 283.
9. Benn, S., Rutledge, R., Folks, T. et al. (1985). Genomic heterogeneity of AIDS retroviral isolates from North America and Zaire. *Science 230*:949-951.

10. Kanki, P. J., Jurth, R., Becker, W. et al. (1985). Antibodies to simian T-lymphotropic virus type III in African green monkeys and recognition of STLV-III viral proteins by AIDS and related sera. *Lancet 1*:1330-1332.

11. Barin, F., M'Boup, S., Denis, F. et al. (1985). Serological evidence for a virus related to simian T-lymphotropic retrovirus III in residents of West Africa. *Lancet 2*:1387-1390.

12. Franchini, G., Gurgo, C., Guo, H. G. et al. (1987). Sequence of the simian immunodeficiency virus and its relationship to the human immunodeficiency viruses. *Nature 328*:539-543.

13. Kanki, P. J. (1987). West African human retroviruses related to STLV-III. *AIDS 1*:141-145.

14. Clavel, F., Guétard, D., Brun-Vézinet, F. et al. (1986). Isolation of a new human retrovirus from West African patients with AIDS. *Science 233*:343-346.

15. Clavel, F. (1987). HIV-2, the West African AIDS virus. *AIDS 1*:135-140.

16. Clumeck, N., Van de Perre, P., Carael, M., Rouvroy, D., and Nzaramba, D. (1985). Heterosexual promiscuity among African patients with AIDS. *N. Engl. J. Med. 313*:182.

17. Van de Perre, P., Clumeck, N., Carael, M., Robert-Guroff, M., Freyens, P., Gallo, R. C., Nzabihimana, E., De Mol, P., Butzler, J. P., and Kanyamupira, J. B. (1985). Female prostitutes: A risk group for infection with human T-cell lymphotropic virus type III. *Lancet 2*:524-526.

18. Kreiss, J. K., Koech, D., Plummer, F. A., Holmes, K. K., Lightfoote, M., Piot, P., Ronald, A. R., Ndinya-Achola, J. O., D'Costa, L. J., Roberts, P., Ngugi, E. N., and Quinn, T. C. (1986). AIDS virus infection in Nairobi prostitutes: Spread of the epidemic to East Africa. *N. Engl. J. Med. 314*:521-523.

19. Quinn, C. T., Mann, J. M., Curran, J. W., and Piot, P. (1986). AIDS in Africa: An epidemiologic paradigm. *Science 234*:955-963.

20. Ayehunie, S., Britton, S., Yemane-Berhane, T., and Fehninger, T. (1987). Prevalence of human immunodeficiency virus (HIV) antibodies in prostitutes and their colients in Addis Ababa, Ethiopia. *Abstr. Int. Conf. AIDS*. June 1987, Washington, D.C., p. 45.

21. Piot, P. and Mann, J. M. (1986). Transmission patterns of HTLV-III/LAV: Evidence for heterosexual transmission. *Abstr. II Int. Conf. AIDS*. June 1986, Paris, France, p. 107.

22. Wikoff, R. (1985). Female to male transmission of the AIDS agent. *Lancet 2*: 1017-1018.

23. Vittecoq, D., May, T., Roue, R. T., Stern, M., Mayaud, C., Chavanet, P., Borsa, F., Jeantils, P., Armengaud, M., Modai, J., Autran, B., and Rey, F. (1987). Acquired immunodeficiency syndrome after travelling in Africa: An epidemiological study in seventeen Caucasian patients. *Lancet 1*:612-614.

24. Clumeck, N., Hermans, P., Taelman, H., Roth, D., Zissis, G., and De Wit, S. (1987). Cluster of heterosexual transmission of HIV in Brussels. *Abstr. III Int. Conf. AIDS*. June 1987, Washington, D.C., p. 76.

25. Linke, U. (1986). AIDS in Africa. *Science 231*:203.

26. Burton, M. (1986). AIDS and female circumcision. *Science 231*:1236.

27. Van de Perre, P., Clumeck, N., Steens, M., Zissis, G., Carael, M., Lagasse, R., De Wit, S., Lafontaine, T., De Mol, P., and Butzler, J. P. (1987). Seroepidemiological study on sexually transmitted diseases and hepatitis B in African promiscuous heterosexuals in relation to HTLV-III infection. *Eur. J. Epidemiol. 3*: 14-18.

28. Hira, S. K., Perine, P. L., Redfield, R. R., Chikamata, D. M., Wadhawan, D., Mwendafilumba, D. et al. (1986). The epidemiology and clinical manifestations of acquired immune deficiency syndrome (AIDS) and its related complex (ARC) in Zambia. *Abstr. Int. Conf. AIDS.* June 1986, Paris, France, p. 101.

29. Greenblatt, R. M., Lukehart, S. L., Plummer, F. A., Quinn, T. C., Critchlow, C. W., D'Costa, L. J. et al. (1987). Genital ulceration as a risk factor for human immunodeficiency virus infection in Kenya. *Abstr. III Int. Conf. AIDS.* June 1987, Washington, D.C., p. 174.

30. Clumeck, N., Hermans, P., De Wit, S., Lee, F., Van de Perre, P., and Nahmias, A. (1987). Herpes type II (HSV₂): A possible co-factor of HIV infection among Central African heterosexual patients. *Abstr. 27th Intersci. Conf. Antimicrob. Agents Chemother.* October 1987, New York.

31. Vogt, M. W., Witt, D. J., Craven, D. E., Byington, R., Crawford, D. F., Schooley, R. T., and Hirsch, M. S. (1986). Isolation of HTLV-III/LAV from cervical secretions of women at risk for AIDS. *Lancet 1*:525-527.

32. Wofsy, C. B., Cohen, J. B., Hauer, L. B., Padian, N. S., Michaelis, B. A., Evans, L. A., and Levy, J. A. (1986). Isolation of AIDS-associated retrovirus from genital secretions of women with antibodies to the virus. *Lancet 1*:527-529.

33. Kraus, S. J. (1984). Genital ulcer adenopathy syndrome. In *Sexually Transmitted Diseases.* (Holmes, K. K., Mardh, P. A., Sparling, P. F., and Wiesner, P. J., eds.). New York, McGraw-Hill, pp. 706-714.

34. Piot, P. and Meheus, A. (1983). Epidemiologie des maladies sexuellement transmissibles dans les pays en développement. *Ann. Soc. Belge Méd. Trop. 63*:87-110.

35. Cates, W., Farley, T. M. M., and Rowe, P. J. (1985). Worldwide patterns of infertility: Is Africa different? *Lancet 2*:596-598.

36. Romaniuk, A. (1969). Infertility in tropical Africa. In *The Population of Tropical Africa.* (Caldwell, J. C. and Onkojo, C., eds.). London, Langmans, pp. 214-224.

37. Muir, D. G. and Belsey, M. A. (1980). Pelvic inflammatory disease and its consequences in the developing world. *Am. J. Obstet. Gynecol. 138*:913-928.

38. Conant, M., Hardy, D., Sernatinger, J., Spicer, D., and Levy, J. A. (1986). Condoms prevent transmission of AIDS-associated retrovirus. *JAMA 225*:1706.

39. Mann, J. M., Quinn, T. C., Piot, P., Bosenge, N., Nzilambi, N., Kalala, M., Francis, H., Colebunders, R. L., Byers, R., Kasa Azila, P., and Curran, J. W. (1986). Condom use and HIV infection among prostitutes in Zaire. *N. Engl. J. Med. 316*:345.

40. Hicks, D. R., Martin, L. S., Getchell, J. P., Heath, J. L., Francis, D. P., McDougal, J. S., Curran, J. W., and Voeller, B. (1985). Inactivation of HTLV-III/LAV-infected cultures of normal human lymphocytes by nonoxynol-9 in vitro. *Lancet 2*:1422-1423.

41. Biggar, R. J., Johnson, B. K., Musoke, S., Masembe, J. B., Silverstein, D. M., Warshow, M. M., and Alexander, S. (1986). Severe illness associated with appearance of antibody to human immunodeficiency virus in an African. *Br. Med. J. 293*:000-000.

42. Clumeck, N., Hermans, P., and De Wit, S. (1987). Some epidemiological and clinical characteristics of African AIDS. *Antibiotics Chemother. 38*:41-51.

43. Pape, J. W., Liautaud, B., Thomas, F., Mathurin, J. R., St. Amand, M. M. A., Boncy, M., Pean, V., Pamphile, M., Laroche, C., Dehovitz, J., and Johnson, W. D. (1985). The acquired immunodeficiency syndrome in Haiti. *Ann. Intern. Med. 103*:674-678.

44. Colebunders, R., Francis, H., Izaley, L., Kabasele, K., Nzilambi, N., Van Der Groen, G., Vercauteren, G., Mann, J. M., Bila, K., Kakonde, N., Ifoto, L., Quinn, T. C., Curran, J. W., and Piot, P. (1987). Evaluation of a clinical case-definition of acquired immunodeficiency syndrome in Africa. *Lancet 1*:492-494.

45. Serwadda, D., Mugerwa, R. D., Sewankambo, N. K., Lwegaba, A., Carswell, J. W., Kirya, G. B., Bayley, A. C., Downing, R. G., Tedder, R. S., Clayden, S. A., Weiss, R. A., and Dalgleish, A. G. (1985). Slim disease: A new disease in Uganda and its association with HTLV-III/LAV infection. *Lancet 2*:849-852.

46. De Cock, K. M. (1984). AIDS: An old disease from Africa? *Br. Med. J. 289*: 306-308.

47. Weber, J. (1984). Is AIDS an epidemic form of African Kaposi's sarcoma? Discussion paper. *J. R. Soc. Med. 77*:572-576.

48. Taylor, J. I., Templeton, A. C., Vogel, C. L., Ziegler, J. L., and Kyalwazi, S. K. (1971). Kaposi's sarcoma in Uganda: A clinico-pathological study. *Int. J. Cancerol. 8*:122-135.

49. Biggar, R. J., Melbye, M., Kestems, L. et al. (1984). Kaposi's sarcoma in Zaire is not associated with HTLV-III infection. *N. Engl. J. Med. 16*:1051.

50. Bayley, A. C. (1984). Aggressive Kaposi's sarcoma in Zambia, 1983. *Lancet 1*: 1318-1320.

51. Odio, W., Kapita, B., Mbendi, N., Kayembe, K., Ndangi, K., Muyembe, T., Mazebo, P., Izzia, K., Lurhuma, Z., Sansa, A., Declercq, D., Henry, M. C., Mbongo, M., McCormick, J. B., Taelman, H., and Piot, P. (1985). Le syndrome d'immunodéficience acquise (SIDA) à Kinshasa, Zaïre: Observations cliniques et épidémiologiques. *Ann. Soc. Belge Méd. Trop. 65*:357-361.

52. Safai, B., Johnson, K. G., Myskowski, P. L., Koziner, B., Yang, S. Y., Cunningham-Rundles, S., Bodbold, J. H., and Dupont, B. (1985). The natural history of Kaposi's sarcoma in the acquired immunodeficiency syndrome. *Ann. Intern. Med. 103*:744-750.

53. Mann, J., Snider, D. E., Francis, H., Quinn, T. C., Colebunders, R. L., Piot, P., Curran, J. W., Nzilambi, N., Bosenge, N., Malonga, M., Kalunga, D., Mu Nzingg, M., and Bagala, N. (1986). Association between HTLV-III/LAV infection and tuberculosis in Zaire. *JAMA 256*:346.

54. Mann, J. M., Quinn, T. C., Francis, H., Miatudila, M., Piot, P., Curran, J. et al. (1986). Sexual practices associated with LAV/HTLV-III seropositivity among

female prostitutes in Kinshasa, Zaire. *Abstr. Int. Conf. AIDS.* June 1986, Paris, France, p. 105.

55. De Cock, K. M., Nzilambi, N., Forthal, D., Ryder, R., Piot, P., McCormick, J. B. et al. (1987). Stability of HIV infection prevalence over 10 years in a rural population of Zaire. *Abstr. III Int. Conf. AIDS.* June 1987, Washington, D.C., p. 117.

56. Denis, F., Barin, F., Gershy-Damet, G. et al. (1987). Prevalence of human T-lymphotropic retrovirus type III (HIV) and type IV in Ivory Coast. *Lancet 1*: 408-411.

57. Neequarye, A. R., Neequaye, J., Mingle, J. A., and Ofori Adjei, D. (1986). Preponderance of females with AIDS in Ghana. *Lancet 2*:978.

58. Durand, J. P., Merlin, M., Josse, R., Garrigue, G., Kaptue Noche, L. et al. (1987). AIDS survey in Cameroon. *Abstr. III Int. Conf. AIDS.* June 1987, Washington, D.C., p. 123.

59. Beth Giraldo, E., Giraldo, G., Gharbi, R. M., Ceparano, M. L., Ceparano, S., and Monaco, M. (1986). AIDS-associated retrovirus (ARV) infection in Tunisia. *Abstr. Int. Conf. AIDS.* June 1986, Paris, France, p. 128.

60. Hardy, A. M., Selik, R. M., Starcker, E. T., Morgan, W. M., and Allen, J. R. (1985). AIDS trends in the United States. *Abstr. 25th Intersci. Conf. Antimicrob. Agents Chemother.*, Minneopolis, 1985, Abstr. No. 222.

3
Defects in Host Defenses in HIV Infection and AIDS: Characteristics and Pathogenesis

James P. Steinberg and John P. Phair *Northwestern University Medical School, Chicago, Illinois*

The human immunodeficiency viruses (HIV-1, HIV-2, and possibly others) are now established as the cause of the acquired immunodeficiency syndrome (AIDS). The marked selective depletion of the CD4 (T4) lymphocyte subset seen in AIDS along with the pivotal role of the CD4 cell in the integrity of the immune system suggested that the causative agent would directly affect these cells. With the discovery of HIV-1 (1,2), a retrovirus cytopathic for CD4 cells, a unifying hypothesis of infection followed by impairment and depletion of CD4 cells followed by immunodeficiency seemed plausible. It is now known that HIV can infect many other cells including macrophages (3) and B cells (4). Primary infection of these cells may be important in the development of the immunodeficiency characteristic of AIDS.

This chapter reviews the characteristics and the pathogenesis of the immunologic abnormalities in AIDS. In addition, some of the opportunistic pathogens seen in AIDS are discussed in the context of the observed immune dysfunction.

T-LYMPHOCYTE DEFECTS

Quantitative Abnormalities

Patients with AIDS have a marked decrease in the number of circulating lymphocytes bearing the CD4 molecule (T4 or helper/inducer lymphocytes).

The CD4 molecule is customarily identified by binding to fluorochrome-conjugated monoclonal antibodies (e.g., OKT4, Leu3). The reduced "helper/suppressor" or CD4/CD8 ratio is primarily due to depletion of CD4 cells; the CD8 lymphocyte number is variable, but it is often increased early in the course of HIV infection. In HIV-infected individuals, a decreased number of CD4 cells is a marker of disease progression. Asymptomatic seropositive individuals have a near normal CD4 lymphocyte count (normal = 1000 ± 200/mm^3), whereas progressively fewer circulating CD4 lymphocytes are found in patients with lymphadenopathy, AIDS related symptoms, Kaposi's sarcoma, and in patients with AIDS-defining opportunistic infections (OI). Patients with OI usually have a CD4 cell count of fewer than 100/mm^3. The number of CD4 cells is also a predictor of progression of HIV infection; over a 2-year period close to 50% of infected individuals with fewer than 400/mm^3 cells, and about 85% with fewer than 200/mm^3 cells develop AIDS. With use of monoclonal antibodies that identify subsets of the CD4 lymphocyte population, a pattern of CD4 cell loss emerges. The CD4 lymphocyte subset which binds Leu8 monoclonal antibody (CD4+ Leu8+) is decreased in lymphadenopathy patients and in AIDS patients. This subset induces suppressor cell function. The CD4+ Leu8− subset, which provides help for B cells, is preserved in lymphadenopathy patients but is also decreased in AIDS patients (5).

The mechanism(s) of CD4 cell depletion in AIDS is not clear. Although HIV infection can cause syncytium formation and cell death in vitro, the direct cytopathic effect of HIV alone probably does not account for the CD4 cell depletion in vivo, because in situ hybridization studies can detect productive virus infection in only 1:20,000 to 1:100,000 CD4 lymphocytes (6). A cell expressing the HIV envelope glycoprotein could form syncytia with uninfected CD4 cells, leading to cell death, potentially explaining the loss of uninfected CD4 cells (7). The cytopathic effect of HIV may be dependent on a high density of CD4 molecules on the cell surface. Infection of monocytes and B cells, cells that have a low density of surface CD4 molecules, does not lead to cell death. Immune destruction of CD4 cells may result from a humoral or cellular response directed against viral antigens bound to the CD4 molecule or present elsewhere in the lymphocyte envelope. Another postulated mechanism is the selective loss of a subset of cells critical to CD4 cell propagation.

Functional Abnormalities

The opportunistic infections seen in AIDS patients provide clear evidence of functional inadequacy of cell-mediated immunity, which is orchestrated by T lymphocytes. Delayed-type hypersensitivity (DTH) to common antigens is almost always absent in AIDS patients with OI, and represents in vivo evidence of impaired cellular immunity. Some AIDS patients with only Kaposi's sarcoma are not anergic. Many in vitro T-cell functional defects have been reported in AIDS, including decreased proliferative responses to mitogens and antigens, abnormal lymphokine production, a qualitative defect in providing B-cell help, and defective cytotoxic T-lymphocyte function (8).

The abnormal proliferative response to pokeweed mitogen seen in mononuclear cell preparations from peripheral blood of AIDS patients is due to the quantitative depletion of CD4 lymphocytes rather than a qualitative deficit in CD4 funciton. Lane et al. (9) showed that purified CD4 populations from HIV-infected patients responded normally to mitogenic stimulation. Response to soluble antigen (tetanus toxoid), however, was significantly reduced in purified CD4 preparations. This deficient response to tetanus toxoid was also demonstrated in cell preparations from asymptomatic seropositive men with normal numbers of circulating CD4 lymphocytes, suggesting a qualitative abnormality in CD4 cells (10). An alternative possibility was the selective depletion of the subset of CD4 cells that respond to protein antigen. In addition, defective antigen presentation by monocytes/macrophages could account for the observed results, because antigen presentation in conjunction with the major histocompatibility complex (MHC) class II receptor complex is necessary for CD4 cell response to soluble antigen but not to nonspecific mitogens. This possibility is especially intriguing now that it has been shown that HIV can infect macrophages. In this situation, and in several others, the issue of qualitative versus quantitative abnormalities has not been resolved nor has the potential contribution (or lack of contribution) from other arms of the immune system been excluded. Thus, the mechanism of defective response to soluble antigen has not been definitively explained.

Interleukin 2 (IL-2) production by T cells in response to mitogens has been reported to be diminished in AIDS patients. As with proliferative responses, however, IL-2 production by standard numbers of CD4 cells from HIV seropositive patients after mitogenic stimulation is not reduced (11). The IL-2 production in response to soluble antigen (purified protein derivative; PPD) is decreased in CD4 preparations, paralleling the proliferative response to soluble antigen. Spontaneous IL-2 production is decreased in HIV-infected men without AIDS (12).

Epstein et al. found that interferon (IFN) production by T lymphocytes in response to cytomegalovirus (CMV) antigen was impaired, whereas near-normal levels of IFN were produced following mitogenic stimulation (13). In this study, lymphocyte proliferation and IFN production were similarly reduced in AIDS patients with CMV viremia compared with those without, suggesting that the abnormalities were not due to immunosuppression from coexisting CMV infection. Other investigators reported subnormal IFN-γ production by unfractionated T lymphocytes in response to mitogens (14). Interleukin 2 may be an important stimulus for IFN-γ production in the intact immune system, and defective IL-2 production in AIDS could account for the abnormal IFN response to antigen. However, after recombinant IL-2 stimulation, AIDS patient's lymphocytes produce on average 13- to 14-fold less IFN-γ than controls (15). Thus, deficient IL-2 alone does not explain the abnormal IFN generation.

The CD4 cells from AIDS patients do not help normal allogeneic B cells produce immunoglobulin when incubated with pokeweed mitogen (16). Suppression of immunoglobulin production by CD8 (T8 or suppressor/cytotoxic) cells from AIDS patients is identical with normal controls. In general, suppressor cell function in patients with HIV infection appears to be qualitatively normal. The activated CD8 cells seen with AIDS probably represent a secondary response to coexistent viral infections.

Lymphocytes from AIDS patients have defective in vitro cytotoxic T-lymphocyte (CTL) responses to CMV and influenza virus-infected cells and to HLA alloantigens (17,18). The CTL response can be increased by the addition of IL-2, evidence that the defect is in CD4 help and not in the cytotoxic T-effector cells. Interleukin 2 does not restore CTL function in all AIDS patients, however, suggesting that other mechanisms for decreased CTL response, such as a true defect in CTL precursors, might exist.

Generation of a CTL response to virus-infected cells requires presentation of viral antigens in conjunction with MHC class II antigens on monocytes/macrophages. The CTL response to HLA alloantigens, in contrast, is not MHC class II restricted. Shearer et al. demonstrated that patients with AIDS-related complex (ARC) and some AIDS patients have absent CTL response to influenza virus-infected cells but retain normal CTL response to HLA alloantigens, whereas most other AIDS patients have defective CTL responses to both stimuli (19). They observed that patients with recently diagnosed AIDS often had selective loss of anti-influenza CTL response, whereas more advanced cases lost CTL response to alloantigens as well. Thus, it appears that a selective defect in CTL responses precedes a more generalized one, possibly because of an early depletion of the CD4 cell subset responsible for MHC class II antigen recognition or to a qualitative defect in CD4 cells. Alternatively, a defect in the antigen-presenting cells (monocytes/macrophages) could explain the loss of MHC-restricted CTL response.

NATURAL KILLER CELL ACTIVITY

Natural killer (NK) cells are large granular lymphocytes that appear to be responsible for immune surveillance against neoplastic cells. They also are capable of lysing virus-infected cells and mediate antibody-dependent cell-mediated cytotoxicity (ADCC). The number of circulating NK cells in AIDS patients has been reported to be normal but also has been reported to decrease with disease progression (20). In vitro, NK cells from patients with generalized lymphadenopathy and AIDS are deficient in their ability to lyse the K562 tumor cell line, a standard measure of NK cell function (20). However, the magnitude of this defect is small and some AIDS patients have normal NK activity. The defect appears to be the trigger for release of the cytotoxic factors responsible for target cell lysis (21). Interleukin 2 supplementation can partially restore cytolytic function, suggesting that the underlying problem is a lack of T-cell inductive signal.

MONOCYTE/MACROPHAGE FUNCTION

Tissue macrophages of the reticuloendothelial system (RES) are responsible for clearance of particulate antigen from the blood stream and are important in the killing of intracellular organisms, including many of the opportunistic pathogens common in AIDS patients. Splenic macrophages clear IgG-sensitized autologous erythrocytes from the circulation, and measuring the rate of clearance of IgG-sensitized ^{51}Cr-labeled erythrocytes is an in vivo estimate of Fc receptor-mediated macrophage function. With use of this assay, 11 of 15 AIDS patients were found to have defective clearance (22). The mean clearance halftime for the AIDS patients was significantly longer than the control group (73.2 min vs 26.6 min). Patients with AIDS-related illness had an intermediate halftime of 37.1 min. As mentioned previously, monocytes and macrophages serve as antigen-presenting cells to CD4 lymphocytes, and defects in CD4 cell response to antigen may be due to defective antigen presentation. The effect of HIV infection on this function of monocytes and macrophages has not yet been thoroughly investigated. However, there is preliminary in vitro evidence from studies on identical twins suggesting that monocyte dysfunction alone is not responsible for defective CD4 cell response to tetanus toxoid (10). In these studies, the impaired blastogenic response to tetanus toxoid of CD4 cells from a patient with AIDS could not be restored by the addition of monocytes from his seronegative twin.

Monocyte chemotaxis, phagocytosis, and killing have been reported as defective (8,23) and as normal (24). Alveolar macrophages from AIDS patients undergoing diagnostic bronchoscopy respond normally to lymphokines including recombinant IFN-γ by inhibiting the replication of *Toxoplasma gondii* and *Chlamydia psittaci* (25). Thus, there is no consensus on the ability of monocytes and macrophages to function in their effector roles. Alternatively, mononuclear cells from various compartments may be altered differently in HIV infection. Spontaneous secretion of IL-1 and defective IL-1 production in response to inducers of IL-1 has been observed, suggesting that monocytes are in a preactivated state and, consequently, are unable to respond to normal signals. In contrast, other investigators have reported decreased IL-1 production by unstimulated adherent mononuclear cells (12). These abnormalities could be a direct effect of HIV infection in monocytes or could be due to defective stimulation from CD4 lymphocytes. Macrophages, when infected with HIV in vitro, produce a substance that suppresses IL-1 activity (26). The significance of this "contra IL-1" is unknown.

B-LYMPHOCYTE FUNCTION

Infection with HIV leads to elevated serum levels of immunoglobulins (IgG and IgA) and to the presence of circulating immune complexes and autoantibodies. The increased immunoglobulin level was initially thought to be reactive and reflect a humoral immune system that was intact. Subsequent work has shown that the hypergammaglobulinemia is the result of an intense polyclonal activation of B cells (16). In AIDS, there is a marked increase in the number of lymphocytes spontaneously secreting immunoglobulin, but there is a failure of B cells to increase immunoglobulin production after stimulation with mitogens. Thus, AIDS patients appear to lack unactivated B cells, those normally responsive to activation signals. In vivo, AIDS patients do not mount appropriate antibody responses after immunization with protein or polysaccharide antigens (27). The inability to produce antibody in response to new antigens has clinical relevance in that it limits the utility of serologic tests in the diagnosis of new infections. Patients with AIDS rarely produce IgM antibody to CMV or *T. gondii*, even with active infection.

Multiple mechanisms are probably responsible for the polyclonal B-cell activation described earlier. AIDS patients are almost invariably infected with Epstein-Barr virus (EBV), which transforms and activates B lymphocytes. Indeed, the number of spontaneously outgrowing B cells, a measurement of the number of circulating EBV-infected B cells, is increased in AIDS patients (28). However, the estimated number of EBV-infected cells is far fewer than the number of B cells in AIDS that spontaneously produce antibody, which is between 0.1% to 1% of circulating lymphocytes. Secondly, some B cells from AIDS patients spontaneously secrete antibody to HIV, contributing to the observed hypergammaglobulinemia. This antibody production is probably a consequence of chronic antigenic stimulation. A third and possibly the major cause of the polyclonal B-cell activation is direct activation by HIV. Incubating B cells from seronegative donors with HIV for only 1 hr induces marked T-cell-independent proliferative responses and immunoglobulin secretion (29). The responses to HIV are of the same order of magnitude as responses to potent B-cell mitogens, suggesting that they could account for the hypergammaglobulinemia observed in AIDS patients.

POLYMORPHONUCLEAR LEUKOCYTE FUNCTION

Patients with AIDS have increased susceptibility to cutaneous infections with *Staphlyococcus aureus*, suggesting a defect in polymorphonuclear (PMN) cell function. Comparatively little data is available on PMN function in AIDS. Two studies reported that PMN chemotaxis was depressed in AIDS patients (24,30). The PMN phagocytosis and killing was found to be normal in homosexuals with AIDS, but it was defective in intravenous drug abusers with AIDS. Seronegative drug abusers also had abnormal PMN phagocytosis and killing, suggesting that the defect was related to the IV drug use and not to HIV. This finding raises an important issue that might explain some of the conflicting data in the literature on the immunologic defects in AIDS. Immunologic abnormalities have been described in homosexual males, intravenous drug abusers, and hemophiliacs, unrelated to infection with HIV. These groups differ somewhat in exposure to other infectious agents and to other antigenic stimulation that could be immunosuppressive. Consequently, the underlying AIDS risk group examined could influence the results of a study, underscoring the need to use controls from the same high-risk group.

SUPPRESSOR SUBSTANCES

Sera from AIDS patients can suppress IL-2 production by T cells and large granular lymphocytes from normal hosts (31). The suppressive factor(s) is stable at 60 °C and is not inactivated by ether and, therefore, is not HIV. Because IL-2 is essential for normal cytotoxic T-cell and NK-cell activity, this putative suppressor substance may be important in the pathogenesis of AIDS. In addition, supernatants from mononuclear cell cultures of AIDS patients can interfere with antigen and mitogen (phytohemagglutinin, pokeweed mitogen, and concanavalin A)-induced T-cell proliferative responses (32). The relative molecular mass of the suppressive factor from these cell cultures is about 47,000 Da.

Soluble immunosuppressive substances have been found in other retroviral infections. The best characterized is p15E, which is part of the protein envelope of feline leukemia virus. Recently, the large envelope protein of HIV (gp120) was shown to suppress phytohemagglutinin-induced lymphocyte blastogenesis but not T-cell responses to concanavalin A or pokeweed mitogen (33). Recombinant gp120 in concentrations greater than 1 μg/ml suppresses tetanus toxoid-induced lymphocyte proliferative responses (34). It is postulated that the binding of gp120 to the CD4 molecule prevents the CD4 molecule from interacting with the MHC class II antigens of monocytes/macrophages during antigen presentation. It is not known if the amount of HIV or gp120 present in vivo during HIV infection is sufficient to cause immunosuppresion by this mechanism.

PATHOGENESIS

A simplified representation of the immunologic abnormalities resulting from infection with HIV is presented in Figure 1. Although impairment of CD4 cells can account for most of the immunodeficiency, direct effects of

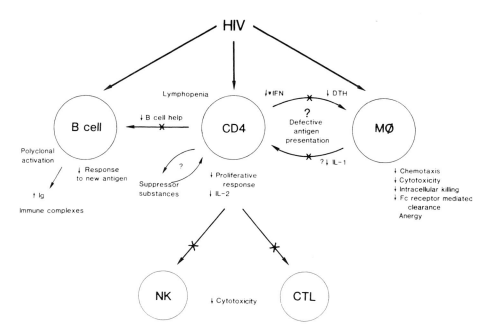

FIGURE 1   Schematic representation of the alterations in the immune system in AIDS. Abnormal effector cell functions of B cells and monocyte/macrophages (MØ) may be a direct consequence of HIV infection or be caused by lack of CD4 cell induction, or both. Deficient CD4-inductive signals impair the cytotoxic function of natural killer (NK) and cytotoxic T cells (CTL). Antigen processing and presentation to CD4 cells by macrophages has not been studied in depth, but abnormalities in these macrophage functions could contribute to the observed CD4 cell defects. Immunosuppressive substances produced by HIV-infected cells may play a role in the pathogenesis of AIDS.

HIV on monocyte/macrophages and B cells, and the existence of soluble suppressor substances may be essential to the development of immunodeficiency. Factors that influence the course of infection with HIV are currently poorly understood. Clinically, infection may be latent and asymptomatic for months or years, or result in the profound immunodeficiency characteristic of AIDS. At the cellular level, HIV can establish latency in CD4 cells and, upon activation, replicate rapidly and produce a lytic infection. In monocytes and macrophages, HIV can enter a state of limited replication that is not cytopathic, perhaps because the cytopathic effect of HIV is dependent upon high levels of surface CD4 molecules (7). The importance of genetic and environmental factors and coinfections in the development of progressive HIV infection and immunodeficiency is not known. In vitro, T-cell activation is necessary to produce active infection. The clinical correlation with this observation may be that coinfections or immune stimulators, such as IL-2, that activate T cells could convert a latent HIV infection into an active infection.

CLINICAL CONSEQUENCES

The clinical consequences of the profound immunosuppression seen in AIDS are unrelenting infections with a wide range of opportunistic pathogens and "opportunistic tumors" such as Kaposi's sarcoma. The opportunistic infections are typically those associated with defective cell-mediated immunity (Table 1). These organisms are primarily intracellular pathogens that can escape or are unaffected by the antimicrobial actions of antibody and complement.

TABLE 1 Defects in Host Defenses, Degree of Impairment in AIDS, and Associated Microorganisms

Defect	Impaired in AIDS	Pathogen
T lymphocyte-macrophage	+ + + +	Herpesvirus group, *Listeria*, *Legionella*, *Salmonella*, mycobacteria, *Nocardia*, *Cryptococcus*, *Candida*, *Histoplasma*, *Coccidioides*, *Pneumocystis*, *Toxoplasma*, *Strongyloides*
B-cell		
adults	+	Streptococci including pneumococcus,
children	+ + +	*Haemophilus*
Granulocytes	±	Gram-negative bacilli, staphylococci, *Candida*, *Aspergillus*
Complement	−	*Neisseria*, pneumococci

Host defense against these organisms requires intact antigen processing by monocytes and macrophages, the ability of CD4 cells to proliferate and elaborate lymphokines, and normal effector function of cytotoxic T cells, NK cells, and activated macrophages. Although cellular immunity is often discussed separately from humoral immunity for convenience, the arms of the immune system usually operate in concert. For example, activated macrophages can kill ingested *T. gondii* only if the organisms have been opsonized.

A clear relationship exists between progressive CMV disease and the absence of in vitro cytotoxic T-cell responses to CMV-infected cells. Most AIDS patients have active CMV infections, and CMV viremia is usually present preterminally. Accordingly, cytotoxic T-cell activity toward CMV-infected cells is absent in AIDS patients (35). The spectrum of candidal infections in AIDS patients also correlates well with the observed in vitro immune defects. Mucosal infections with *Candida albicans* are common in AIDS and in other diseases involving cell-mediated immunity such as chronic mucocutaneous candidiasis, whereas disseminated candidiasis, usually associated with prolonged granulocytopenia, is rare in AIDS. Not all pathogens behave as would be suspected, however. *Listeria monocytogenes* is an intracellular organism that replicates in nonactivated macrophages and is a frequent pathogen in other cellular immunodeficiency states. For unknown reasons, listeriosis is rare in AIDS.

Other factors, such as the colonization rate with an organism, are important determinants of the incidence of infection. Histoplasmosis, coccidioidomycosis, and tuberculosis are relatively common infections in AIDS patients from areas endemic for the organisms. Antibody to *Pneumocystis carinii* can be demonstrated in 90% of normal adults, suggesting that this organism is widespread in the environment. The ubiquity of *P. carinii* may help explain the incidence of pneumocystis pneumonitis in AIDS, but the remarkable frequency of infection with this previously uncommon organism also highlights the uniqueness of the immunodeficiency of AIDS. The severity of the immunodeficiency in AIDS is also demonstrated by the high relapse rate of cryptococcal, Salmonella and other infections after therapy that is curative in other hosts. The inability of macrophages from AIDS patients to kill ingested *Mycobacterium avium-intracellulare* is dramatically shown by tissue specimens laden with macrophages engorged with acid-fast bacilli. Finally, the frequency of multiple coexistent opportunistic infections in AIDS is unprecedented and is testimony to the devastation of cell-mediated immunity.

AIDS patients are unable to mount antibody responses to new antigens, yet infections indicative of B-cell dysfunction are not diagnostic of AIDS in adults. In fact, pneumonias caused by *Haemophilus influenzae* and *Streptococcus pneumoniae* do occur at an increased frequency in AIDS patients and are commonly bacteremic (36). Because of past exposure to these organisms, the spontaneously secreting B cells in AIDS patients probably afford some protection against these pathogens. Encapsulated organisms more commonly cause disease in pediatric AIDS patients, possibly because of the lack of prior exposure to these bacteria and the absence of spontaneously produced protective antibody. Adults infected with HIV should receive vaccines to encapsulated organisms before the development of immunodeficiency. Gamma globulin therapy has been used in pediatric AIDS patients to prevent recurrent bacterial infections; a controlled trial to document efficacy is currently underway. Finally, although a clear-cut defect in PMN function has not been delineated, there are reports of serious staphylococcal infections, including pneumonia and cellulitis, complicating the course of patients with Kaposi's sarcoma.

SUMMARY

The recent medical literature is replete with studies on the immunological abnormalities in AIDS. Some of the data is in apparent conflict, complicating attempts to understand the nature of the disease. The use of different methodologies and the small size of populations studied are partial explanations. In addition, patient populations may not be comparable from study to study. AIDS patients with OI are dramatically more immunocompromised than patients with Kaposi's sarcoma. In patients with OI, it may be difficult to separate the effects of HIV from coexisting and potentially immunosuppressive infections such as CMV. Finally, immunologic defects unrelated to HIV infection exist in homosexual males, hemophiliacs, and intravenous drug abusers and can confound comparison of data.

Notwithstanding these obstacles, the understanding of the immunopathogenesis of AIDS has progressed rapidly over the past several years. It is now recognized that HIV infects and alters the function of B cells and macrophages. Accordingly, the schematic representation of HIV's effect on the immune system presented in this review differs from previously published models that attribute the entire spectrum of immunologic abnormalities to CD4 cell dysfunction and depletion. The relative importance of infection of the different cell types in the development of immunodeficiency is not known. Further knowledge of the basic mechanisms by which HIV alters cellular function, and advances in the understanding of immunoregulation, in general, are needed to clarify the immunopathogenesis of AIDS and are undoubtedly forthcoming. At present, prospects of reversing HIV-induced immunodeficiency, once established, are not encouraging. Preventing the progression of immunodeficiency may be a less formidable and, perhaps, a more important challenge considering the large number of individuals who are currently infected and still immunocompetent.

REFERENCES

1. Barre-Sinoussi, F., Chermann, J. C., Rey, F., Nugeyre, M. T., Chamaret, S., Greust, J., Dauguet, C., Axler-Blin, C., Brun-Vezinet, F., Rouzioux, C., Rozenbaum, W., and Montagnier, L. (1983). Isolation of a new T lymphotropic retrovirus from a patient at risk for acquired immune deficiency syndrome (AIDS). *Science 220*:868-871.
2. Gallo, R. C., Salahuddin, S. Z., Popovic, M., Shearer, G. M., Kaplan, M., Haynes, B. F., Palker, T. J., Redfield, R., Oleske, J., Safai, B., White, G., Foster, P., and Markham, P. D. (1984). Frequent detection and isolation of cytopathic retroviruses (HTLV-III) from patients with AIDS and at risk for AIDS. *Science 224*:500-505.
3. Gartner, S., Markovits, P., Markovitz, D. M., Kaplan, M. H., Gallo, R. C., and Popovic, M. (1986). The role of mononuclear phagocytes in HTLV-III/LAV infection. *Science 233*:215-219.
4. Montagnier, L., Gruest, J., Chamaret, S., Daugnet, C., Axler, C., Guetard, D., Nugeyre, M. T., Barre-Sinoussi, F., Chermann, J. C., Brunet, J. B., Klatzmann, D., and Gluckman, J. C. (1984). Adaptation of lymphadenopathy associated virus (LAV) to replication in EBV-transformed B lymphoblastoid cell lines. *Science 225*:63-66.
5. Nicholson, J. K. A., McDougal, J. S., and Spira, T. J. (1985). Alternations of functional subsets of T helper and T suppressor cell populations in acquired immunodeficiency syndrome (AIDS) and chronic unexplained lymphadenopathy. *J. Clin. Immunol. 5*:269-274.
6. Harper, M. E., Marselle, L. M., Gallo, R. C., and Wong-Staal, F. (1986). Detection of lymphocytes expressing human T-lymphotrophic virus type III in lymph nodes and peripheral blood from infected individuals by in situ hybridization. *Proc. Natl. Acad. Sci. USA 83*:772-776.
7. Sodroski, J., Goh, W. C., Rosen, C., Campbell, K., and Haseltine, W. A. (1986). Role of the HTLV-III/LAV envelope in syncytium formation and cytopathicity. *Nature 322*:470-474.
8. Bowen, D. L., Lane, H. C., and Fauci, A. S. (1985). Immunopathogenesis of the acquired immunodeficiency syndrome. *Ann. Intern. Med. 103*:704-709.
9. Lane, H. C., Depper, J. M., Greene, W. C., Whalen, G., Waldmann, T. A., and Fauci, A. S. (1985). Qualitative analysis of immune function in patients with the acquired immunodeficiency syndrome. *N. Engl. J. Med. 313*:79-84.
10. Fauci, A. S. (1987). AIDS: Immunopathogenic mechanisms and research strategies. *Clin. Res. 35*:503-510.
11. Antonen, J. and Krohn, K. (1986). Interleukin 2 production is HTLV-III/LAV infection: Evidence of defective antigen-induced, but normal mitogen-induced IL-2 production. *Clin. Exp. Immunol. 65*:489-496.

12. Goldsmith, J. M., Huprikar, J., Wu, S. J. Y., and Phair, J. P. (1986). Interleukin 1 and 2 production in homosexual men: A controlled trial of Therafectin (SM-1213), a possible immunomodulator. *J. Immunopharm. 8*:1-14.
13. Epstein, J. S., Frederick, W. R., Rook, A. H., Jackson, L., Manischewitz, J. F., Mayner, R. E., Masur, H., Enterline, J. C., Djeu, J. Y., and Quinnan, C. V. (1985). Selective defects in cytomegalovirus- and mitogen-induced lymphocyte proliferation and interferon release in patients with acquired immunodeficiency syndrome. *J. Infect. Dis. 152*:727-733.
14. Murray, H. W., Rubin, B. Y., Masur, H., and Roberts, R. B. (1984). Impaired production of lymphokines and immune (gamma) interferon in the acquired immunodeficiency syndrome. *N. Engl. J. Med. 310*:883-889.
15. Murray, H. W., Welte, K., Jacobs, J. L., Rubin, B. Y., Mertelsmann, R., and Roberts, R. B. (1985). Production of and in vitro response to interleukin 2 in the acquired immunodeficiency syndrome. *J. Clin. Invest. 76*:1959-1964.
16. Lane, H. C., Masur, H., Edgar, L. C., Whalen, G., Rook, A. H., and Fauci, A. S. (1983). Abnormalities of B-cell activation and immunoregulation in patients with the acquired immunodeficiency syndrome. *N. Engl. J. Med. 309*:453-458.
17. Rook, A. H., Manischewitz, J. F., Frederick, W. R., Epstein, J. S., Jackson, L., Gelmann, E., Steis, R., Masur, H., and Quinnan, G. V. (1985). Deficient, HLA-restricted cytomegalovirus-specific cytotoxic T cells and natural killer cells in patients with the acquired immunodeficiency syndrome. *J. Infect. Dis. 152*: 627-630.
18. Sharma, B. and Gupta, S. (1985). Antigen-specific primary cytotoxic T lymphocyte (CTL) responses in acquired immune deficiency syndrome (AIDS) and AIDS-related complexes (ARC). *Clin. Exp. Immunol. 62*:296-303.
19. Shearer, G. M., Bernstein, D. C., Tung, K. S. K., Via, C. S., Redfield, R., Salahuddin, S. Z., and Gallo, R. C. (1986). A model for the selective loss of major histocompatibility complex self-restricted T cell immune responses during the development of acquired immune deficiency syndrome (AIDS). *J. Immunol. 137*:2514-2521.
20. Creemers, P. C., Stark, D. F., and Boyko, W. J. (1985). Evaluation of natural killer cell activity in patients with persistent generalized lymphadenopathy and acquired immunodeficiency syndrome. *Clin. Immunol. Immunopathol. 36*:141-150.
21. Bonavida, B., Katz, J., and Gottlieb, M. (1986). Mechanism of defective NK cell activity in patients with acquired immunodeficiency syndrome (AIDS) and AIDS-related complex. *J. Immunol. 137*:1157-1163.
22. Bender, B. S., Frank, M. M., Lawley, T. J., Smith, W. J., Brickman, C. M., and Quinn, T. C. (1985). Defective reticuloendothelial system Fc-receptor function in patients with acquired immunodeficiency syndrome. *J. Infect. Dis. 152*: 409-412.
23. Smith, P. D., Ohura, K., Masur, H., Lane, H. C., Fauci, A. S., and Wahl, S. M. (1984). Monocyte function in the acquired immune deficiency syndrome. *J. Clin. Invest. 74*:2121-2128.

24. Nielsen, H., Kharazmi, A., and Faber, V. (1986). Blood monocyte and neutrophil functions in the acquired immune deficiency syndrome. *Scand. J. Immunol.* *24*:291-296.

25. Murray, H. W., Gellene, R. A., Libby, D. M., Rothermel, C. D., and Rubin, B. Y. (1985). Activation of tissue macrophages from AIDS patients: In vitro response of AIDS alveolar macrophages to lymphokines and interferon-gamma. *J. Immunol.* *135*:2374-2377.

26. Crowe, S., Heinzel, F., McGrath, M., Mills, J., and Locksley, R. (1987). Production of contra interleukin I by HIV-infected macrophages. *Abstracts 27th Intersci. Conf. Antimicrob. Agents Chemother.* New York, American Society for Microbiology.

27. Ammann, A. J., Schiffman, G., Abrams, D., Volberding, P., Ziegler, J., and Conant, M. (1984). B-cell immunodeficiency in acquired immunodeficiency syndrome. *JAMA 251*:1447-1449.

28. Yarchoan, R., Redfield, R. R., and Broder, S. (1986). Mechanisms of B cell activation in patients with acquired immunodeficiency syndrome and related disorders. *J. Clin. Invest.* *78*:439-447.

29. Schnittman, S. M., Lane, H. C., Higgins, S. E., Folks, T., and Fauci, A. S. (1986). Direct polyclonal activation of human B lymphocytes by the acquired immune deficiency syndrome virus. *Science 233*:1084-1086.

30. Lazzarin, A., Uberti Foppa, C., Galli, M., Mantovani, A., Poli, G., Franzetti, F., and Novati, R. (1986). Impairment of polymorphonuclear leukocyte function in patients with acquired immunodeficiency syndrome and with lymphadenopathy syndrome. *Clin. Exp. Immunol.* *65*:105-111.

31. Siegel, J. P., Djeu, J. Y., Stocks, N. I., Masur, H., Gelman, E. P., and Quinnan, G. V. (1985). Sera from patients with the acquired immunodeficiency syndrome inhibit production of interleukin-2 by normal lymphocytes. *J. Clin. Invest.* *75*:1957-1964.

32. Laurence, J. and Mayer, L. (1984). Immunoregulatory lymphokines of T hybridomas from AIDS patients: Constitutive and inducible suppressor factors. *Science 225*:66-69.

33. Mann, D. L., Lasane, F. L., Popovic, M., Arthur, L. O., Robey, W. G., Blattner, W. A., and Newman, M. J. (1987). HTLV-III large envelope protein (gp120) suppresses PHA-induced lymphocyte blastogenesis. *J. Immunol.* *138*:2640-2644.

34. Shalaby, M. R., Krowka, J. F., Gregory, T. J., Hirabayashi, S. S. E., McCabe, S. M., Kaufman, D. S., Stites, D. P., and Ammann, A. J. (1987). The effects of human immunodeficiency virus recombinant envelope glycoprotein and immune cell function in vitro. *Cell. Immunol.* *110*:140-148.

35. Quinnan, G. V., Siegel, J. P., Epstein, J. S., Manischewitz, J. F., Barnes, S., and Wells, M. A. (1985). Mechanisms of T-cell functional deficiency in the acquired immunodeficiency syndrome. *Ann. Intern. Med.* *103*:710-714.

36. Polsky, B., Gold, J. W. M., Whimbey, E., Dryjanski, J., Brown, A. E., Schiffman, G., and Armstrong, D. (1986). Bacterial pneumonia in patients with the acquired immunodeficiency syndrome. *Ann. Intern. Med.* *104*:38-41.

4

Clinical and Laboratory Features Associated with Acute Human Immunodeficiency Virus Infection

Suzanne Crowe   *San Francisco General Hospital, San Francisco, California*

Infection with human immunodeficiency virus (HIV), the primary causal agent of the acquired immunodeficiency syndrome (AIDS), results in a wide spectrum of clinical manifestations. These include an acute illness associated with seroconversion (acute HIV), an asymptomatic carrier state, persistent generalized lymphadenopathy and other AIDS-related conditions (ARC), and the production of a severe immunodeficiency that ultimately results in severe opportunistic infections and malignancies characteristic of AIDS. This chapter discusses the acute illness associated with HIV infection, herein termed *HIV mononucleosis*.

This acute illness may present as a syndrome resembling infectious mononucleosis (1-3) or, less commonly, solely as an acute neurologic illness—meningitis (4), encephalitis (5), polyneuropathy (6), or myelopathy (7). It is uncertain why the acute illness associated with HIV infection was not recognized and reported until December 1984, 3-½ years after AIDS was initially described. Perhaps the diffuse and often nonspecific nature of the symptoms associated with acute HIV infection passed unnoticed amidst the clinical and diagnostic drama produced by the sudden epidemic of unusual infections and malignancies in a young and previously healthy population. Alternatively, the illness may have been mistaken for atypical Epstein-Barr virus (EBV) or cytomegalovirus (CMV) infection.

The pathogenesis of HIV mononucleosis has not been established. It is most probably related to HIV infection and replication within the reticuloendothelial system. This acute illness is part of the clinical spectrum of disease associated with HIV infection and should be considered in the differential diagnosis of infectious mononucleosislike syndromes and acute neurologic disorders.

EPIDEMIOLOGY

Prevalence and Incidence

The prevalence of HIV mononucleosis is not accurately known. In an early Australian study, 11 of 12 men who seroconverted were retrospectively questioned and reported an infectious mononucleosislike illness (2). In a recent Scandinavian study, three individuals who were infected through sexual contact with an HIV carrier all developed HIV mononucleosis (8). In a third study of seroconversion in intravenous drug abusers in Italy, 16 of 17 individuals were symptomatic (9). In other studies in which subjects may have been less closely questioned or examined, only a few individuals have developed an acute illness before seroconversion, and most individuals have remained asymptomatic during this early phase of HIV infection (10,11).

Human immunodeficiency mononucleosis has been described in all groups at risk for HIV infection. It was first described in a female health care worker infected by a needle-stick exposure (1). It has since been recognized in homosexual and bisexual men (2), sexually active heterosexual African men (12), intravenous drug abusers (4,9), hemophiliacs receiving factor VIII (13-15), recipients of blood transfusions (14), renal transplant recipients (16), in the female sexual partner of a bisexual man (6) and in the lesbian sexual partner of a female intravenous drug abuser (17), and in health care workers after parenteral and nonparenteral workplace exposure to infected materials (18-20). There have been no reports of HIV mononucleosis occurring in children, other than in a 14-year-old hemophiliac (13). Regions in which the syndrome has been documented include Australia, the United Kingdom, New Zealand, Scandinavia, United States, Europe, and Africa (1,2,8,9,12,21).

Risk Factors

A reduction in the number of sexual partners by homosexual men in San Francisco from a median number of 16 per year in 1978 to one in 1985 has effectively reduced the seroconversion rate from over 10% per year (1980/1984) to less than 1% per year during 1986 (22). When compared with seronegative controls, homosexual men in San Francisco who seroconverted between 1983 and 1987 statistically had a greater number of male partners, a higher incidence of receptive anal intercourse within the preceding year, and were more likely to have used cocaine, amphetamines, or hallucinogens during sexual activity (23). Anal sexual contact has also correlated with seroconversion in a recent study from the Netherlands (10).

A recent study of risk factors for HIV infection in sexually active women in San Francisco indicates that a sexual relationship with an intravenous drug abuser or bisexual male carries a higher risk of HIV infection than multiple partner exposure (24). This risk factor is obviously dependent upon the seroprevalence of heterosexual males within the community, which is currently low in San Francisco. Condom use has been demonstrated to reduce HIV infection among spouses of patients with AIDS and ARC, from 82% to 17% over an 18-month period, indicating effective but incomplete protection (25).

Incubation Period

The date of exposure to HIV through sexual contact or intravenous drug abuse is often not known or is imprecise. However, health care workers who have accidental exposure to HIV and recipients of contaminated blood transfusions have provided more reliable data about the incubation period of acute HIV infection.

The reported time interval from infection to onset of illness has varied from 6 days to 6 weeks (1,4). There have been infrequent instances in which the incubation period is much longer, up to 6 months (9,26); however, the documentation of exposure is less reliable in these reports.

CLINICAL FEATURES OF ACUTE HIV

The symptoms of HIV mononucleosis may be nonspecific; however, the syndrome is usually manifest as an illness resembling infectious mononucleosis or as an acute neurologic disorder. The illness begins with the abrupt onset of a constellation of symptoms, including fever, sweats, rigors, malaise, fatigue, myalgia, neuralgia, arthralgia, headaches, and gastrointestinal disturbances (2; Table 1).

Approximately three-quarters of patients complain of a sore throat (2) and difficulty swallowing (8,12); this is usually associated with pharyngeal and buccal erythema (7). There may be shallow ulcers on palatal and gingival mucosa and exudate over the tonsillar fossae (3,12). Routine bacterial throat cultures are negative (8).

A macular, erythematous rash develops during the course of the illness in about half of the symptomatic individuals (2). Initially, the eruption is more

TABLE 1 Comparison of Clinical Features of HIV Mononucleosis and EBV Mononucleosis

	Percentage of patients with indicated findings	
Feature	HIV[a] (%)	EBV[b] (%)
Fever/sweats	92	76
Myalgia/arthralgia	92	20
Malaise/lethargy	83	57
Lymphadenopathy	75	94
Sore throat	75	82
Anorexia/nausea/vomiting	67	21
Headaches/photophobia	58	51
Rash	50	10

Sources: [a]Ref. 2; [b]Ref. 27.

prominent on the face, neck, and chest, later spreading to involve the extremities, including palms and soles in some patients (3). The rash may be morbilliform (8) or resemble that of roseola (28,29), but in general the individual lesions are sparse and somewhat larger than those associated with common viral exanthemata, being up to 1 cm in diameter (3; Fig. 1). The rash usually fades within 5 to 7 days leaving no pigmentation of the skin. Other reported dermatologic manifestations associated with HIV mononucleosis include urticaria (4), alopecia (21), genital ulceration (12), desquamation of palms and soles (2,21), and the sudden appearance of seborrheic dermatitis (30).

Lymphadenopathy develops during HIV mononucleosis in about three-quarters of individuals, and often persists after resolution of other symptoms (12). In a recent study, lymphadenopathy was the sole manifestation of HIV mononucleosis in individuals who subsequently seroconverted (14). The lymphadenopathy is generalized and often accompanied by mild splenomegaly. Lymph node biopsy, if performed, will show nonspecific reactive hyperplasia (12).

Acute anicteric hepatitis has been described in association with HIV mononucleosis, often occurring later in the illness (up to 4 weeks after onset of the first clinical manifestation). Liver biopsy shows mild cytolysis and portal inflammation. The hepatitis resolves spontaneously, with liver function returning to normal within 10 weeks. In most patients there is no clinical evidence of hepatitis, despite mild to moderate elevation of hepatic transaminases (12,28,31).

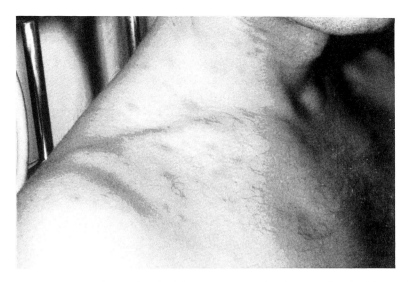

FIGURE 1   Rash associated with HIV mononucleosis. (Reprinted with permission from Dr. R. Lucas and Dr. H. Newton-John, Fairfield Hospital, Melbourne, New South Wales, Australia.)

Human immunodeficiency virus has been isolated from brain tissue, and neurologic disease may be the only clinical manifestation of HIV mononucleosis. However the neurologic disease is generally accompanied by the febrile illness associated with the other components of HIV mononucleosis (4,7). Despite headaches and photophobia occurring in over 50% of patients with HIV mononucleosis, laboratory-documented acute lymphocytic meningitis has been reported in very few patients (4). The virus can be isolated simultaneously from the cerebrospinal fluid and plasma (32).

Acute and subacute encephalopathy are also rare consequences of HIV mononucleosis, characterized by a nonspecific febrile prodromal period lasting up to 2 weeks (5,12). This is followed by the development of mood changes, confusion, progressive obtundation, incontinence, and seizures. Neurologic examination reveals an altered mental status without focal signs. In the reported cases, the individuals recovered spontaneously with no short-term neurologic sequelae (5,12).

The abrupt onset of facial palsy and peripheral sensory-motor neuropathy has been described in one patient with acquisition of HIV (6). Recently, an acute myelopathy has been reported in one individual, characterized by an increasingly unsteady gait, paraparesis, and hyperreflexia of the upper limbs; sensation was normal. This disorder was associated with shaking spasms of the legs and severe lancinating back pain (7). Two months after presentation obvious neurologic signs persisted and his gait remained unsteady. A burning sensation in the lower limbs in the absence of objective neurologic signs has also been described (21).

Significant depression develops in some patients during acute HIV infection and may persist for several months (3). Other reported features of acute HIV infection include conjuctivitis (7), sacral hyperesthesia, and major weight loss (21). Recurrent nasopharyngeal infection (33) and immune thrombocytopenic purpura (33) have been noted at seroconversion. This illness is usually severe; the duration of acute symptoms generally ranges from 15 to 66 days (2,3,9), and continuing lethargy, malaise, low-grade fever, and depression may incapacitate the individual for an additional 2 to 3 months (12).

LABORATORY FINDINGS

At the onset of HIV mononucleosis there is initially a lymphopenia and thrombocytopenia followed by a lymphocytosis coincident with the development of atypical lymphocytes (2,3,31). Some patients develop an absolute polymorphonuclear leukocytosis, rather than a lymphopenia during the acute illness (4,6). There is usually no overall change in numbers of T4 (CD4) cells before and after seroconversion (2), although the number of T4 cells falls transiently within the first week of illness (3,14). A marked proliferation of T8 (CD8) suppressor cells occurs, reaching a peak about 2 weeks after the onset of illness, and causing an inversion of the T4/T8 (CD4/CD8) ratio (3). Recovery from HIV mononucleosis is associated with a gradual and incomplete resolution of the T8 lymphocytosis, with sustained inversion of T4/T8 ratio (12). Generally, the erythrocyte sedimentation rate is elevated and the hematocrit level is normal (4).

There is often a modest elevation of hepatic transminases (two to three times normal; 6); less commonly this elevation is marked and prolonged (21). Peak aspartate transaminase and alanine transaminase may reach 18 times normal, with alkaline phosphatase rarely exceeding twice normal levels (34). Lactate dehydrogenase levels may be markedly elevated (21), and bilirubin concentration is invariably normal (3). Liver function test results return to normal within 10 weeks (31,34). Although hepatitis A and B, and EBV- and CMV-associated hepatitis can be excluded by appropriate testing, hepatic dysfunction resulting from simultaneous acquisition of HIV with non-A, non-B hepatitis agent(s) remains a possibility.

The cerebrospinal fluid (CSF) of patients with meningitis has been reported to show between 20 to 100 lymphocytes/mm^3, with normal protein and glucose levels (4). The HIV has been cultured from CSF (32). In a report of three patients who presented with encephalopathy, the CSF pressure was normal, there was a mild pleocytosis (0 to 30 lymphocytes/mm³) and the protein concentration was elevated (up to 1 g/L) with a normal glucose level (5). Computed tomography of the brain was unremarkable but electroencephalography showed diffuse slow-wave changes compatible with encephalitis (5).

Immunologic testing has generally shown cutaneous anergy to multiple antigens (31), a low mitogenic response to phytohemagglutinin (31), an increase in C1Q binding (35), and polyclonal elevation of serum IgG (14,21) during HIV mononucleosis.

DIFFERENTIAL DIAGNOSIS OF HIV MONONUCLEOSIS

Acute HIV infection should be considered as part of the differential diagnosis of any infectious mononucleosislike or influenzalike illness, or acute neurologic disorder. It produces a constellation of symptoms similar to those induced by a variety of other infectious agents. Depending on the presentation, infection with Epstein-Barr virus, cytomegalovirus, *Toxoplasma gondii*, *Treponema palladum*, herpes simplex virus, and hepatitis B virus, should be considered (see Table 1). Heterophil antibody test, VDRL, and viral serology are negative (4,5).

DIAGNOSIS

Antibodies to HIV generally appear from 8 days to 10 weeks after the onset of clinical illness in adults (2). In infants, the period between infection and seroconversion is not known (see Chap. 9). Antibodies directed against the various retroviral components do not develop simultaneously; antibodies directed against core proteins (p24, p55) may be detected up to 4 weeks before those directed against transmembrane proteins (p41) and viral enzymes (p34, p53/68; 4,36). The antibody response to envelope glycoproteins (gp 160/gp 120) appears to be more variable. It is possible that different assay techniques might give different results. For example, the western blot technique is relatively insensitive for detection of envelope antibodies, which may explain the temporal difference in core and envelope antibody appearance (36,37).

The whole-virus (first generation) enzyme-linked immunosorbent assay (ELISA) is the usual screening test performed by most laboratories to detect HIV infection. Several investigators have found it to be a less sensitive assay than the western blot, which in general detects antibody to HIV several weeks earlier than the ELISA (29,36). In some individuals there is a window period lasting up to 16 weeks during which the ELISA is negative but a western blot (if performed) will detect specific antibodies (29,37). A typical pattern observed in sequential serum samples during early seroconversion is an ELISA that is initially negative in the presence of a weakly reactive western blot, or western blot that is positive for only p24. Over the next few weeks, there will be an increasing signal/cutoff ELISA ratio, with acquisition of antibodies to additional HIV antigens detected by western blot (14).

Immunoglobulin M antibody production is not clearly correlated with either the IgG antibody response or the clinical manifestations of acute HIV infection. The IgM antibodies to HIV are generally detected less commonly in the sera of HIV-infected individuals (38), are found in lower titer than the IgG antibodies, and may persist longer than 1 year (39). However, in one recently published study of eight homosexual men with acute HIV infection, IgM antibody (tested by an immunofluorescent assay) consistently developed before the IgG response. Anti-HIV IgM was detected at a mean of 5 ($\pm$ 3) days after the onset of acute illness, peaking at 24 ($\pm$ 17) days, and disappearing by 81 ($\pm$ 27) days. Antibody to IgG was first detected at 11 ($\pm$ 3)

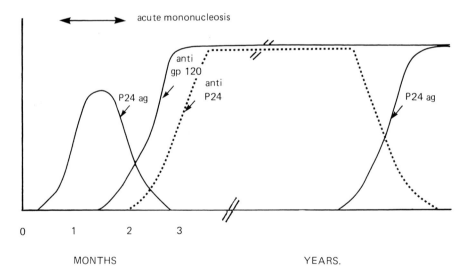

FIGURE 2 Development of HIV antigens and antibodies in relation to symptoms of HIV mononucleosis. P24 antigen (p24 ag) is first detected coincident with clinical symptoms. The initial antibody to appear in the serum is directed towards HIV envelope glycoprotein gp120 (anti-gp120) and this usually remains elevated throughout the course of the disease. Antibody directed against core protein p24 (anti p24) appears in the serum coincident with a decline in 24 antigen. The reappearance of p24 antigen and associated decline in anti p24 is a marker of disease progression.

days, and the titer peaked at 133 (± 63) days, persisting thereafter (40). In a second study, from Switzerland, of six individuals after serconversion, IgM antibodies directed against HIV viral proteins were detected by western blot 18 to 114 days before development of IgG (41).

The development of commercial antigen capture assays to detect HIV p24 core antigen in serum may allow earlier detection of HIV infection (Fig. 2). Whereas seroconversion uncommonly occurs during HIV mononucleosis, HIV antigenemia can be demonstrated as soon as 2 weeks after infection (33), providing an earlier definitive diagnosis of HIV infection. The HIV p24 antigen can be transiently detected before or at the time of seroconversion (42). In a recently reported study, sequential samples of serum from 35 men who seroconverted revealed HIV antigen in five individuals up to 16 weeks before seroconversion (43). In a second study, 9 of 14 individuals had detectable HIV p24 antigen before seroconversion. Some individuals remain antigenemic; however, HIV antigenemia usually disappears within 3 to 5 months (33) (it often recurs late in the disease, when p24 antibody levels decline). It is possible that at seroconversion p24 antigen becomes complexed with antibody and is, thus, no longer detectable. The loss of detectable antigen may also reflect a decrease in viral replication or the development of a latent phase of HIV infection.

The presence of HIV p24 antigen in CSF has been described (43); HIV p24 was detected in the CSF of an individual during seroconversion, before the appearance of CSF antibodies. Persistence of p24 antigen within CSF is considered to reflect severe CNS disease (43).

In patients with HIV mononucleosis, HIV can also be isolated from serum or peripheral blood lymphocytes before the development of antibody. However, HIV culture is much less suitable as a diagnostic tool because it is labor- and reagent-intensive and, therefore, much more expensive than commercially available antigen detection assays. A comparison between antigen detection and virus isolation in eight patients with acute HIV infection showed that during the first 2 weeks of illness both HIV antigen and virus were detected, with a decreasing titer in antigen concentration occurring over this time. Thereafter, HIV antigen was not detectable, despite continued isolation of HIV from plasma (44).

SUMMARY AND CONCLUSIONS

Symptomatic acute HIV infection (HIV mononucleosis) is a nonspecific febrile illness, usually resembling infectious mononucleosis but that occasionally presents as an acute neurologic disorder (as can also be seen rarely in acute EBV infection) and, thus, should be considered in the differential diagnosis of these conditions. The illness is often accompanied by an initial lymphopenia and thrombocytopenia, with the development of atypical lymphocytes and an inverted T4/T8 (T-helper/T-suppressor) ratio later during the course.

The data regarding the proportion of patients infected with HIV who develop HIV mononucleosis are conflicting, with no data on large studies available. The incubation period between infection and onset of illness is generally from 6 days to 6 weeks, with seroconversion usually occurring within 10 weeks from commencement of symptoms. Although antibodies directed against HIV are not detected during the early phase of this illness, the development of HIV antigen assays may permit earlier diagnosis. If available, viral cultures from lymphocytes, serum, or cerebrospinal fluid may also aid in early diagnosis. There is now no indication that individuals who develop symptoms associated with acute infection have a long-term prognosis that differs from those who have asymptomatic infection.

REFERENCES

1. Editorial (1984). Needlestick transmission of HTLV III from a patient infected in Africa. *Lancet 2*:1376-1377.
2. Cooper, D. A., Gold, J., Maclean, P. et al. (1985). Acute AIDS retrovirus infection. *Lancet 1*:537-540.
3. Biggs, B. and Newton-John, H. (1986). Acute HTLV III infection. *Med. J. Aust. 144*:545-546.
4. Ho, D. D., Sarngadharan, M. A., Resnick, L. et al. (1985). Primary human T lymphotropic virus type III infection. *Ann. Intern. Med. 103*:880-883.
5. Carne, C. A., Tedder, R. S., Smith, A. et al. (1985). Acute encephalopathy coincident with seroconversion for anti-HTLV III. *Lancet 2*:1206-1208.
6. Piette, A. M., Tusseau, F., Vignon, D. et al. (1986). Acute neuropathy coincident with seroconversion for anti-LAV/HTLV III. *Lancet 1*:852.
7. Denning, D. W., Anderson, J., Rudge, P. et al. (1987). Acute myelopathy associated with primary infection with human immunodeficiency virus. *Br. Med. J. 294*:143-144.
8. Valle, S. (1987). Febrile pharyngitis as the primary sign of HIV infection in a cluster of cases linked by sexual contact. *Scand. J. Infect. Dis. 19*:13-17.
9. Pristeria, R., Seebacher, C., Casini, M. et al. (1987). Acute infection by HIV in drug addicts. *Abstr. III Int. Conf. AIDS*, Washington, D.C., 1987, Abstr. THP89.
10. Coutinho, R. A., Krone, W. J., Smit, L. et al. (1986). Introduction of lymphadenopathy associated virus or human T lymphotropic virus (LAV/HTLVIII) into the male homosexual community in Amsterdam. *Genitourin. Med. 62*:38-43.
11. Fox, R., Eldred, L. J., Fuchs, E. J. et al. (1987). Clinical manifestations of acute infection with human immunodeficiency virus in a cohort of gay men. *AIDS 1*: 35-38.

12. Biggar, R. J., Johnson, B. K., Musoke, S. S. et al. (1986). Severe illness associated with appearance of antibody to human immunodeficiency virus in an African. *Br. Med. J. 293*:1210-1211.

13. *Lancet* (1985). HTLV III infection associated with glandular-fever like illness in a hemophiliac. *1*:585.

14. AIDS-Hemophilia French Study Group (1986). Natural history of primary infection with LAV in multitransfused patients. *Blood 68*:89-94.

15. White, A. C., Mathews, T. J. Weinhold, K. J. et al. (1986). HTLV III seroconversion associated with heat-treated factor VIII concentrate. *Lancet 1*:611-612.

16. Kumar, P., Pearson, J. E., and Martin, D. H. (1987). Transmission of human immunodeficiency virus by transplantation of a renal allograft with development of the acquired immunodeficiency syndrome. *Ann. Intern. Med. 106*:244-245.

17. Marmor, M., Weiss, L. R., Lyden, M. et al. (1986). Possible female-to-female transmission of human immunodeficiency virus. *Ann. Intern. Med. 105*:969.

18. Stricof, R. L. and Morse, D. (1986). HTLV III/LAV seroconversion following a deep intramuscular needlestick injury. *N. Engl. J. Med. 314*:1115.

19. Oksenhendler, E., Harzic, M., LeRoux, J. M. et al. (1986). HIV infection with seroconversion after a superficial needlestick injury to the finger. *N. Engl. J. Med. 315*:582.

20. CDC (1987). Update: Human immunodeficiency virus infections in health care workers exposed to blood of infected patients. *MMWR 36*:285-289.

21. Romeril, K. R. (1985). Acute HTLV III infection. *N.Z. Med. J. 22*:401.

22. Werdegan, D., O'Malley, P., Bodecker, T. et al. (1987). Self-reported changes in sexual behavior among homosexual and bisexual men from the San Francisco City Clinic Cohort. *MMWR 36*:187-189.

23. Greenblatt, R. M., Samuel, M., Osmond, D. et al. (1987). Risk factors for seroconversion with human immunodeficiency virus among homosexual men in San Francisco 1983-1987. *Abstr. III Int. Conf. AIDS.* Washington, D.C., 1987, Abstr. THP47.

24. Cohen, J., Hauer, L. B., Poole, L. E. et al. (1987). Sexual and other practices and risk of infection in a cohort of 450 sexually active women in San Francisco. *Abstr. III Int. Conf. AIDS.* Washington, D.C., 1987, Abstr. WP57.

25. Fischl, M. A., Diskiman, G. M., Segal, A. et al. (1987). Heterosexual transmission of human immunodeficiency virus: Relationship of sexual practices to seroconversion. *Abstr. III Int. Conf. AIDS.* Washington, D.C., 1987, Abstr. THP92.

26. Matheron, S., Dormont, D., Rey, M. A. et al. (1987). Kinetics of HIV infection after IV exposure to blood from an AIDS patient. *Abstr. III Int. Conf. AIDS.* Washington, D.C., 1987, Abstr. TP27.

27. Schooley, R. and Dolin, E. (1985). Epstein-Barr virus (IM). In *Principles and Practice of Infectious Diseases.* (Mandell, A. L., Douglas, R. G., and Bennett, J. E., eds.). New York, John Wiley & Sons, pp. 971-982.

28. Lindskov, R., Orskov-Lindhardt, B., Weismann, K. et al. (1986). Acute HTLV III infection with roseola-like rash. *Lancet 1*:447.

29. Marlink, R. A., Allan, J. S., McLane, M. F. et al. (1986). Low sensitivity of ELISA testing in early HIV infection. *N. Engl. J. Med. 315*:1549.

30. Ranki, A., Anonen, J., Valle, S. et al. (1987). Characterization of the latent period and development of neutralizing antibodies in early sexually transmitted HIV infection. *Abstr. III Int. Conf. AIDS.* Washington, D.C., 1987, Abstr. MP119.

31. Buchanan, J. A., Goldwater, P. N., and Somerfield, S. D. (1986). Mononucleosis-like syndrome associated with acute AIDS retrovirus infection. *N. Z. Med. J. 11*:405-407.

32. Holander, H. and Levy, J. A. (1987). Neurologic abnormalities and recovery of human immunodeficiency virus from cerebrospinal fluid. *Ann. Intern. Med. 106*:692-695.

33. Allain, J. P., Laurian, Y., Paul, D. A. et al. (1986). Serological markers in early stages of human immunodeficiency virus infection in hemophiliacs. *Lancet 2*: 1233-1236.

34. Giraud, P. M., Matheron, S., Rey, M. A. et al. (1987). Acute hepatitis during human immunodeficiency virus primary infection. *Abstr. III Int. Conf. AIDS.* Washington, D.C., 1987, Abstr. ThP169.

35. McLeod, A. W., Schecter, M. T., Boyko, W. J. et al. (1987). Primary infection with human immunodeficiency virus: Clinical and laboratory features of 73 cases. *Abstr. III Int. Conf. AIDS.* Washington, D.C., 1987, Abstr. MP111.

36. Ulstrup, J. C., Skaug, K., Figenschau, K. J. et al. (1986). Sensitivity of Western blotting (compared with ELISA and immunofluorescence) during seroconversion after HTLV III infection. *Lancet 1*:1151-1152.

37. Johnson, S., Maskill, W. T., Waters, M. J. et al. (1987). The acquisition of anti HIV markers during seroconversion observed in 40 high risk males. *Abstr. III Int. Conf. AIDS.* Washington, D.C., 1987, Abstr. THP31.

38. Tan, S. L., Eymard, D., Gilmore, N. et al. (1987). IgM antibodies to HIV in sera from HIV infected homosexual men in Montreal. *Abstr. III Int. Conf. AIDS.* Washington, D.C., 1987, Abstr. THP96.

39. Epstein, J., Gregg, R., Saah, A. et al. (1987). Western blot analysis of serial IgA, IgM and IgA responses to the human immunodeficiency virus (HIV) in recent seroconverters. *Abstr. III Int. Conf. AIDS.* Washington, D.C., 1987, Abstr. WP129.

40. Cooper, D. A., Imrie, A. A., and Penny, R. (1987). Antibody response to human immunodeficiency virus infection after primary infection. *J. Infect. Dis. 155*:1113.

41. Joeller-Jemelka, H. I., Joller, P. W., Muller, F. et al. (1987). Anti-HIV IgM antibody analysis during early manifestation of HIV infections. *AIDS 1*:45-48.

42. Wall, R. A., Denning, D. W., and Amos, A. (1987). HIV antigenaemia in acute HIV infection. *Lancet 1*:566.

43. Goudsmit, J., deWolf, F., Paul, D. A. et al. (1986). Expression of human immunodeficiency virus antigen (HIV-Ag) in serum and cerebrospinal fluid during acute and chronic infection. *Lancet 2*:177-180.

44. Gaines, H., Albert, J. von Sydow, M. et al. (1987). HIV antigenaemia and virus isolation from plasma during primary HIV infection. *Lancet 1*:1317-1318.

Part II
Clinical Approach to
the HIV-Infected Patient

5
General Approach to the Human Immunodeficiency Virus-Infected Patient

Michael Clement   *San Francisco General Hospital, San Francisco, California*

The intention of this chapter is to provide a general framework with which a practitioner may evaluate an actual or suspected human immunodeficiency virus (HIV)-infected individual. Because there is no "AIDS test," the clinician must rely upon a constellation of pertinent findings from the history and physical examination and from selected laboratory tests to arrive at an HIV-related diagnosis.

CLINICAL MANIFESTATIONS OF HIV INFECTION

The Centers for Disease Control (CDC) classification system for HIV infection (May 1986) (1) is based upon the documentation of HIV infection and the manifestations of disease (Table 1). There are four major groups, each of which is mutually exclusive. In the fourth group there are five subgroups that are not mutually exclusive. In fact, many patients could have diagnoses in one or more of those subgroups concurrently. The classification system is hierarchical; that is, once a patient is diagnosed with a specific HIV group infection, he is not reclassified into a prior group even if symptoms of an infection or malignancy resolve.

   Group I includes patients with an acute mononucleosislike syndrome that occurs after initial infection with HIV.

   Group II consists of asymptomatic HIV-infected ("seropositives") who constitute the vast majority of persons infected by HIV. In the United States, it is estimated that somewhere between 1 and 2 million people are asympto-

TABLE 1   CDC Classification of HIV Infections

Group I	Acute HIV infection
Group II	Asymptomatic infection
Group III	Persistent generalized lymphadenopathy[a]
Group IV	Other disease
	Subgroup A Constitutional disease
	Subgroup B Neurologic disease
	Subgroup C Secondary infectious disease
	Category C-1 Specified secondary infectious diseases listed in the CDC surveillance for AIDS[b]
	Category C-2 Other specified infectious diseases
	Subgroup D Secondary cancers[b]
	Subgroup E Other conditions (e.g., LIP)

[a]Patients in Groups II and III may be subclassified on the basis of a laboratory evaluation.
[b]Includes those patients whose clinical presentation fulfills the definition of AIDS used by the CDC for national reporting.

matic "seropositives." In Africa, the number is much higher and estimates range from 5 to 10 million (2).

Group III consits of those persons with persistent generalized lymphadenopathy. This is not a subtle clinical finding. On the average, 10 different lymph node groups are enlarged counting left and right separately (3). It is very common to find people with enlarged pre-, post-, and infra-auricular lymph nodes, scalene, axillary, epitrochlear, and inguinofemoral lymph nodes.

Group IV includes those persons with symptomatic disease other than lymphadenopathy. It contains five subgroups. *Subgroup A* consists of those persons with constitutional symptoms, such as weight loss greater than 15% of baseline weight, persistent diarrhea with no identifiable infectious cause, persistent fatigue, night sweats, and fevers. *Subgroup B* consists of those persons with neurologic disease primarily related to HIV infection. These persons may have peripheral neuropathy manifested as painful dysesthesia of the distal extremities, or may suffer from the acquired immunodeficiency syndrome (AIDS) dementia complex. Early manifestations of the AIDS dementia complex include depression, social withdrawal and apathy; the condition relentlessly progresses to global dementia frequently associated with incontinence and paraparesis (4). *Subgroup C* consists of those with opportunistic infections classically diagnostic of AIDS, the principal focus of this text. *Subgroup D* consists of patients with HIV-associated malignancies including Kaposi's sarcoma (5) and non-Hodgkin's lymphoma (6), as well as primary lymphoma of the brain (7). Kaposi's sarcoma in AIDS patients is declining in incidence, whereas non-Hodgkin's lymphoma appears to be increasing. *Subgroup E* includes a hodgepodge of other conditions, presumed to be infections, such as the lymphoid interstitial pneumonitis (LIP) seen in children and adults (8). Note that confirmation of lymphoid interstitial pneumonitis in a person under 12 years of age constitutes a diagnosis of AIDS.

CLINICAL EVALUATION OF PATIENTS WITH SUSPECTED SYMPTOMS OF HIV INFECTION

History

In evaluating a patient with suspected HIV infection, assessment of the risk of infection is best made by inquiring about factors that might have led to such infection. The main risk groups in the United States and Western Europe include homosexual and bisexual men, intravenous drug users, transfusion recipients, hemophiliacs who have received blood factor concentrates contaminated with HIV, sexual partners of those in the aforementioned groups, and children congenitally infected by women in these groups (Table 2).

When establishing a person's sexual orientation, one may approach the patient with open-ended questions, for example: "What is your sexual preference?" or directly ask, "Do you prefer sex with women, men, or both?" or "Do you consider yourself heterosexual, homosexual, or bisexual?" Previously, much emphasis was placed upon ascertaining specific sexual practices, for example, whether or not the person engaged in receptive anal intercourse. However, it is more important to ask whether or not someone has been sexually active with a known AIDS patient or someone who subsequently developed AIDS.

Intravenous drug use per se does not contribute to the spread of HIV infection, but the sharing of needles with people who are infected is a definite risk factor. Group needle use ("shooting galleries") appears to be a particularly high risk. Because blood and blood products were not routinely screened for HIV before 1985, patients who received transfusions between 1975 and

TABLE 2 Risk Groups for HIV Infection

Homosexual or bisexual men
Intravenous drug users
Transfusion recipients
Hemophiliacs
Sexual partners of the above groups
Children congenitally infected by HIV infected mothers

1985 are at risk for HIV infection. Because of the high prevalence of HIV infection in certain metropolitan areas, such as New York, Los Angeles, San Francisco, and Miami, it is important to ask where a person has lived for the last 10 years and whether or not they were sexually active during that period.

Review of Systems

The review of systems is used to elicit manifestations of immune deficiency. Certain symptoms, especially constellations of symptoms, are particularly characteristic of the immunodeficiency of HIV infection.

Fevers and drenching night sweats are common complaints of HIV-infected individuals. Fever can be as high as 40 °C without detectable opportunistic infection. The night sweats are usually drenching and require changing bed clothing. Fatigue is common and can be so severe people are unable to work. Many patients complain they barely get through their day's work before needing to sleep 14 to 16 hr. Unintentional weight loss is a frequent historical finding; however, unintentional weight gain can occur as physical activity decreases because of fatigue.

Persistent sinus congestion (with or without evidence of acute sinusitis); recurrent or persistent sore throat, tongue, or mouth; gingivitis, and dental abscesses are all more common in HIV-infected individuals (9). Blurring or loss of vision may occur from retinitis (10).

The pulmonary review of systems may be negative. However, patients with *Pneumocystis carinii* pneumonia (PCP) will complain of dyspnea on exertion and ultimately at rest (11). A persistent dry cough, especially with a deep breath, usually occurs later in the course of PCP. This disease is often preceded by a long history of constitutional symptoms before the osnet of pulmonary symptoms.

Common gastrointestinal symptoms include odynophagia or dysphagia consistent with esophagitis; cramping abdominal pain with diarrhea, suggesting small-bowel enteritis; or diarrhea associated with tenesmus, suggestive of proctitis. Rectal herpes is common in homosexual men, and they may also have a past history of multiple enteric parasite infections (e.g., *Giardia lamblia, Entamoeba histolytica*), or a history of bacterial bowel infections with *Shigella* species or *Salmonella* species, pointing to a markedly increased risk of HIV infection (12,13).

The most common neuropsychiatric symptom is depression, which may be the first manifestation of AIDS-related dementia (4), or it may simply reflect the patient's awareness of symptomatic HIV infection. Other early manifestations of HIV-related dementia include becoming apathetic, socially withdrawn, and isolated. Patients may complain of a loss of concentration and of an inability to read, or will lose track of dates and need to write messages to themselves to keep appointments. In some patients, progression of HIV-related dementia can result in ataxia, incontinence and, eventually, an awake, vegetative state. Distal paresthesias suggest an HIV-related peripheral neuropathy. Isolated limb weakness has also been reported with HIV neuropathy.

The skin is almost uniformly affected by HIV infection (14). A seborrhea-like rash involving the scalp, eyebrows, malar eminences, and mustache or beard is seen commonly. Some patients will complain of severe itching with or without evidence of folliculitis. This itching can be severe enough to interrupt sleep. Recurrent fungal infections of the skin (e.g., tinea pedis), extensive or frequently recurrent mucocutaneous herpes simplex virus infection, or a history of recurrent varicella-zoster (shingles) are also common. Likewise, extensive or recurrent warts (genital or cutaneous) or molluscum contagiosum are frequent in HIV-infected patients. Persistent or enlarging painless red to purple nodules are suggestive of Kaposi's sarcoma and warrant a biopsy.

Physical Examination

Patients often appear older than their stated age, and evidence of recent weight loss (10-15% of baseline body weight) is also common. Male-pattern baldness with greying and thinning of the hair accompanies this wasted, prematurely aged appearance.

On examination of the mouth, white curdlike patches sometimes associated with erythema are very suggestive of oral candidiasis (see Chap. 8). Inspections of the lateral aspects of the tongue can reveal ridged, furrowed, white, velvety patches known as hairy leukoplakia (15; see Chap. 8). The mouth is a common site for the initial lesions of Kaposi's sarcoma (KS), which will present as flat, purple, infiltrating lesions, or as nodular red to purple lesions of the hard palate, soft palate, or gingiva. Angular cheilitis suggests an oral candidal infection and painful, shallow necrotic ulcers are consistent with herpes labialis or recurrent aphthous stomatitis (9).

A fundoscopic examination should be part of every initial evaluation of a suspected HIV-infected patient. Cotton wool spots are common in HIV-infected patients (16). Patients may also have edema, hemorrhage, and exudate that are consistent with cytomegalovirus retinitis (10). Any kind of ophthalmologic abnormality should be evaluated further by a qualified ophthalmologist, because cytomegalovirus retinitis may be difficult to distinguish from benign cotton wool spots.

Scars from previous varicella-zoster infections, folliculitis, and excoriations are common. In gay and bisexual men, raised, asymptomatic nodular, nonblanching red to purple lesions are very suggestive of KS, and biopsies should be taken (14).

Lymph nodes may be normal, diffusely enlarged (3) or greatly shrunken and not palpable. A disproportionately enlarged node suggests an infiltrative opportunistic infection, for example, *Mycobacterium avium* complex or a tumor, either a non-Hodgkin's lymphoma or Kaposi's sarcoma. Biopsy is indicated for the disproportionately enlarged or rapidly enlarging lymph node. Biopsy is generally not indicated in a patient with persistent generalized lymphadenopathy (Group III HIV infection). Lymph node biopsy of Group III patients most often yields benign follicular hyperplasia (3). Diagnostic efforts in these patients should be directed toward identifying treatable causes of generalized lymphadenopathy (e.g., syphilis).

Results of the chest examination are usually normal, except when a patient has an intercurrent opportunistic pulmonary infection or a coexisting disease (e.g., asthma). The most common finding on cardiovascular examination is sinus tachycardia. Gallops and rubs are uncommon but do occur with cardiomyopathy and pericardial disease. In one study, the most common cardiac abnormality associated with HIV infection was a lymphocytic myocarditis of unknown etiology (17). Pericardial disease may be secondary to opportunistic infection with mycobacterial, fungal, or viral diseases, or it may be secondary to lymphoma or Kaposi's sarcoma.

Abdominal pain and tenderness can be a sign of cytomegalovirus colitis (10). Abdominal examination may reveal hepatosplenomegaly resulting from an infiltrative opportunistic infection, such as *M. avium* complex, or a tumor, such as non-Hodgkin's lymphoma or Kaposi's sarcoma. Splenomegaly may be seen with persistent generalized lymphadenopaty (3). Otherwise, the abdominal examination is usually nonspecific.

Genitourinary examination may reveal lesions of Kaposi's sarcoma, evidence of previous herpetic or varicella infection, or condyloma acuminata. Opportunistic infections of the epididymis or prostate have been reported (18).

Although patients with HIV-related neurologic disease may appear to have a normal mental status upon cursory neurologic examination, upon more in-depth testing of recent memory and cognitive abilities, as many as 87% of patients with an AIDS diagnosis will have evidence of neurologic involvement on neuropsychologic testing (19). Patients may have focal findings consistent with central nervous system toxoplasmosis or lymphoma. Mononeuropathies may result in isolated limb weakness or cranial neuropathies. Distal limb paresthesias and pain can be secondary to HIV peripheral neuropathy (7). Patients with a stiff neck (possibly with a Kernig or a Brudzinski sign) should be evaluated for meningitis with a lumbar puncture.

LABORATORY EXAMINATION

Hematology

A mild normocytic, normochromic anemia is common in HIV-infected individuals; iron studies usually show a pattern consistent with anemia of chronic disease (20). Macrocytic anemia can be seen in patients receiving zidovudine, usually after 8 to 12 weeks of continuous administration (21). The administration of dihydrofolate reductase inhibitors (e.g., pyrimethamine) without replacement of folinic acid can also cause macrocytic anemia.

Lymphopenia with a reversed T-lymphocyte helper/suppressor ratio, the result of depletion of the T4 (CD4) helper lymphocytes (22,23), is common. Neutropenia is also common and may be due to an autoimmune process (24), to zidovudine administration (21), or to therapy for opportunistic infections with sulfonamides (25), ganciclovir (10), or pentamidine (26). Mild thrombocytopenia (100 to 140 $\times$ 10^3 platelets/mm^3) is common, and idiopathic thrombocytopenic purpura has been described secondary to a platelet-specific IgG (27). The presence of pancytopenia should suggest bone marrow invasion by lymphoma cells, mycobacteria, or fungi.

Coagulation studies may reveal a prolonged partial thromboplastin time, which is usually not associated with an increased frequency of thrombosis or hemorrhage. A lupuslike anticoagulant composed of an IgG-IgM complex has been identified in these patients. It has been noted that a prolonged partial thromboplastic time is common in persons with an acute opportunistic infection and reverts to normal with treatment of the underlying opportunistic infection (28).

Serology

Previously, the prevalence of syphilis was high in gay and bisexual men. Therefore, it is reasonable as a screening test to do a VDRL or RPR on these patients. Recent literature suggests that people with a past history of syphilis who have developed symptomatic HIV infection may be at risk for developing reactivation of latent syphilis (29,30). The prevalence of hepatitis is also very high in gay and bisexual men, and hepatitis serology as an initial screening examination is reasonable in these patients to identify those patients chronically infected by hepatitis B virus (31).

Testing for HIV infection per se (HIV antibody or p24 antigen) is not useful except in some specific instances. Persons not in an identified risk group with an unexplained immunodeficiency or opportunistic infection deserve HIV antibody testing. These patients may not have volunteered historical information that would have identified them as a member of a risk group. It is also important to test for HIV infection in patients with non-Hodgkin's lymphoma. Persons who are HIV antibody-positive and have non-Hodgkin's lymphoma have a worse prognosis and a lower response rate to therapy.

CHEMISTRY

Because of polyclonal stimulation of B cells, patients often have a nonspecific hypergammaglobulinemia (32). Hypoalbuminemia, as well as marked hypocholesterolemia, is probably related to nutritional deficiency. An addisonian-like adrenal insufficiency state has been described in HIV-infected patients. Therefore, the presence of hyponatremia and associated hyperkalemia should prompt one to measure cortisol levels and consider a cosyntropin (Cortrosyn) stimulation test (33). Elevated liver enzyme levels are seen in patients with chronic active hepatitis as well as in patients receiving therapy (especially sulfonamides) for certain opportunistic infections (34). A disproportionate elevation in the alkaline phosphatase concentration relative to other liver enzymes suggests either an infiltrative process in the liver (lymphoma or mycobacterial infection) or papillary stenosis caused by cytomegalovirus or cryptosporidium (35). Renal complications occur in AIDS patients and may be the result of a focal and segmental glomerulosclerosis, the etiology of which is unknown. Additionally, renal insufficiency can develop from a number of drugs used to treat opportunistic infections including pentamidine and amphotericin. Fluid and electrolyte abnormalities can result from fever, vomiting, diarrhea, adrenal insufficiency, and renal tubular acidosis (36,37).

SPECIFIC CLINICAL PRESENTATIONS OF HIV-INFECTED PATIENTS

Fever

Fever is one of the most common complaints of HIV-infected persons. Although HIV infection itself can cause fever, this is a diagnosis of exclusion, and other infectious processes or malignancies must be ruled out. Routine blood cultures are indicated to exclude infection with encapsulated bacteria (*Haemophilus influenzae* or *Streptococcus pneumoniae*; 38) or infection with other bacteria related to indwelling central venous catheters. Salmonellae can cause recurrent bacteremia (presumably from an intestinal source) requiring long-term suppressant therapy with antimicrobials (39). Viral blood cultures are rarely indicated. Many AIDS patients will have cytomegalovirus viremia, and unless specific organ abnormality is present a positive blood culture for cytomegalovirus appears to be clinically irrelevant (10). Adenoviruses and enteroviruses are occasionally recovered from blood of AIDS patients, and again, the clinical significance is unclear.

Mycobacterial blood cultures (*M. avium* complex or *M. tuberculosis*) are useful in the evaluation of persistent fever and night sweats or pancytopenia (40). Although no drug regimen has been shown to be effective for *M. avium* complex infection, some persons will respond symptomatically to routine tuberculosis therapy (40) or to nonsteroidal anti-inflammatory agents.

If results of the initial set of blood cultures in the febrile HIV-infected patient are negative, repeat blood cultures are rarely indicated unless there is a

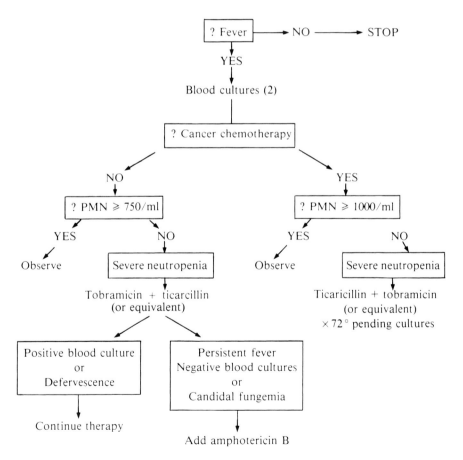

FIGURE 1 Algorithm for treatment of a febrile neutropenic patient with AIDS.

dramatic change in the patient's condition. Our experience also has shown that results of routine blood cultures are rarely positive in a febrile neutropenic patient who has not received chemotherapy for an AIDS-related malignancy. Neutropenia in AIDS patients can occur secondary to an autoimmune process, to antibiotic therapy (sulfanomides, pentamidine, ganciclovir), to antiretroviral therapy (zidovudine), or to an infiltrative bone marrow process (disseminated fungal or mycobacterial infection or lymphoma). None of these processes specifically predispose the febrile neutropenic patient to bacterial infection. This is in contrast to HIV-related lymphoma patients who have received chemotherapy for their malignancy. These chemotherapeutic agents can cause mucous membrane ulceration and neutrophil dysfunction, with resultant gram-negative, anaerobic, or gram-positive bacteremias (41). Figure 1 illustrates a reasonable approach to the febrile neutropenic AIDS patient.

The HIV-related malignancies can cause fever in AIDS patients. Non-Hodgkin's lymphoma can present with persistent high fevers, cytopenias, elevated erythrocyte sedimentation rate, and elevated lactate dehydrogenase levels. A recently enlarged, painful, hard lymph node, hepatosplenomegaly, or soft-tissue mass can be the initial clinical manifestation of lymphoma (6). Kaposi's sarcoma can cause fever if there is visceral involvement.

Neisseria gonorrhoeae, Treponema pallidum, and chlamydial infections were all common infections in homosexual and bisexual men before the AIDS epidemic and should be considered in a differential of fever.

Adrenal insufficiency in AIDS patients has been described and can present with fever, hypotension, hyponatremia, and hyperkalemia (33). If suspected, a patient should have a baseline cortisol level drawn and a synthetic ACTH (Cortrysin) stimulation test performed.

Lymphadenopathy

Persistent generalized lymphadenopathy (PGL; Group III infection) is common in HIV-infected patients and is usually due to HIV alone. No biopsy is necessary in the setting of asymptomatic HIV-infected patients with PGL because previous studies have shown benign follicular hyperplasia on biopsy (3). However, 50% of non-Hodgkin's lymphoma patients will have a prior history of persistent generalized lymphadenopathy (6). Therefore, in patients with recently symptomatic lymphadenopathy, rapidly enlarging nodes, marked nodal asymmetry, constitutional symptoms (fevers, night sweats), or an elevated erythrocyte sedimentation rate, a biopsy should be considered. The biopsy is also useful for excluding lymphoma, lymphadenopathic Kaposi's sarcoma and infiltrative fungal or mycobacterial disease.

Diarrhea

Copious watery stools, which may or may not contain undigested food and are associated with cramping, suggest an upper small-bowel source of diarrhea. Bright red blood and tenesmus suggest a colonic source.

Initial laboratory evaluation should include culture for bacterial causes of enteritis: *Salmonella, Shigella, Yersinia,* and *Campylobacter* (including species other than *C. jejuni*). Stool should be examined concurrently for fecal leukocytes; if these are present, bacterial dysentery is likely.

Three sequential ova and parasite examinations for *Giardia lamblia, Entamoeba histolytica,* and the so-called nonpathogenic ameba should be done (see Chap. 20 for comment on nonpathogenic amebas). Special testing procedures are employed to detect *Cryptosporidium* spp. and *Isospora belli.* The laboratory should be alerted if these pathogens are suspected.

If results from all initial cultures and stool examinations are negative, sigmoidoscopy with biopsy is indicated. Cytomegalovirus can cause ulcerative colitis with associated submucosal hemorrhage mimicking Kaposi's sarcoma of the bowel. If the biopsy reveals viral inclusions, or if viral cultures are positive for cytomegalovirus, therapy with ganciclovir relieves symptoms in about 70% of patients (10; see Chap. 11).

Histologic examination and biopsy of the sigmoid mucosa are also useful in diagnosing disease due to *M. avium* complex, chlamydia, herpes simplex virus, lymphoma, and cryptosporidiam.

Perirectal Pain

Perirectal pain in HIV-infected patients can be due to infections or to malignant processes. Recurrent herpes simplex virus proctitis is common and presents with exquisitely tender, shallow, irregularly bordered ulcerations anywhere in the perineal area. Culture results for herpes simplex virus will frequently be positive. While awaiting these results, empiric acyclovir therapy is indicated at a dose of 200 mg (one capsule) orally five times a day. Pain and symptoms will dramatically decrease within 48 to 72 hr of beginning therapy.

Perirectal abscesses are common in homosexual and bisexual men (42) and can present with perirectal pain and fever simulating symptoms of gonococcal, syphilitic, or chlamydial proctitis. Digital rectal examination or sigmoidoscopy may be necessary to make a definitive diagnosis.

Non-Hodgkin's lymphoma can present as a perirectal mass simulating perirectal abscess (6). Therefore, biopsy is indicated during the incision and drainage procedure. Squamous cell carcinoma of the rectum in homosexual men can also present with perirectal pain, and this entity is seen with in-

creased frequency in homosexual men who practice receptive anal intercourse (43).

Dysphagia

The most common cause of dysphagia or odynophagia in HIV—infected
persons is esophagitis caused by candida, by cytomegalovirus, or by herpes
simplex virus (12,13). It was once thought that dysphagia alone occurred
more commonly with esophageal candidiasis, whereas cytomegalovirus and
herpes simplex virus more commonly caused odynophagia. Although the
most common cause of esophagitis—C. albicans—can be diagnosed on the
basis of response to empiric ketoconazole therapy (400 mg/day), we prefer
to confirm the diagnosis of esophagitis by a barium esophogram or esopha-
goscopy. The latter study (if accompanied by biopsy) will provide definitive
diagnostic information. Suspected herpes simplex esophagitis may also be
treated empirically, but treatment of suspected cytomegalovirus esophagitis
should not be undertaken without biopsy confirmation.

Cutaneous Processes

Pruritus with or without folliculitis is an extremely common complaint of
HIV-infected patients. Frequently, no cause for pruritus can be found. Patients respond symptomatically to 0.25% menthol plus 0.125% phenol in a
lubricating lotion. Antihistamines and topical 1% hydrocortisone lotion are
variably effective. If folliculitis coexists, benzoyl peroxide washes, followed by
1% hydrocortisone lotion may be beneficial. If secondary infection is present, a short course of antistaphylococcal therapy is indicated (see Chap. 7).

Red to purple, asymptomatic, nonblanching, cutaneous nodules suggest
Kaposi's sarcoma. Biopsy should be performed on suspected KS lesions because secondary syphilis, postinflammatory hyperpigmentation, and der-
matofibromas can all mimic cutaneous KS.

Extensive mucocutaneous herpes simplex virus is common in HIV-infected
individuals. Extensive dermatomal or disseminated varicella-zoster virus
(VZV) is also common in HIV-infected persons (44,45). Nonhealing cutaneous ulcers can be caused by invasive fungi, for example, cryptococcosis or
sporotrichosis. A biopsy for histologic examination and culture should be
performed.

Dyspnea

Dyspnea on exertion and, ultimately, at rest is associated with P. carinii pneumonia (PCP) and frequently follows a long history of constitutional complaints. Patients complain of persistent fevers, night sweats, weight loss,

fatigue, diarrhea, and then ultimately shortness of breath and dyspnea on exertion. Patients may or may not have a dry cough. This cough typically worsens with deep inspiration resulting in painful spasmodic coughing with associated increased shortness of breath. Patients attempt to suppress this cough with a rapid shallow pattern of breathing. On physical examination, the patient is typically febrile, tachycardic, and dyspneic, and has a rapid, shallow pattern of respiration. Chest auscultation can reveal decreased breath sounds in the bases, clear breath sounds, or mild diffuse crackles. Prominent, diffuse crackles are heard with severe *P. carinii* pneumonia.

The chest radiograph is abnormal in 90% of patients with PCP, most commonly with a diffuse interstitial pattern (46). However, PCP can present radiographically as solitary nodules, lobar consolidation, or cavitary lesions (47,48). Pleural effusions are very uncommon with PCP. After chest radiography, arterial blood gases should be evaluated to help define the severity of the illness. Arterial blood gas examination usually reveals a respiratory alkalosis; hypoxemia can be severe but is quite variable. Patients with an abnormal chest radiograph or arterial blood gases should have a diagnostic procedure for PCP (see Chap. 17). If chest radiographs or arterial blood gases are normal, the next step is pulmonary function tests with a diffusing capacity for carbon monoxide (DLCO). These tests usually reveal a mild restrictive pattern of breathing with a decreased DLCO consistent with an interstitial process (49). Gallium scanning can also be performed in patients with clinically equivocal chest x-ray, arterial blood gases, and pulmonary function tests. The gallium scan is very sensitive (100%) but not particularly specific (20%) for PCP (50,51). Patients with decreased DLCO or increased pulmonary gallium uptake should be evaluated for *P. carinii* pneumonitis (see Chaps. 17 and 21).

Blindness

Persons infected with HIV are subject to a wide variety of pathogens that can affect the eye. Any complaint of loss of vision, decreased visual acuity, or eye pain should be taken seriously and evaluated with dilated fundoscopic examination. Cytomegalovirus retinitis is the most common cause of visual symptoms and signs as well as blindness in AIDS patients. This can present abruptly and progress rapidly to total blindness. Fundoscopic examination reveals areas of hemorrhage, exudate, and edema. Any suggestion of these findings on examination merits referral to an ophthalmologist experienced with a diagnosis of cytomegaloviral retinitis. Ganciclovir therapy preserves the remaining vision and prevents progression of disease in 75% of patients (10). Other treatable causes of eye disease in AIDS patients include parasitic disease (*T. gondii*), fungal disease (*C. albicans, Cryptococcus neoformans*), viral disease (HSV, VZV), and bacterial disease (*T. pallidum*).

SUMMARY

This chapter is designed as a general overview of the complex clinical presentations seen in HIV-infected patients. Virtually no organ system is left untouched either directly or indirectly by this disease. Patients infected with the HIV may be symptomatic as a direct result of the retrovirus (e.g., HIV encephalopathy) or resulting from secondary opportunistic infections (e.g., PCP), or malignancies (e.g., KS). These diverse clinical presentations and diagnostic possibilities warrant a thorough history and physical examination. Specific clinical scenarios then direct the laboratory evaluation.

REFERENCES

1. CDC (1986). Classification system for human T-lymphotrophic virus type III-lymphadenopathy associated virus infection. *MMWR 20*:334-339.
2. Quinn, T. C., Mann, J. M., Curran, J. W. et al. (1986). AIDS in Africa: An epidemiologic paradigm. *Science 234*:955-963.
3. Abrams, D. I., Lewis, B. J., Beckstead, J. H. et al. (1984). Persistent diffuse lymphadenopathy in homosexual men: Endpoint or prodrome? *Ann. Intern. Med. 100*:801-808.
4. Navia, B. A., Jordan, B. D., and Price, R. W. (1986). The AIDS dementia complex clinical features. *Ann. Neurol. 19*:517-524.
5. Groopman, J. E. (1987). AIDS-related Kaposi's sarcoma: Therapeutic modalities. *Semin. Hematol. 24*:55-58.
6. Ziegler, J. L., Beckstead, J. A., Volberding, P. A. et al. (1984). Non-Hodgkin's lymphoma in 90 homosexual men; relation to generalized lymphadenopathy and the acquired immunodeficiency syndrome. *N. Engl. J. Med. 311*:565-570.
7. Levy, R. M., Bredesen, D. E., and Rosenblum, M. L. (1985). Neurological manifestations of the acquired immunodeficiency syndrome: Experience at UCSF and review of the literature. *J. Neurosurg. 62*:475-495.
8. Morris, J. C., Rosen, M. J., and Marchevsky, A. et al. (1987). Lymphocytic interstitial pneumonia in patients at risk for the acquired immune deficiency syndrome. *Chest 91*:63-67.
9. Schioat, M. and Pindborg, J. J. (1987). AIDS and the oral cavity; epidemiology and clinical oral manifestations of human immune deficiency virus infection: A review. *Int. J. Oral Maxillofac. Surg. 16*:1-14.
10. Jacobson, M.A. and Mills, J. (1988). Serious cytomegalovirus disease in the acquired immunodeficiency syndrome (AIDS); clinical findings, diagnosis, and treatment. *Ann. Intern. Med. 108*:585-594.
11. Hopewell, P.C. and Luce, J. M. (1985). Pulmonary involvement in the acquired immunodeficiency syndrome. *Chest 87*:104-112.

12. Weber, J. (1986). Gastrointestinal disease in AIDS. *Clin. Immunol. Allergy 6*: 519-541.
13. Santangelo, W. C. and Krejs, G. J. (1986). Southwestern Internal Medicine Conference: Gastrointestinal manifestations of the acquired immunodeficiency syndrome. *Am. J. Med. Sci. 292*:328-334.
14. Warner, L. C. and Fisher B. K. (1986). Cutaneous manifestations of the acquired immunodeficiency syndrome. *Int. J. Dermatol. 25*:337-349.
15. Greenspan, D., Greenspan, J. S., Hearst, N. G. et al. (1987). Relation of oral hairy leukoplakia to infection with the human immunodeficiency virus and the risk of developing AIDS. *J. Infect. Dis. 155*:475-481.
16. Humphrey, R. C., Weber, J. N., and Marsh, R. J. (1987). Ophthalmic findings in a group of ambulatory patients infected by human immunodeficiency virus (HIV): A prospective study. *Br. J. Ophthalmol. 71*:565-569.
17. Roldan, E. O., Moskowitz, L., Hensley, G. T. (1987). Pathology of the heart in the acquired immunodeficiency syndrome. *Arch. Pathol. Lab. Med. 111*:943-946.
18. Lief, M. and Sarfarazi, F. (1986). Prostatic cryptococcosis in acquired immunodeficiency syndrome. *Urology 28*:318-319.
19. Grant, I., Atkinson, J. H., Hesselink, J. R. et al. (1987). Evidence for early central nervous system involvement in the acquired immunodeficiency syndrome and other human immunodeficiency virus (HIV) infections. *Ann. Intern. Med. 107*:828-836.
20. Costella, A., Croxson, T. S., Mildvan, D. et al. (1985). The bone marrow in AIDS, a histologic hematologic and microbiologic study. *Am. J. Clin. Pathol. 84*:425-432.
21. Richman, D. D., Fischl, M. A., Grieco, M. H. et al. (1987). The toxicity of azidothymidine in the treatment of patients with AIDS and AIDS-related complex. *N. Engl. J. Med. 317*:192-197.
22. Seligman, M., Pinching, A. J., Rosen, F. S. et al. (1987). Immunology of human immunodeficiency virus infection and the acquired immunodeficiency syndrome, an update. *Ann. Intern. Med. 107*:234-242.
23. Spirak, J. L., Bender, B. S., Quinn, T. C. et al. (1984). Hematologic abnormalities in the acquired immune deficiency syndrome. *Am. J. Med. 77*:224-228.
24. Murphy, M. F., Metcalf, P., Waters, A. H. et al. (1987). Incidence and mechanism of neutropenia and thrombocytopenia in patients with human immunodeficiency virus infection. *Br. J. Haematol. 66*(3):337-340.
25. Wofsy, C. B. (1987). Use of trimethoprim sulfamethoxazole in treatment of *Pneumocystis carinii* pneumonia in patients with acquired immunodeficiency syndrome. *Rev. Infect. Dis. 9*(suppl 2):S184-S194.
26. CDC (1984). Severe neutropenia during pentamidine treatment of *Pneumocystis carinii* pneumonia in patients with AIDS. *MMWR 33*:65-67.
27. Schneider, P. A., Abrams, D. I., Rayner, A. A. et al. (1987). Immune deficiency-associated thrombocytopenic purpura (IDTP), response to splenectomy. *Arch. Surg. 122*:1175-1178.
28. Bloom, E. J., Abrams, D. I., and Rodgers, G. (1986). Lupus anticoagulant in the acquired immunodeficiency syndrome. *JAMA 256*:491-493.

29. Johns, D. R., Tierney, M., and Felsenstein, D. (1987). Alteration in the natural history of neurosyphilis by concurrent infection with the human immunodeficiency virus. *N. Engl. J. Med. 316*:1569-1572.

30. Berry, C. D., Hooton, T. M., Collier, A. C. et al. (1987). Neurologic relapse after benzathine penicillin therapy for secondary syphilis in a patient with HIV infection. *N. Engl. J. Med. 316*:1587-1589.

31. Schneiderman, D. J., Arenson, D. M., Cello, J. P. et al. (1987). Hepatic disease in patients with the acquired immunodeficiency syndrome (AIDS). *Hepatology 7*:925-930.

32. Crapper, R. M., Dean, D. R., and MacKay, I. R. (1987). Paraproteinemias in homosexual men with HIV infection, lack of association with abnormal clinical or immunologic findings. *Am. J. Clin. Pathol. 88*:348-351.

33. Biglieri, E. G. (1988). Adrenocortical function in the acquired immunodeficiency syndrome. *West. J. Med. 148*:70-73.

34. Wharton, M., Coleman, D. L., Fitz, G. et al. (1986). Trimethoprim-sulfamethoxazole or pentamidine for *Pneumocystis carinii* pneumonia in the acquired immunodeficiency syndrome. *Ann. Intern. Med. 105*:37-44.

35. Schneiderman, D. J., Cello, J. P., and Laing, F. C. (1987). Papillary stenosis and sclerosing cholangitis in the acquired immunodeficiency syndrome. *Ann. Intern. Med. 106*:546-549.

36. Humphreys, M. H. and Schoenfeld, P. Y. (1987). Renal complications in patients with the acquired immune deficiency syndrome. *Am. J. Nephrol. 7*:1-7.

37. Rao, T. K. S., Friedman, E. A., and Nicastri, A. D. (1987). The types of renal disease in the acquired immunodeficiency syndrome. *N. Engl. J. Med. 316*:1062-1068.

38. Witt, D. J., Craven, D. E., and McCabe, W. R. (1987). Bacterial infections in adult patients with the acquired immune deficiency syndrome and AIDS-related complex. *Am. J. Med. 82*:900-906.

39. Jacobs, J. L., Gold, J. W., Murray, H. W. et al. (1985). Salmonella infections in patients with the acquired immunodeficiency syndrome. *Ann. Intern. Med. 102*:186-188.

40. CDC (1987). Diagnosis and management of mycobacterial infection and disease in persons with human immunodeficiency virus infection. *Ann. Intern. Med. 106*:254-256.

41. Schimpff, S. C. (1985). Overview of empiric antibiotic therapy for the febrile neutropenic patient. *Rev. Infect. Dis. 7*:S734-740.

42. Wexner, S. D., Smithy, W. B., Milsom, J. W. et al. (1986). The surgical management of anorectal disease in AIDS and pre-AIDS patients. *Dis. Colon Rectum 29*:719-723.

43. Croxson, T., Chabon, A. B., Rorat, E. et al. (1986). Intraepithelial carcinoma of the anus in homosexual men. *Dis. Colon Rectum 29*:503-506.

44. Quinnan, G. V., Masur, H., Rook, A. H. et al. (1984). Herpes virus infections in the acquired immunodeficiency syndrome. *JAMA 252*:72-77.

45. Friedman-Kien, A. E., Lafleur, F. L., Gendler, E. et al. (1986). Herpes zoster: A possible early clinical sign for development of acquired immunodeficiency syndrome in high risk individuals. *J. Am. Acad. Dermatol. 14*:1023-1028.

46. Goodman, P. C., Broaddus, V. C., and Hopewell, P. C. (1984). Chest radiographic patterns in the acquired immunodeficiency syndrome. *Am. Rev. Resp. Dis. 129*:36.
47. Barrio, J. L., Suarez, M., Rodriguez, J. L. et al. (1986). *Pneumocystis carinii* pneumonia presenting as cavitating and noncavitating solitary pulmonary nodules in patients with the acquired immunodeficiency syndrome. *Am. Rev. Respir. Dis. 134*:1094-1096.
48. Barter, S. (1986). Radiological features of AIDS. *Clin. Immunol. Allergy 6*: 601-625.
49. Coleman, D. L., Dodek, P. M., Golden, J. A. et al. (1984). Correlation between serial pulmonary function tests and fiberoptic bronchoscopy in patients with *Pneumocystis carinii* pneumonia and the acquired immune deficiency syndrome. *Am. Rev. Respir. Dis. 129*:491-493.
50. Tuazon, C. U., Delaney, M. D., Simon, G. I. et al. (1985). Use of gallium-67 scintigraphy and bronchial washings in the diagnosis and treatment of *Pneumocystis carinii* pneumonia in patients with the acquired immunodeficiency syndrome. *Am. Rev. Respir. Dis. 132*:1087-1092.
51. Coleman, D. L., Hattner, R. S., Luce, J. M. et al. (1984). Correlation between gallium lung scans and fiberoptic bronchoscopy in patients with suspected *Pneumocystis carinii* pneumonia and the acquired immune deficiency syndrome. *Am. Rev. Respir. Dis. 130*:1166-1169.

6
Neurologic Disease in the Acquired Immunodeficiency Syndrome

Robert M. Levy   *Northwestern University Medical School, Chicago, Illinois*

Dale E. Bredesen and Mark L. Rosenblum   *University of California, San Francisco, California*

Neurologic dysfunction in patients with acquired immunodeficiency syndrome (AIDS) has been reported from the beginning of the AIDS epidemic (1,2). However, only recently have the frequency and breadth of the neurologic manifestations of AIDS become apparent (Table 1; 3,4). The demonstration that these neurologic illnesses arise not only from opportunistic infections and cancers but also from primary human immunodeficiency virus type 1 (HIV-1) infection of the nervous system is of great importance (5-7). Additionally, primary infection with HIV-1 can produce a number of previously unrecognized neurologic illnesses (8,9). As the AIDS epidemic spreads and the number of patients increases dramatically, physicians must become familiar with the broad spectrum of the neurologic manifestations of this disease.

INCIDENCE OF HIV-1-RELATED
CENTRAL NERVOUS SYSTEM ILLNESS

Epidemiologic data concerning the incidence of HIV-1-related CNS illness is only now being obtained. Data collected by the Centers for Disease Control (CDC) for the United States do not yet provide incidence figures because in over 90% of cases there is no follow-up data available after the initial report. Reliable institutional data have been collected at the University of

TABLE 1   Illnesses Affecting the Central Nervous System in AIDS

Primary viral (HIV-1)
  HIV-1 encephalopathy
  HIV-1 meningitis
  vacuolar myelopathy
Secondary viral (encephalitis, retinitis, vasculitis)
  cytomegalovirus
  herpes simplex virus types 1 and 2
  varicella-zoster virus
  papovavirus (progressive multifocal leukoencephalopathy)
Nonviral infections (encephalitis, meningitis, abscess)
  Toxoplasma gondii
  Cryptococcus neoformans
  Candida albicans
  Coccidioides immitis
  Aspergillus fumigatus
  Histoplasma capsulatum
  Mycobacterium avium complex
  Mycobacterium tuberculosis
  Listeria monocytogenes
  Nocardia asteroides
  Treponema pallidum
Neoplasms
  primary CNS lymphoma
  metastatic systemic lymphoma
  metastatic Kaposi's sarcoma
Cerebrovascular
  infarction
  hemorrhage
  vasculitis
Complications of Systemic AIDS therapy

California, San Francisco and the San Francisco General Hospital (UCSF); of 1286 patients with AIDS or the AIDS-related complex (ARC) evaluated at UCSF by June 1986, 482 (37%) had findings of neurologic illness (4). In these 482 patients, 553 neurologic diseases were identified, of which 474 affected the central nervous system and 79 affected the peripheral nervous system (Tables 1 & 2). Sixty-five patients had multiple neurologic illnesses. The incidence of HIV-1-related neurologic illness in patients evaluated at UCSF has more than doubled in each of the past 6 years.

Of the 37% of AIDS patients with neurologic illness, about one-third had neurologic complaints as the initial manifestation of AIDS. Thus, approximately 10% of all AIDS patients were first seen with symptoms of neurologic

TABLE 2 AIDS-Related CNS Disease: Clinical Profile

	n	Mean age (yrs)	CNS[a] 1st (%)	Length Sx (days)	CT findings (%)				Mean CSF			Mean survival (days)
					Neg	Atrophy	Lesion	H/C[b]	Prot (mg/dl)	Gluc (mg/dl)	WBC (cc³)	
HIV-1 encephalopathy	100	38.8	16	48	44	48	5	3	62	53	3	93
Secondary viral encephalitis	28	36.2	11	19	50	32	18	5	95	63	64	48
PML	8	40.3	38	14	20	0	80	0	69	46	4	c
Toxoplasmosis	53	40.0	44	22	4	8	88	0	97	58	6	79
Cryptococcosis	68	38.0	34	21	53	31	8	4	82	43	49	95
Primary CNS lymphoma	25	37.0	48	42	4	4	86	0	81	57	9	53

[a]CNS disease was the presenting AIDS diagnosis.
[b]Hydrocephalus.
[c]Inadequate data.
Source: Data from UCSF series, Ref. 4.

illness. A similar incidence of overall AIDS-related neurologic illness (1,10) and neurologic illness at presentation with AIDS (11) has been reported in other groups of AIDS patients. The incidence of AIDS-related neuropathology is much higher in autopsy series, which suggests that 75% of AIDS patients have nervous system abnormalities on postmortem evaluation (4, 12,13).

EPIDEMIOLOGY OF AIDS-RELATED CENTRAL NERVOUS SYSTEM ILLNESS

Recent epidemiologic studies (11) have confirmed the empiric observation that the risk of contracting AIDS-related neurologic illnesses varies with the AIDS risk group and geographic location. Toxoplasmosis occurs most frequently in Florida, in both Haitian and non-Haitian AIDS patients. In general, Haitian AIDS patients are more frequently reported to have CNS complications than are patients in other risk groups. Cryptococcal meningitis is reported most frequently in New Jersey, possibly because of the higher percentage of AIDS patients in that state who are black or intravenous drug users. Progressive multifocal leukoencephalopathy (PML) and primary CNS lymphoma do not appear to occur preferentially in any single risk group or geographic location.

AIDS-RELATED CENTRAL NERVOUS SYSTEM SYNDROMES

Central nervous system syndromes associated with AIDS or ARC may arise from HIV-1 infection itself or from secondary opportunistic infections or cancers. Neurologic disease may occur alone or as part of a diffuse systemic illness and may reflect nonfocal, diffuse CNS involvement; focal involvement by a space-occupying lesion; or obstructive hydrocephalus. Central nervous system syndromes include focal or diffuse encephalopathy, myelopathy, meningitis, cranial neuropathy, and retinopathy.

Table 3 lists the frequency with which many of the more common signs and symptoms are present in AIDS patients with neurologic illness. Disorders of consciousness or cognition, including dementia, are most common, being evident in 68% of patients with neurologic findings. Headaches are only slightly less frequent, being present in 55%. Also common are complaints of focal weakness (18%), incoordination (18%), and seizures (17%). Less frequently, patients present with aphasia (12%), incontinence (10%), cranial neuropathies (9%), sensory loss (8%), and visual disturbances (8%).

The presence of focal weakness or sensory loss is suggestive of a focal process, such as toxoplasmosis or primary CNS lymphoma. The presence of

TABLE 3 AIDS-Related CNS Disease: Signs and Symptoms

Neurologic finding	Overall	HIV-1	2° Viral	PML[a]	Toxo	Crypto	Lymphoma
			(% of patients exhibiting the given finding)				
Headaches	55	39	50	75	45	85	40
Altered mental status	68	90	50	75	70	42	64
Incoordination	18	18	21	0	21	10	32
Aphasia	12	17	17	0	8	5	16
Seizures	17	12	17	0	24	13	32
Incontinence	10	9	4	0	13	3	32
Hemiparesis	18	9	21	50	38	3	44
Hemisensory loss	8	3	13	25	11	3	16
Visual disturbances	8	5	0	25	8	6	20
Cranial neuropathies	9	3	21	0	11	6	20
Pain	1	0	0	0	4	2	0

[a]Data from three patients.
Source: Data from UCSF series, Ref. 4.

cranial neuropathies is suggestive of lymphoma or infection with opportunistic viruses such as herpes simplex or cytomegalovirus (CMV; 4). Because there is a noteable overlap in the clinical profiles of HIV-1-related neurologic diseases, clinical findings are, however, of little value in the differential diagnosis of these illnesses.

HIV-1-RELATED CENTRAL NERVOUS SYSTEM DISEASES

The spectrum of diseases known to affect the CNS in AIDS is listed in Table 1.

Primary Viral Infection

HIV-1 Encephalopathy

The most common CNS illness associated with AIDS is associated with HIV-1 infection of the brain. First reported by Snider et al. (1) as "subacute encephalitis," this potentially fatal dementing illness has also been called "AIDS encephalopathy" and the "AIDS dementia complex." The first step toward understanding the pathogenesis of this illness was made by Shaw et al. (14), who demonstrated HIV-1 RNA in the brains of demented AIDS patients by in situ hybridization. Ho and co-workers (5) subsequently demonstrated that HIV-1 could be recovered from CSF and neural tissues of patients with AIDS-related neurologic syndromes. Levy et al. (15) also isolated HIV-1 from the brains and CSF of AIDS patients with neurologic disease. At the same time, Resnick and colleagues (7) demonstrated the intra-blood-brain barrier synthesis of HIV-1-specific IgG in 10 of 11 patients with AIDS-related mental status alterations. Sharer and co-workers (16) reported the presence of multinucleated giant cells and HIV-1 in patients with AIDS encephalopathy and, more recently, Wiley and co-workers (17) and Koenig et al. (18) detected HIV-1 within macrophages in brain tissue from patients with HIV-encephalopathy. Thus, it appears that HIV-1 encephalopathy results from primary infection of the brain by HIV-1 and the predominant cells containing this virus appear to be of macrophage origin. The precise mechanism whereby this infection results in dementia remains to be elucidated.

Price and his co-workers have carefully studied the clinical profile of these patients. This HIV-1-related encephalopathy may be the presenting or sole manifestation of HIV-1 infection (19), or it may occur in the setting of other AIDS-related illnesses. All patients initially are seen with cognitive impairment. The syndrome is characterized by a progressive dementia, often first appearing as a confusional state and frequently accompanied by fever or mild metabolic derangement. Less commonly, patients demonstrate weakness (34%), personality change (38%), transient dysarthrias, or movement disorders (7%).

Patients typically complain of forgetfulness, slowness, poor concentration, and difficulties with problem-solving and reading. They may appear apathetic and exhibit reduced spontaneity and social withdrawal. Bedside mental status examination demonstrates inattention, psychomotor slowing, impaired memory, and impairment of complex processing. Physical examination often reveals tremor, impaired rapid repetitive movements, imbalance, ataxia, hypertonia, generalized hyperreflexia, frontal release signs, and impaired pursuit and saccadic eye movements. Formal neuropsychologic testing reveals multiple abnormalities on a variety of tests including primarily those that measure performance under time constraints, problem-solving, visual scanning, perceptual and visual motor integration, learning, memory, and alternation between two or more performance rules or sets.

Point prevalence data on AIDS patients from a number of studies indicate that the prevalence of HIV-1 encephalopathy ranges between 8% and 16% (1,4,21). In an autopsy-based series of patients referred to a neurology service, 66% of AIDS patients had this disorder, whereas an additional 15% had some lesser degree of dementia (21).

The characteristic radiologic finding of HIV-1 encephalopathy is diffuse cerebral atrophy (22). Brain atrophy and, less commonly, white matter changes can be evident on CT or MRI (8). A characteristically abnormal pattern of regional brain glucose metabolism has been identified by positron emission tomography in patients with HIV-1 encephalopathy (23). The HIV-1 virus can be recovered from blood, brain, or CSF of patients with HIV-1 encephalopathy (24). Cerebrospinal fluid examination usually reveals normal glucose and white blood cell concentrations and mildly elevated protein concentration, but CSF mononuclear pleocytosis has been observed (25). Neuropathologic studies reveal diffuse white matter changes characterized by multinucleated cell and macrophage infiltrates.

There is no effective therapy for HIV-1 encephalopathy at the present time. Trials of zidovudine, formerly known as azidothymidine (AZT), an antiviral compound that crosses the blood brain barrier, are currently underway. There is strong evidence that zidovudine may be beneficial for patients with HIV-1 encephalopathy (26,94). HIV-1 encephalopathy is rapidly progressive and usually fatal; mean survival after diagnosis is currently about 3 months (4).

HIV-1 Meningitis

An acute "aseptic" meningitis that occurs shortly after seroconversion to HIV-1 appears to represent a primary response of the nervous system to HIV-1 infection. Symptoms compatible with acute meningeal inflammation occur commonly and include headache, retro-orbital pain, meningismus, fever, photophobia, and cranial neuropathies. A more indolent variant of HIV-1-related meningitis, with only headache and persistent low-grade CSF pleocytosis, has been recognized. This type of meningitis is attributed to HIV-1 infection after the exclusion of other potential causes. The diagnosis of HIV-1 meningitis is made in light of these clinical findings, HIV-1 seropositivity, and a CSF white blood cell count of greater than $5/mm^3$. Typically, the acute symptoms are self-limited, require no special treatment, and resolve within 1 month.

An atypical meningitis, characterized by chronicity and recurrence, has also been reported in association with HIV-1 infection (2). Although it was initially called "atypical aseptic meningitis," recent studies have demonstrated that HIV-1 can be cultured from the CSF of most patients with this disorder (5,15). Although both are associated with HIV-1 infection of the CNS, aseptic meningitis presents clinically in an entirely different manner from HIV-1 encephalopathy. Common features include headache, fever, and meningeal signs. Patients with atypical meningitis often have associated long tract findings or cranial neuropathies, especially of the fifth, seventh, and eighth cranial nerves. They may have evidence of elevated intracranial pressure and all, by definition, have CSF pleocytosis. Cerebrospinal fluid findings are otherwise similar to those of patients with HIV-1 encephalopathy.

The clinical course of atypical meningitis is also different from that of HIV-1 encephalopathy, being self-limited or recurrent, rather than progressive. It has been suggested that the occurrence of HIV-1 encephalopathy or atypical meningitis as a manifestation of HIV-1 infection may be a reflection of the patient's degree of immunosuppression (1,3). Both illnesses, however, have been seen in otherwise asymptomatic patients (19), and autopsy findings indicate remarkable histopathologic similarities between these two clinical entities.

Vacuolar Myelopathy

Vacuolar myelopathy, first reported by Snider et al. (1) and Goldstick et al. (27) and further characterized by Petito and co-workers (9), appears to be a third unique HIV-related CNS syndrome. Recent studies (5,15) have demonstrated that HIV-1 can be cultured from the spinal cords of many of these patients, which suggests that primary HIV-1 infection is required for the development of this syndrome.

The most common symptoms associated with vacuolar myelopathy include leg weakness and incontinence (9,28). Neurologic examination often reveals paraparesis, spasticity and ataxia. Berger and Resnick (28) note that hyperreflexia and extensor plantar responses may be detected in the absence of weakness. They observe that muscle stretch reflexes are occasionally absent, presumably owing to concomitant peripheral neuropathy. Patients with vacuolar myelopathy frequently present with acute myelopathy and undergo either myelography or magnetic resonance imaging (MRI) before their diagnosis.

Vacuolar myelopathy was first described as a pathologic abnormality. Petito et al. (9) detected this degenerative disorder, most severe in the lateral and posterior columns of the thoracic spinal cord, in 20 of 89 patients with AIDS upon autopsy (22%). Pathologically, this syndrome resembled closely the subacute combined degeneration of vitamin B_{12} deficiency, with loss of myelin and spongy degeneration of the cord substance. Clinical neurologic findings were present more frequently in those patients with more severe pathologic changes; these clinical findings were present in 12 of the 20 patients initially reported. Interestingly, 14 of these patients (70%) were also demented. There currently is no effective therapy for vacuolar myelopathy.

Opportunistic Viral Infections

Progressive Multifocal Leukoencephalopathy

Progressive multifocal leukoencephalopathy (PML) is an unusual infectious central demyelinating disease caused by the papovavirus JC (29). Miller et al.

(30) first reported PML occurring in an AIDS patient. They described a male homosexual with a T-cell immune deficiency and progressive brain stem dysfunction. The computed tomographic (CT) brain scans revealed a lucent cerebellar lesion that on biopsy, was shown to be PML. Bedri et al. (31) demonstrated papovavirus by electron microscopy in an AIDS patient with PML.

As of August 1986, 172 cases of AIDS-related PML had been reported to the CDC. Clinically, PML in the AIDS patient appears to behave in a fashion similar to PML in other immunocompromised patients. Affected patients present with mental status alterations, blindness, aphasia, hemiparesis, ataxia, and other focal deficits that slowly progress until death (32).

The characteristic CT finding is that of low-density lesions without contrast enhancement, mass effect, or associated edema. Krupp and co-workers (33) detailed seven cases of PML; four of these patients also had AIDS. The clinical findings were usually more severe than the CT abnormalities would suggest. Although lesions were noted to enlarge progressively on CT, these findings lagged behind the rate of clinical evolution.

Autopsy findings in patients with PML reveal focal myelin loss with sparing of axon cylinders and the presence of bizarre astrocytes and enlarged oligodendrocytes containing eosinophilic intranuclear inclusions surrounding these areas of demyelination (34). Survival after diagnosis of PML in the patient with AIDS is extremely short. Several patients have died within 1 month of diagnosis; the longest reported survivor lived for 5 months after biopsy. No effective therapy exists for PML. The early suggestion by Snider et al. (1) that cytosine arabinoside therapy may be effective in these patients has not been confirmed (33).

Other Viral Infections

Infection with herpesviruses, including cytomegalovirus (CMV), herpes simplex viruses type 1 and 2 (HSV-1 and HSV-2) and varicella-zoster virus (VZV), is a major source of central neurologic disease in AIDS patients. Herpes simplex type 1 is the most frequent agent causing sporadic (nonepidemic) viral encephalitis. In immunocompetent patients, HSV-1 produces a hemorrhagic necrotizing encephalitis, usually confined to the medial temporal and inferior frontal lobes (35). Episodes of encephalitic illness have been associated with CMV (36), VZV (37), and HSV-2 (38), although infection with HSV-2 usually produces a benign self-limited meningitis in association with initial genital infection (39).

Several reports of AIDS-related CNS infection with HSV (4,40,41) or HSV combined with CMV (42,43) have recently appeared. In our experience, the severity of inflammation and the rapidity of disease progression are roughly proportional to the degree of immune competence (3). Intravenous acyclovir may be an effective therapy for HSV encephalitis in HIV-1-infected patients, although published data supporting this are lacking.

Cytomegalovirus meningoencephalitis has also been reported in patients with AIDS (44-46). The rigor with which these patients were evaluated for concomitant HIV-1 meningitis or encephalitis is unknown. In a study of 10 patients with CMV encephalitis, Post et al. (47) reported that CMV infection of the CNS was the cause of death in six patients, was superimposed on systemic infection in two patients, and was not clinically evident in two patients. Diffuse cerebral atrophy was evident on CT scans in all cases, although CT studies significantly underestimated the degree of CNS involvement and frequently failed to demonstrate focal abnormalities when they were apparent on autopsy. Very little information is available about the efficacy of ganciclovir [(9-[2-hydroxy-1-(hydroxymethyl)ethoxymethyl]quanine; DHPG] for the treatment of CNS CMV infection.

Varicella-zoster virus is also an important opportunistic central nervous system pathogen in AIDS patients (3,48). Interestingly, Ryder et al. (49) have reported on a patient with AIDS who developed progressive, ultimately fatal, neurologic deficits 12 weeks after a course of cutaneous zoster. Autopsy revealed a diffuse zoster encephalomyelitis. As with HSV, acyclovir might well be an effective therapy for VZV encephalitis in the HIV-1-infected patient, although data supporting this are lacking. On empiric grounds, acyclovir therapy should be implemented as soon as the diagnosis of VZV encephalitis is suspected.

Although viruses other than papovaviruses or herpesviruses are potential opportunistic CNS pathogens in patients with AIDS, very few such cases have been reported. West and co-workers (50) reported the case of a bisexual man with a history of intravenous drug abuse who developed encephalitis. Adenovirus type 2 was isolated from brain tissue obtained by biopsy, whereas systemic infection with Epstein-Barr virus (EBV) was demonstrated. Infection with more than one opportunistic viral pathogen is now a well-recognized entity (3,42,43).

Other Central Nervous System Infections

Toxoplasma gondii

The first report of cerebral toxoplasmosis in a patient with AIDS was that by Rutsaert et al. in 1980 (51). Several series of such patients have since appeared (52-55). Toxoplasmosis in the patient with AIDS almost always involves the CNS and appears to result from the reactivation of latent brain infection with the opportunistic intracellular parasite *T. gondii*. By August 1986, 625 cases of cerebral toxoplasmosis had been reported to the CDC. The prevalence of cerebral toxoplasmosis ranges between 2% and 13% depending upon patient risk group and geographic location. In a significant proportion of AIDS patients with toxoplasmosis, this disease was their first clinical manifestation of illness; overall, however, the percentage of AIDS patients first presenting with toxoplasmosis is small. In 44% of patients at UCSF with toxoplasmosis, this was the initial manifestation of AIDS. This represents 1.8% of all patients with AIDS at UCSF (4). The CDC data suggest that 5.4% of AIDS patients are first seen with CNS toxoplasmosis (11).

Patients with AIDS and cerebral toxoplasmosis most frequently have a short history of headaches and altered mental status (see Chap. 18). Focal weakness and seizures are also commonly observed (see Table 3). Cerebrospinal fluid analysis reveals a mildly elevated protein and few lymphocytes (see Table 2). The CT scans frequently show multiple bilateral contrast-enhancing intracerebral lesions. There is considerable overlap in the radiologic appearance of toxoplasmosis and other AIDS-related CNS diseases, such that specific diagnosis by radiologic criteria is impossible. Magnetic resonance imaging appears to be more sensitive than CT in the detection of brain lesions caused by *T. gondii* and, in virtually all cases, demonstrates multiple intracerebral lesions (56). Thus, in a patient with a single lesion on MRI, the diagnosis of toxoplasmosis is to be questioned.

Several groups have recommended a routine biopsy from all patients with presumed cerebral toxoplasmosis (57,58). Brain biopsy has, in fact, proved to be remarkably sensitive in the diagnosis of toxoplasmosis (59). *Toxoplasma* organisms can be identified by touch preparation, peroxidase-antiperoxidase staining, or by direct visualization on light or electron microscopy. The morbidity from biopsy techniques, however small, and the sheer number of affected patients have led some groups to suggest that empiric therapy be initiated before biopsy (60). In stable patients with strong clinical and radiologic evidence for cerebral toxoplasmosis, an empiric trial of pyrimethamine and sulfadiazine may well establish the diagnosis without the need for cerebral biopsy and should be considered. Antibiotic therapy, without the use of adjunctive steroids unless absolutely necessary, should be initiated after baseline radiologic and clinical examination. Patients should be followed clinically at weekly intervals. After 2 to 3 weeks, a follow-up radiologic study should be obtained. Should patients deteriorate, either radiologically or clinically, during the trial, it should be aborted, and a biopsy should be obtained. Care should be taken to obtain the follow-up radiologic study by use of the same technique as the baseline study. If both radiologic and clinical examinations are improving, then the presumptive diagnosis of toxoplasmosis is made, and the patient is maintained on antibiotic therapy. If either clinical or radiologic examinations are unchanged or have worsened, then a brain biopsy is indicated. Contraindications for this empiric trial include allergy to pyrimethamine or sulfadiazine, unstable neurologic condition, and the uncertainty of the diagnosis of AIDS.

In immunocompetent patients, infection of the CNS with *T. gondii* is extremely rare and produces acute focal or diffuse meningoencephalitis with cellular necrosis, microglial nodules, and perivascular mononuclear inflammation associated with both intra- and extracellular trophozoites (61). Thrombosis of blood vessels causing large areas of coagulation necrosis may produce mass lesions in the brain. In immunodeficient hosts, the lack of cell-mediated immunity may result in a persistent acute infection with severe necrotizing lesions. Pathologic analysis of biopsy specimens from AIDS patients with toxoplasmosis reveals necrotizing granulomas, usually within thin capsules and with little inflammation (62). Encysted *T. gondii* and tachyzoites are usually present.

Early aggressive diagnosis and therapy with pyrimethamine and sulfadiazine often results in a dramatic clinical and radiographic response (52-55). Therapy with pyrimethamine and sulfadiazine must be maintained at maximal doses for life to ensure adequate control of this illness. Meaningful survival of as long as 1 year after diagnosis has been reported.

Cryptococcus neoformans

Cryptococcus neoformans is a soil fungus that causes the most common fungal infection of the CNS. Twelve hundred fifty-two cases of AIDS-related cryptococcal meningitis had been reported to the CDC by August 1986 (see Chap. 15). This data, reflecting best the incidence of cryptococcosis at presentation with AIDS, represents an overall prevalence of approximately 5% of all patients with AIDS. At particular risk are AIDS patients from New Jersey and those who are black or intravenous drug users; these risk factors may increase the risk of contracting cryptococcal meningitis to as high as 10% (11). At UCSF, 68 reliably diagnosed cases of AIDS-related cryptococcal meningitis had been recorded as of June 1986. This represents an institutional incidence of 5.3%. Many AIDS patients who develop cryptococcal meningitis will have this illness as their first clinical sign of AIDS; still, the number of AIDS patients who first appear with cryptococcal maningitis is small. At UCSF, 34% of AIDS patients with cryptococcal meningitis (1.8% of all AIDS patients) had this illness as the initial manifestation of AIDS.

Seventy-nine AIDS patients with cryptococcal meningitis have been reported (1,3,63). Patients most frequently have a short history of decreasing mental status, headache, and signs of meningeal irritation. Cranial CT scans are usually normal (4). The diagnosis of cryptococcosis is made by CSF analysis with cryoptococcal cultures, cryptococcal antigen titers, or direct staining with India ink. In the series of Kovacs and co-workers (63), 7 of 27 patients with AIDS and cryptococcal meningitis had this infection as the initial manifestation of AIDS (26%). Meningitis was the most frequent clinical feature (67%). Studies of CSF frequently revealed a normal leukocyte count, protein and glucose concentrations; CSF cryptococcal antigen; and a positive culture for cryptococci were found in all cases.

Pathologically, cryptococcal meningitis results in a granulomatous meningitis with additional granulomas and cysts that form within the cerebral cortex and deeper brain structures (64). One feature unique to AIDS-related cryptococcal infection of the CNS is the frequency of intraparenchymal cryptococcal lesions. Quite rare in immunocompetent patients, cryptococcomas are found in 10% of AIDS patients with cryptococcal meningitis (4). This observation must be considered in the evaluation of the AIDS patient with cryptococcal meningitis and the appearance of a mass lesion on radiologic studies.

Despite treatment with amphotericin B with or without 5-flucytosine, the mortality of CNS cryptococcal infection in immunocompetent hosts is 40% (64). In the series reported by Kovacs and co-workers (63), only 10 of 24 patients had no evidence of clinical activity of cryptococcal infection after the completion of therapy; 6 of these 10 had either clinical or autopsy demonstrated relapses. The authors concluded, somewhat contrary to our experience, that standard therapy with amphotericin B, with or without additional 5-flucytosine, was ineffective. At UCSF, the more common experience is that patients respond to conventional therapy but require chronic suppressive therapy after treatment of the acute disease. Recurrent cryptococcal meningitis is, however, a significant problem; mean survival after initial diagnosis has been only 2 to 3 months (4).

Other Fungal Infections

Candida albicans Candidiasis, usually associated with diabetes, leukemia, lymphoma and intravenous drug abuse, is a relatively rare CNS pathogen (65). Nine cases of cerebral candidiasis have been reported in patients with AIDS (1,3,4,10,66,67). The combination of surgical abcess excision followed by amphotericin B appears to be the only effective therapy.

Aspergillus fumigatus Infections with the mold *A. fumigatus* are uncommon, even in immunocompromised patients. Aspergillosis infecting the central nervous system may present as meningitis, encephalitis, or abcess. Four cases of AIDS-related CNS aspergillosis have been reported (10,68).

Coccidioides immitis Meningeal infection occurs in nearly one-half of all cases of disseminated coccidioidomycosis. Although most immunocompetent patients with coccidioidal meningitis have a subclinical or chronic, relapsing, meningitis, the disease can present as a rapid, fulminant illness in the immunocompromised patient (69). Treatment involves the long-term administration of intrathecal amphotericin B; frequently, this requires the placement of an Ommaya reservoir (70). Several cases of AIDS-related CNS infection with *C. immitis* have been reported (3,4,71).

Miscellaneous fungal infections   We have treated one child with AIDS and cerebral mucormycosis. Micozzi et al. (72) have reported five cases of mucormycosis and intravenous drug users; these cases may well be AIDS-related. Two cases of cerebral infection with *Rhizopus* spp. and one case of cerebral infection with *Acremonium alabamensis* have been reported by Welti and co-workers (68); these patients also probably had AIDS. There are also scattered case reports of intracranial infection with *Histoplasma capsulatum* (71).

Mycobacterial Infections

Mycobacterium tuberculosis   The clinical features and pathology of *M. tuberculosis* meningitis have been well described (64); mycobacterial infection can result in meningitis, encephalitis, or brain abscess formation. Fifteen patients with AIDS and *M. tuberculosis* infections of the CNS have been reported (73). These patients were uniformly either Haitians or intravenous drug abusers; these reports are consistent with the endemic nature of tuberculosis in the Caribbean basin and with epidemiologic data that indicate that Haitians are at higher risk of contracting any AIDS-related neurologic illness. The clinical features of these patients have not been fully reported; of note is that roughly two-thirds presented with CNS mass lesions, and one-third presented with signs and symptoms of meningitis only. Intracranial tuberculous infection is rare in homosexual men with AIDS; of nearly 1300 patients treated at UCSF (more than 99% homosexual men), we have seen only one case of tuberculous meningitis.

Mycobacterium avium complex   Although *M. avium* complex (MAC) infection is extremely common in the AIDS patient population, CNS infection with MAC is rare. Only 14 such cases have been reported (74); an additional four patients have been treated at UCSF. In contrast to CNS *M. tuberculosis* infection, there does not appear to be a Haitian predisposition for AIDS-related CNS, MAC infection. Of patients reported in the literature, most had disseminated systemic MAC infection before their neurologic presentation with diffuse encephalitis. Meningitis, cranial neuropathy (facial nerve), and peripheral neuropathy have also been reported in association with MAC infection of the CNS. Survival after contracting CNS MAC infection is very short; results with both standard tuberculosis chemotherapeutic agents and experimental regimens have been uniformly poor (75).

One patient with AIDS and CNS infection with *M. kansasii* has been reported (66).

Bacterial Infections

Reports of AIDS-related CNS complications from common bacterial pathogens have been conspicuously absent from the literature. None of the patients in the series presented by Snider et al. (1) or that of Levy et al. (3) had bacterial infections of the CNS. This is surprising considering the high frequency of pneumococcal and *Haemophilus influenzae* infections that are often associated with bacteremia in patients with AIDS. Nervous system infections with opportunistic bacterial pathogens in patients with AIDS have rarely been reported.

Listeria monocytogenes Listeria, the most common cause of bacterial meningitis in other types of immunocompromised patients, has only rarely been the cause of AIDS-related neurologic disease. We have treated three patients with AIDS and listerial infections of the CNS at UCSF. Two patients presented with signs and symptoms of meningitis, and CSF cultures grew listeria; antibiotic therapy cured the acute infection. A third patient presented with lethargy, fevers, and a focal neurologic deficit. The CT brain scans revealed a single contrast-enhancing lesion; blood cultures grew listeria. Antibiotic therapy resulted in both resolution of the abscess on follow-up CT scans and of the neurologic signs and symptoms. Two patients later died nonneurologic deaths from other AIDS-related illnesses; one patient was lost to follow-up.

Nocardia asteroides Nocardial infection of the CNS usually accompanies pulmonary infection in immunosuppressed patients; as with listeria, nocardial CNS infection in the AIDS patient population is extremely rare. Sharer and Kapila (76) reported a single case of nocardial brain abscess in a 34-year-old female intravenous drug abuser with AIDS.

Other bacterial infections One case each of AIDS-related *Escherichia coli* meningitis and meningoencephalitis have been reported (71,77); the clinical profiles of these patients are lacking. Syphilitic meningoencephalitis, relatively resistant to penicillin therapy, has been reported in patients with HIV-1 infection (77,78; see Chap. 13, section on syphilis).

Other HIV-1-Related Central Nervous System Illnesses

In addition to primary and opportunistic infections, there are several other causes of HIV-1-related neurologic illness (see Table 1). These processes, including primary CNS lymphoma, systemic lymphoma with CNS involvement, metastatic Kaposi's sarcoma, and cerebrovascular complications such as hemorrhage, infarction, and vasculitis, are detailed elsewhere (4,79,80). It is important to note that these other diseases may mimic HIV-1-related CNS infection in both their clinical and radiologic presentation. Thus, patients with primary CNS lymphoma may present in the same way as those with cerebral toxoplasmosis, with a short history of lethargy, headaches, and focal weakness. The CSF analysis may be entirely normal or may be remarkable only for a mild lymphocytic pleocytosis. The CT scans often reveal multiple contrast-enhancing intracranial lesions. Not infrequently, these patients undergo empiric therapy for toxoplasmosis; when this fails, the diagnosis of primary CNS lymphoma is made upon brain biopsy.

Several groups have reported neurologic symptoms arising as complications of AIDS therapy; these, too, may mimic the signs or symptoms of HIV-1-related CNS infection. Hollander and co-workers (81) reported the development of extrapyramidal motor symptoms in AIDS patients treated with low-dose antiemetic therapy. Bates et al. (82) have reported acute myelopathy following intrathecal chemotherapy for lymphoma in an AIDS patient. Antiviral therapy in AIDS patients with a nucleoside analog, FIAC, has also been reported to produce startle myoclonus, dysphasia, and delerium (83).

MULTIPLE INTRACRANIAL PATHOLOGIC PROCESSES

The evaluation and treatment of the AIDS patient with neurologic illness has been complicated by the observation that multiple intracranial pathologic processes may be present in patients with AIDS (4,67,84). Of 482 neurologically symptomatic AIDS patients treated at UCSF, 65 patients were identified with multiple intracranial pathologic processes (13.5%). In a more carefully studied group of patients, 29% of AIDS patients with nervous system illness had more than one CNS pathologic process identified at autopsy (4). Of note is that these processes were identified both within the same lesion and within spatially separated lesions, as well as both sequentially and simultaneously.

The high prevalence of multiple intracranial diseases in patients with AIDS has profound implications for the diagnosis and treatment of intracranial lesions in this patient population. The reported frequency of cerebral toxoplasmosis has led some authors to suggest that empiric therapy alone is sufficient for the treatment of AIDS patients with CNS mass lesions. Only 53% of our patients with AIDS and CNS mass lesions had cerebral toxoplasmosis, and only 28% of our patients with multiple, histologically confirmed intracranial diseases had toxoplasmosis. Of the remaining mass lesions, most often including primary CNS lymphomas and cryptococcomas, 67% were potentially treatable. Antibiotic therapy alone, then, may ignore a potentially treatable disease in over half of neurologically symptomatic AIDS patients. Patients treated after biopsy or with a *correct* presumptive diagnosis may also have other intracranial pathologic processes that remain untreated.

Recommendations for the evaluation of AIDS patients with neurologic symptoms are presented in the next section. Because of the high prevalence of multiple intracranial diseases in the AIDS patient population, repeat clinical, CSF, and radiologic studies are indicated at regular intervals during therapy or whenever a patient deteriorates while receiving treatment, even after the diagnosis is confirmed by biopsy. If new lesions appear, or if the response to therapy of other lesions differs from that of the biopsied lesion, the possibility of a second intracranial process must be considered. Repeat biopsy may be indicated and may reveal additional treatable disease.

AIDS-RELATED PERIPHERAL NERVOUS SYSTEM SYNDROMES

Although reported in 9% to 16% of patients with AIDS, peripheral nervous system (PNS) dysfunction is likely to be more common in these patients. A recent study disclosed a 35% prevalence of electrophysiologic abnormalities (85). The frequency of peripheral neuropathies in patients with AIDS-related complex or an otherwise asymptomatic seropositive state is unknown, but in one study, 38% of patients with generalized lymphadenopathy had complaints suggestive of peripheral neuropathy (86).

Peripheral neuropathic complications may occur as a result of many different processes in HIV-1-infected patients. Vincristine-related neuropathy, for example, is a well-recognized entity in this group. Varicella-zoster radiculitis, which may progress to radiculomyelitis, is common, and often precedes other clinical manifestations of AIDS (3). The majority of patients, however, manifest PNS dysfunction with one of four syndromes: distal symmetric peripheral neuropathy (DSPN), chronic inflammatory demyelinating polyradiculoneuropathy (CIDP), mononeuritis multiplex (MM), or progressiove polyradiculopathy. These syndromes differ not only in presentation, treatment and neurologic prognosis, but also in the patients whom they tend to affect and, therefore, in their implications for overall prognosis.

Distal Symmetric Peripheral Neuropathy

Approximately 90% of our patients with HIV-1-related DSPN have had AIDS, with the remainder having ARC (87); however, Janssen found symptoms consistent with DSPN in 38% of unselected ARC patients (86). Paresthesia and hypesthesia, beginning in the feet and spreading proximally, are the most common presenting symptoms. Pain may be a prominent feature of this disorder. Weakness and muscular wasting occur much less frequently than the sensory abnormalities. Reflexes are decreased at the ankles, but may be normal elsewhere, unlike in CIDP. The course is chronic and slowly progressive, although periods of improvement may occur.

The cerebrospinal fluid (CSF) is usually normal, unless a coexistent disease is present. Electromyography and nerve conduction velocity (EMG/NCV) measurements suggest axonal loss and denervation, with fibrillations, reduced sural amplitudes, and reduced compound muscle action potentials in the distal lower extremities. Diagnosis requires ruling out other causes of neuropathy, such as vincristine and ethanol. Nerve biopsy may be nonspecifically abnormal, showing axonal loss with minimal or no inflammation, or may even be normal (1,87,88). The observation, however, that patients with HIV-1-related axonal or demyelinating neuropathies have perineurial IgM (87) may prove helpful in distinguishing HIV-1-related DSPN from the many other causes of axonal neuropathy.

Unfortunately, treatment is only symptomtic in patients with DSPN. Amitriptyline, phenytoin (Dilantin) and carbamazepine (Tegretol) have been used with variable success; plasmapheresis has not proved beneficial for DSPN (89). Ankle-foot orthoses may be useful for foot drop. The effect of zidovudine on DSPN is unknown. Fortunately, DSPN is often mild or is very slowly progressive.

Chronic Inflammatory Demyelinating Polyradiculoneuropathy

Although idiopathic inflammatory demyelinating polyradiculoneuropathy (i.e., Guillain-Barré syndrome) has been reported in association with HIV-1 infection (90), the subacute or chronic form, CIDP, is much more common. Usually, CIDP occurs in patients with ARC or otherwise asymptomatic HIV-1 infection (87,91); it is unusual for the symptoms of CIDP to begin after the appearance of opportunistic infections.

In contrast with DSPN, CIDP produces preponderantly motor signs and symptoms. Weakness may be severe and may result in respiratory failure. All tendon reflexes are usually diminished. Sensory abnormalities are typically restricted to the distal extremities, and vibration sense may be preferentially affected. Facial and bulbar weakness may accompany CIDP, usually at an advanced stage. Clinical manifestations of autonomic dysfunction are usually absent.

The CSF is nearly always abnormal, demonstrating oligoclonal bands, increased immunoglobulin/albumin ratio, and often, increased protein content and mononuclear pleocytosis (87,88). Electromyography and nerve conduction (EMG/NCV) studies suggest both axonal and demyelinating neuropathy. Sural nerve biopsy may be normal, but usually discloses epineurial and endoneurial inflammation, segmental demyelination, and axonal loss without vasculitis. Perineurial IgM has been noted (87).

Plasmapheresis is an effective therapy, especially when demyelination predominates over axonal loss (89). Response to steroids is variable (89,91);

furthermore, the role of such therapy in immunocompromised patients is controversial. The neurologic prognosis in HIV-1-related CIDP is generally good. An, as yet, undetermined fraction of patients will progress to AIDS, but many patients have been stable for months to a few years.

Mononeuritis Multiplex

In some aspects, HIV-1-associated mononeuritis multiplex is similar to CIDP: patients with ARC or otherwise asymptomatic HIV-1 infection are usually affected; EMG/NCV studies suggest axonal and demyelinative abnormalities; and nerve biopsy shows inflammation similar to that in CIDP. Therapeutically, the two groups tend to respond well to plasmapheresis when demyelination outweighs axonal loss.

In other aspects, however, the two conditions are dissimilar. Mononeuritis multiplex affects peripheral nerves in a patchy, rather than a diffuse, manner (sparing some deep tendon reflexes), usually involves sensory and motor function, often causes acute deficits, and leads to cranial neuropathies more often than does CIDP.

Progressive Polyradiculopathy

The syndrome of progressive polyradiculopathy usually occurs in patients with AIDS rather than ARC (87,92). Cytomegalovirus (CMV) has been implicated in some cases by culture or pathology, and in two cases, rashes due to herpes simplex virus have been temporally associated (93). Symptoms usually begin with somewhat asymmetric weakness of the lower extremities, which then progresses subacutely. Pain may accompany the disorder. Sensory deficits, often about the perineum, tend to be less severe than motor deficits. Urinary retention is common. The process may affect the upper extremities and may become a radiculomyelopathy.

The CSF characteristically shows hypoglycorrhachia; of less diagnostic significance is increased CSF protein and mononuclear cell count. Cytomegalovirus may be cultured from the CSF. The EMG/NCV studies suggest denervation. One patient with a positive CMV CSF culture, treated with ganciclovir for concomitant CMV retinitis, had no apparent change in the rate of progression of weakness, despite the arrest of retinitis (Jacobson et al., submitted for publication). Subsequent trials of plasma exchange and foscavnet therapy also had no apparent effect.

DIAGNOSIS OF AIDS-RELATED
CENTRAL NERVOUS SYSTEM ILLNESS

As with other neurologic illnesses, the first diagnostic steps are obtaining a history and physical examination. Because primary neurologic HIV-1 infec-

tion may produce subtle dementia before other signs of systemic or neurologic illness, careful cognitive assessment is critical.

Radiological and cerebrospinal fluid examinations are, then, the mainstays of the diagnosis of AIDS-related nervous system illness. Examination
of CSF may provide a definitive diagnosis in several AIDS-related neurologic diseases, including HIV-1 or other viral infections and cryptococcal
meningitis (see Table 2). Virtually all patients with AIDS and neurologic
disease have a mild elevation of CSF protein, ranging from 62 to 97 mg/dl
(4). Mean CSF glucose concentration is almost invariably within normal
limits, ranging from 43 to 63 mg/dl (4). The CSF cell count is usually normal in patients with HIV-1 encephalopathy, PML, and toxoplasmosis. Some
patients with HIV-1 encephalopathy, however, have been reported with CSF
pleocytosis (25). A minimal pleocytosis is noted in patients with primary
CNS lymphoma, whereas more marked CSF pleocytoses are noted in patients
with cryptococcal meningitis and opportunistic viral infections (4). The CSF
white blood cells were almost exclusively monocytes or lymphocytes. Thus,
in those patients with nonfocal radiologic studies and no CSF pleocytosis,
the diagnosis of HIV-1 encephalopathy is suggested.

Tests for cryptococcal meningitis are very sensitive in patients with AIDS;
cryptococcal antigen, culture, and India ink staining are positive in over
90% of cases (63). Although the presence of a positive toxoplasma titer is
not a reliable indicator of active toxoplasma infection (94), a negative IgG
titer may be of negative predictive value. Tests for HIV-1 infection (e.g.,
antibody, p24 core antigen, or culture) indicate only exposure to the AIDS
virus and not active disease. Quantitative measurement of HIV-1 antigen
may better reflect active neurologic illness in these patients (21).

Computed tomographic brain scans are the most widely used radiologic
examination in AIDS patients with neurologic signs or symptoms. In a review
of 200 patients with AIDS, cranial CT scans were normal in 39.5% of cases,
revealed focal lesions in 25.5%, and demonstrated diffuse cerebral atrophy
in 35% (95). These findings were of some prognostic value· patients with
diffuse cerebral atrophy were three times more likely than patients with normal CT scans to manifest neurologic progression and to subsequently demonstrate CNS structural abnormalities.

In patients without focal CT abnormalities, cryptococcal meningitis was
by far the most frequent diagnosis (28%). Although these studies report an
incidence of CMV and HIV-1 encephalitis in 11% and 3% of these patients,
respectively, this probably reflects a lack of rigor in defining these diagnoses.
It appears that more than one-third of neurologically symptomatic AIDS
patients with nonfocal CT scans actually have HIV-1 encephalitis, whereas
CMV encephalitis is rare.

Patients with focal abnormalities on CT scans were subsequently shown to have toxoplasmosis (50-70%), primary CNS lymphoma (10-25%), progressive multifocal leukoencephalopathy (PML) (10-22%) or had either non-diagnostic biopsies (10%) or other disease (9%) (22,95).

Computerized tomographic scans are of limited value in the specific differential diagnosis of AIDS-related neurologic illness. The presence or absence of focal lesions on CT is, however, of some diagnostic value. As a rule, nonfocal examinations are obtained in patients with HIV-1 encephalopathy, opportunistic viral infection, and cryptococcal meningitis. Focal CT abnormalities are often identified in patients with toxoplasmosis, primary CNS lymphoma, and PML (22,95). Within this latter group, patients with low-density lesions that demonstrate little or no enhancement after the administration of iodinated contrast material tend to have PML or primary CNS lymphoma. Restriction of these lesions to the white matter suggests the diagnosis of PML, whereas the presence of mass effect suggests lymphoma. The demonstration of ring-enhancing lesions, especially within the basal ganglia, suggests the diagnosis of toxoplasmosis. Unfortunately, there are many cases in which ring-enhancing lesions are proved to be primary CNS lymphomas and in which toxoplasmal brain abscesses do not enhance. Thus, CT scans alone cannot provide a definitive diagnosis in AIDS-related CNS disease.

Magnetic resonance imaging (MRI) is more sensitive than CT for the detection of intracranial pathology in the patient with AIDS and neurologic symptoms (56). It also more accurately reflects the extent and distribution of histologically verified CNS disease. This increased sensitivity and accuracy has been demonstrated to have a significant impact on the evaluation and therapy of patients with AIDS-related CNS illness, including indication for and the direction of brain biopsy, plus alterations in both chemotherapeutic and radiation therapy protocols. Interestingly, in all but the rare case, MRI demonstrates multiple bilateral intracranial abnormalities in patients with toxoplasmosis (56). Thus, a single lesion on MRI probably reflects an illness other than toxoplasmosis.

ALGORITHMS FOR THE EVALUATION OF THE PATIENT WITH AIDS AND NEUROLOGIC SYMPTOMS

The evaluation and treatment of the AIDS patient with central neurologic illness is a difficult challenge. Algorithms to assist in the evaluation of the neurologically symptomatic AIDS patient are included in Figures 1 through 3. Close attention must be paid to subtle neurologic complaints and careful neurologic examination is warranted in all AIDS patients. Once the patient

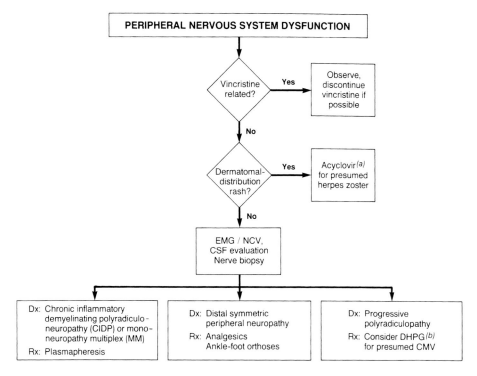

FIGURE 1 Algorithm for the evaluation and treatment of PNS dysfunction in patients infected with HIV-1. a = Acyclovir is recommended because of the high incidence of herpes zoster complications in patients with HIV-1 infection. b = Ganciclovir (DHPG) is currently in experimental use for cytomegalovirus (CMV) retinitis; efficacy has not been shown for progressive polyradiculopathy due to CMV. EMG = electromyography. NCV = nerve conduction velocity. CSF = cerebrospinal fluid.

complains of neurologic dysfunction, or a neurologic abnormality is identified on examination, a careful workup is indicated. For patients with evidence of peripheral nervous system dysfunction, neurologic examination is usually followed by EMG/NCV studies. Occasionally, nerve biopsy may be necessary to establish a diagnosis. Inflammatory peripheral neuropathies (those with predominant demyelinative, rather than axonopathic features) may respond to plasmapheresis. For the other peripheral neurologic diseases, the only treatments are symptomatic.

The current recommendation for the initial evaluation of the patient with central neurologic symptoms is MRI. If this is not readily available, then CT brain scanning should be performed. If the neuroradiologic study is

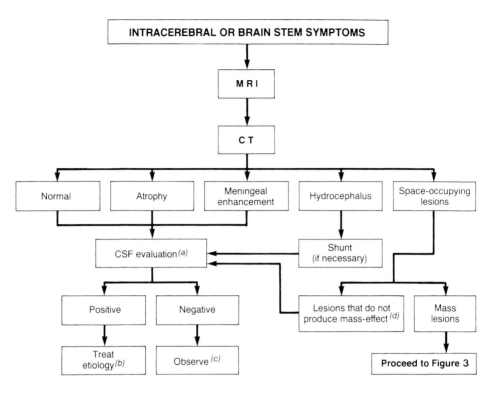

FIGURE 2 Algorithm for the evaluation and treatment of intracerebral or brain stem symptoms in patients infected with HIV-1. a = Cerebrospinal fluid (CSF) should be analyzed for cells, glucose levels, bacteria, fungi, tuberculous organisms, and viruses. b = Refer to sections on the treatment of specific diseases. c = If neurologic symptoms persist, MRI or CT studies and the CSF evaluation are repeated monthly. If significant neurologic deterioration occurs or if new symptoms or signs develop, immediate MRI or CT studies are warranted. d = Space-occupying lesions that do not produce mass effect are usually seen on CT scans as areas of low density that do not enhance after the administration of contrast material; on T2-weighted MRI scans, these lesions are seen as areas of high-signal intensity. Most are due to HIV-1, CMV, PML, and strokes (from Rosenblum, M. L., Levy, R. M., and Bredesen, D. E., eds. (1987). *AIDS and the Nervous System*, Chap. 19. New York, Raven Press, with permission).

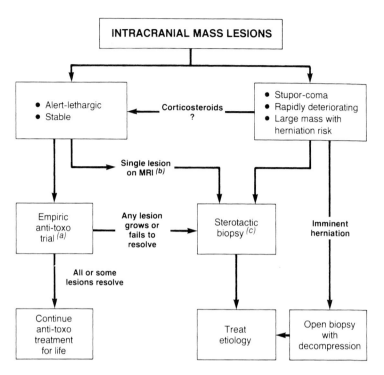

FIGURE 3 Algorithm for the evaluation and treatment of intracranial mass lesions in patients infected with HIV-1. a = Two to three week course of sulfadiazine and pyrimethamine (see text). b = Because most of the single-mass lesions on MRI are not caused by *T. gondii*, a biopsy is recommended. c = Stereotactic biopsies are guided by CT or by real-time ultrasonography; the only absolute contraindication to stereotactic biopsy is a noncorrectable bleeding diathesis (from Rosenblum, M. L., Levy, R. M., and Bredesen, D. E., eds. (1987). *AIDS and the Nervous System*, Chap. 19. New York, Raven Press, with permission).

normal or reveals diffuse cerebral atrophy only, then cerebrospinal fluid examination should be performed. In addition to routine chemistry, cytology, and culture evaluations, CSF examination should include viral cultures. Treatment should be initiated based upon these findings. If no diagnosis is made, then careful, regular clinical and radiologic follow-up is indicated.

Those patients with focal lesions on MRI are divided into those who are stable (alert or lethargic) or those who are deteriorating. In stable patients a trial of empiric therapy for toxoplasmosis with pyrimethamine and sulfadiazine is initiated. If there is clear radiologic and clinical response after 2 to

3 weeks of therapy, maximal antibiotic therapy is continued for life (although in some centers, a reduced dosage maintenance regimen for life is given after 6 weeks of full-dose therapy). If the patient fails to respond, then stereotaxic biopsy is indicated. In patients who are neurologically unstable, stereotaxic biopsy should be performed directly. Open craniotomy is reserved for only those patients with large mass lesions who are at risk of herniation and require emergent decompression.

Specific diagnosis is thus made on the basis of CSF findings, response to empiric therapy, or biopsy. These patients must then be followed with great diligence to evaluate the response to therapy. The very real possibility of multiple treatable intracranial pathologic processes may necessitate a repetition of the patient's diagnostic evaluation and the institution of additional therapies. Although such a diagnostic and therapeutic program requires extreme care and diligence, it is only with such an approach that we may optimally treat the patient with AIDS-related neurologic illness.

ACKNOWLEDGMENTS

The authors would like to thank Dr. Ravi Gupta, clinical research assistant, whose efforts have made this work possible. Some of the information in this chapter has appeared in Rosenblum, M. L., Levy, R. M., and Bredesen, D. E. (eds.), (1988). *AIDS and the Nervous System.* New York, Raven Press.

REFERENCES

1. Snider, W. D., Simpson, D. M., Nielsen, S., Gold, J. W. M., Metroka, C. E., and Posner, J. B. (1983). Neurological complications of acquired immune deficiency syndrome: Analysis of 50 patients. *Ann. Neurol. 14*:403-148.
2. Bredesen, D. E. and Messing, R. (1983). Neurological syndromes heralding the acquired immune deficiency syndrome. *Ann. Neurol. 14*:141.
3. Levy, R. M., Bredesen, D. E., and Rosenblum, M. L. (1985). Neurological manifestations of the acquired immunodeficiency syndrome (AIDS): Experience at UCSF and review of the literature. *J. Neurosurg. 62*:475-495.
4. Levy, R. M. and Bredesen, D. E. (1988). Central nervous system dysfunction in acquired immunodeficiency syndrome. In *AIDS and the Nervous System.* (Rosenblum, M. L., Levy, R. M., and Bredesen, D. E., eds.). New York, Raven Press, pp. 29-63.
5. Ho, D. D., Rota, T. R., Schooley, R. T., Kaplan, J. C., Allan, J. D., Groopman, J. E., Resnick, L., Felsenstein, D., Andrews, C. A., and Hirsch, M. S. (1985). Isolation of HTLV-III from cerebrospinal fluid and neural tissues of patients with neurologic syndromes related to the acquired immunodeficiency syndrome. *N. Engl. J. Med. 313*:1493-1497.

6. Meyenhofer, M. F., Epstein, L. G., Cho, E.-K., and Sharer, L. R. (1987). Ultrastructural morphology and intracellular production of human immunodeficiency virus (HIV) in brain. *J. Neuropathol. Exp. Neurol. 46*:474-484.

7. Resnick, L., DiMarzo-Veronese, F., Schupbach, J., Tourtellotte, W. E., Ho, D. D., Muller, F., Shapshak, P., Vogt, M., Groopman, J. E., Markham, P. D., and Gallo, R. C. (1985). Intra-blood-brain-barrier synthesis of HRLC-III-specific IgG in patients with neurologic symptoms associated with AIDS or AIDS-related complex. *N. Engl. J. Med. 313*:1498-1504.

8. Navia, B. A., Jordan, B. D., and Price, R. W. (1986). The AIDS dementia complex: I. Clinical features. *Ann. Neurol. 19*:517-524.

9. Petito, C. K., Navia, B. A., Eun-Sook, C., Jordan, B. D., George, D. C., and Price, R. W. (1985). Vacuolar myelopathy pathologically resembling subacute combined degeneration in patients with the acquired immunodeficiency syndrome. *N. Engl. J. Med. 312*:874-879.

10. Koppel, B. S., Wormser, G. P., Tuchma, A. J., Maayan, S., Hewlett, D. Jr., and Daras, M. (1985). Central nervous system involvement in patients with acquired immune deficiency syndrome (AIDS). *Acta. Neurol. Scand. 71*:337-351.

11. Levy, R. M., Janssen, R. S., Bush, T. J., and Rosenblum, M. L. (1987). Neuroepidemiology of acquired immunodeficiency syndrome. In *AIDS and the Nervous System*. (Rosenblum, M. L., Levy, R. M., and Bredesen, D. E., eds.). New York, Raven Press, pp. 13-27.

12. Urmacher, C. and Nielsen, S. (1985). The histopathology of the acquired immune deficiency syndrome. *Pathol. Annu. 20*:197-220.

13. Moskowitz, L. B., Hensley, G. T., Chan, J. C., Gregorios, J., and Conley, F. K. (1984). The neuropathology of acquired immune deficiency syndrome. *Arch. Pathol. Lab. Med. 108*:867-872.

14. Shaw, G. M., Harper, M. E., Hahn, B. H. et al. (1985). HTLV-III infection in brains of children and adults with AIDS encephalopathy. *Science 227*:177-182.

15. Levy, J. A., Shimabukuro, J., Hollander, H., Mills, J., and Kaminsky, L. (1985). Isolation of AIDS associated retroviruses from cerebrospinal fluid and brain of patients with neurological symptoms. *Lancet 2*:586-588.

16. Sharer, L. R., Cho, E.-S., and Epstein, L. G. (1985). Multinucleated giant cells and HTLV-III in AIDS encephalopathy. *Hum. Pathol. 16*:760.

17. Wiley, C. A., Oldstone, M. B. A., and Nelson, J. A. (1987). Pathogenesis of AIDS encephalitis. *J. Neuropathol. Exp. Neurol. 46*:348.

18. Koenig, S., Gendelman, H. E., Orenstein, J. M., Dal Canto, M. C., Pezeshkpour, G. H., Yungbluth, M., Janotta, F., Aksamit, A., Martin, M. A., and Fauchi, A. S. (1986). Detection of AIDS virus in macrophages in brain tissue from AIDS patients with encephalopathy. *Science 233*:1089-1093.

19. Navia, B. A. and Price, R. W. (1987). The acquired immunodeficiency dementia complex as the presenting or sole manifestation of human immunodeficiency virus infection. *Arch. Neurol. 44*:65-69.

20. McArthur, J. and Becker, J. (1988). Neuropsychological findings in HIV-1 infection: A preliminary report of the Multicenter AIDS Cohort study (MACS). Presented at the World Health Organization Special Consultation on the Neuropsychiatric Aspects of HIV-1 Infection, Geneva, Switzerland, March 1988.

21. Price, R. W., Brew, B., Sidtis, J., Rosenblum, M., Scheck, A. C., and Cleary, P. (1988). The brain in AIDS: Central nervous system HIV-1 infection and AIDS dementia complex. *Science* 239:586-592.

22. Delapaz, R. and Enzmann, D. (1987). Neuroradiology of acquired immunodeficiency syndrome. In *AIDS and the Nervous System*. (Rosenblum, M. L., Levy, R. M., and Bredesen, D. E., eds.). New York, Raven Press, pp. 121-153.

23. Rottenberg, D. A., Moeller, J. R., Strother, S. C. et al. (1987). The metabolic pathology of the AIDS dementia complex. *Ann. Neurol.* 22:700.

24. Navia, B. A., Cho, E.-S., Petito, C. K. et al. (1986). The AIDS dementia complex: II. Neuropathology. *Ann. Neurol.* 19:525-535.

25. Hollander, H., and Levy, J. (1987). Neurologic abnormalities and recovery of human immunodeficiency virus from cerebrospinal fluid. *Ann. Intern. Med.* 106:692-695.

26. Fischl, M. A., Richman, D. D., Grielo, M. H. et al. (1987). The efficacy of azidothymidine (AZT) in the treatment of patients with AIDS and AIDS related complex. *N. Engl. J. Med.* 317:185-191.

27. Goldstick, L., Mandybur, T. I., and Bode, R. (1985). Spinal cord degeneration in AIDS. *Neurology* 35:103-106.

28. Berger, J. R. and Resnick, L. (1987). HTLV-III/LAV-related neurological disease. In *AIDS: Modern Concepts and Therapeutic Challenges*. (Broder, S., ed.). New York, Marcel Dekker, pp. 263-283.

29. Nayaran, O., Penny, J. B., Johnson, R. T., Herndon, R. M., and Weiner, L. P. (1973). Etiology of progressive multifocal leukoencephalopathy. Identification of papovavirus. *N. Engl. J. Med.* 289:1278-1282.

30. Miller, J. R., Barrett, R. E., Britton, C. B., Tapper, M. L., Bahr, G. S., Bruno, P. J., Marquardt, M. D., Hays, S. P., McMurtry, J. G., Weissman, J. B., and Bruno, M. S. (1982). Progressive multifocal leukoencephalopathy in a male homosexual with T-cell immune deficiency. *N. Engl. J. Med.* 307:1436-1438.

31. Bedri, J., Weinstein, W., and DeGregorio, P. (1983). Progressive multifocal leukoencephalopathy in acquired immunodeficiency syndrome. *N. Engl. J. Med.* 309:492-493.

32. Astrom, K. E., Mancall, E. L., and Richardson, E. P. (1958). Progressive multifocal leukoencephalopathy: A hitherto unrecognized complication of chronic lymphatic leukaemia and Hodgkin's disease. *Brain* 81:93-111.

33. Krupp, L. B., Lipton, R. B., Swerdlow, M. L., Leeds, N. E., and Llena, J. (1985). Progressive multifocal leukoencephalopathy: Clinical and radiographic features. *Ann. Neurol.* 17:344-348.

34. ZuRhein, G. M. (1969). Association of papovavirions with a human demyelinating disease (progressive multifocal leukoencephalopathy). *Prog. Med. Virol.* 11:185-247.

35. Baringer, J. R. and Swoveland, P. (1973). Recovery of herpes-simplex virus from human trigeminal ganglions. *N. Engl. J. Med.* 288:648-650.

36. Bale, J. F. (1984). Human cytomegalovirus infection and disorders of the nervous system. *Arch. Neurol.* 41:310-320.

37. McKendall, R. R. and Klawas, H. L. (1978). Nervous system complications of varicella-zoster virus. In *Handbook of Clinical Neurology*, Vol. 34. (Vinken, P. J. and Bruyn, G. W., eds.). Amsterdam, North-Holland, pp. 161-183.

38. Dix, R. D., Waitzman, D. M., Follansbee, S. et al. (1985). HSV type 2 encephalitis in two homosexual men with persistent lymphadenopathy. *Ann. Neurol.* *17*:203-206.

39. Baringer, J. R. (1978). Herpes simplex infection of the nervous system. In *Handbook of Clinical Neurology*, Vol. 34. (Vinken, P. J. and Bruyn, G. W., eds.). Amsterdam, North-Holland, pp. 145-159.

40. Britton, C. B., Mesa-Tejeda, R., Fenoglio, C. M., Hays, A. P., Garvey, G. G., and Miller, J. R. (1985). A new complication of AIDS: Thoracic myelitis caused by herpes simplex. *Neurology* *35*:1071-1074.

41. Dix, R. D., Bredesen, D. E., Erlich, K. S., and Mills, J. (1985). Recovery of herpesviruses from cerebrospinal fluid of immunodeficient homosexual men. *Ann. Neurol.* *18*:611-614.

42. Pepose, J. S., Hilborne, L. H., Cancilla, P. A., and Foos, R. Y. (1984). Concurrent herpes simplex and cytomegalovirus retinitis and encephalitis in the acquired immune deficiency syndrome (AIDS). *Ophthalmology* *91*:1669-1677.

43. Tucker, T., Dix, R. D., Katzen, C., Davis, R. J., and Schmidley, J. W. (1985). Cytomegalovirus and herpes simplex virus ascending myelitis in a patient with acquired immune deficiency syndrome. *Ann. Neurol.* *18*:74-79.

44. Hawley, D. A., Schaefer, J. F., Schulz, D. M., and Muller, J. (1983). Cytomegalovirus encephalitis in acquired immunodeficiency syndrome. *J. Clin. Pathol.* *80*:874-877.

45. Vital, C., Vital, A., Vignoly, B., Dupon, M., Lacut, J. Y., Gbikpi-Benissan, G., and Cardinaud, J. P. (1985). Cytomegalovirus encephalitis in a patient with acquired immunodeficiency syndrome. *Arch. Pathol. Lab. Med.* *109*:105-106.

46. Edwards, R. H., Messing, R., and McKendall, R. R. (1985). Cytomegalovirus meningoencephalitis in a homosexual man with Kaposi's sarcoma: Isolation of CMV from CSF cells. *Neurology* *35*:560-561.

47. Post, M. J. D., Hensley, G. T., Moskowitz, L. B., and Fischl, M. (1986). Cytomegalic inclusion virus encephalitis in patients with AIDS: CT, clinical and pathologic correlation. *Am. J. Neurol. Radiol.* *7*:275-280.

48. Cole, E. L., Meisler, D. M., Calabrese, L. H., Holland, G. N., Mondino, B. J., and Conant, M. A. (1984). Herpes zoster ophthalmicus and acquired immune deficiency syndrome. *Arch. Ophthalmol.* *102*:1027-1029.

49. Ryder, J. W., Croen, K., Kleinschmidt-DeMasters, B. K., Ostrove, J. M., Straus, S. E., and Cohn, D. L. (1986). Progressive encephalitis three months after resolution of cutaneous zoster in a patient with AIDS. *Ann. Neurol.* *19*:182-188.

50. West, T. E., Papsian, C. J., Park, B. H., and Parker, S. W. (1985). Adenovirus type-2 encephalitis and concurrent Epstein-Barr virus infection in an adult man. *Arch. Neurol.* *42*:815-817.

51. Rutsaert, J., Melot, C., Ectors, M., Cornil, A., De Prez, C., and Flament-Durand, J. (1980). Complications infectieuses pulmonaires et neurologiques d'un sarcome de Kaposi. *Ann. Anat. Pathol.* (*Paris*) *25*:125-138.

52. Chan, J. C., Moskowitz, L. B., Olivella, J., Hensley, G. T., Greenman, R. L., and Hoffman, T. A. (1983). Toxoplasma encephalitis in recent Haitian entrants. *South. Med. J.* *76*:1211-1215.

53. Handler, M., Ho, K. V., Whelan, M., and Budzilovich, G. (1983). Intracerebral toxoplasmosis in patients with acquired immune deficiency syndrome. *J. Neurosurg.* *59*:994-1001.
54. Post, J. D., Hensley, G. T., Sheldon, J. J., Chan, J. C., Soila, K., Tobias, J., Quencer, R. M., and Moskowitz, L. B. (1984). CNS disease in AIDS: A CT-MR pathologic correlation. *Radiology 153*:55-56.
55. Luft, B. J., Conley, F., and Remington, J. S. (1983). Outbreak of central-nervous-system toxoplasmosis in Western Europe and North America. *Lancet 1*: 781-783.
56. Levy, R. M., Mills, C., Posin, J., Moore, S., Rosenblum, M., and Bredesen, D. (1986). The superiority of MR to CT in the detection of intracranial pathology in the acquired immunodeficiency syndrome (AIDS). Second International Conference on AIDS, Paris, France, 1986.
57. Levy, R. M., Pons, V. G., and Rosenblum, M. L. (1984). Central nervous system mass lesions in the acquired immunodeficiency syndrome (AIDS). *J. Neurosurg.* *61*:9-16.
58. Rodan, B. A., Cohen, F. L., and Bean, W. J. (1984). CT biopsy of cerebral toxoplasmosis in AIDS. *J. Fla. Med. Assoc.* *71*:158-160.
59. Chan, J. C., Hensley, G. T., and Moskowitz, L. B. (1984). Toxoplasmosis in the central nervous system. *Ann. Intern. Med.* *100*:615-616.
60. Wong, B., Gold, J. W. M., Brown, A. E., Lange, M., Gried, R., Grieco, M., Mildvan, D., Giron, J., Tapper, M. L., Lerner, C. W., and Armstrong, D. (1984). Central-nervous-system toxoplasmosis in homosexual men and parenteral drug abusers. *Ann. Intern. Med.* *100*:36-42.
61. Remington, J. S. and Desmonts, G. (1976). Toxoplasmosis. In *Infectious Disease of the Fetus and Newborn Infant.* (Remington, J. S. and Klein, J. O., eds.). Philadelphia, W.B. Saunders, pp. 191-332.
62. Sher, J. H. (1983). Cerebral toxoplasmosis. *Lancet 1*:1225.
63. Kovacs, J. A., Kovacs, A. A., Polis, M., Wright, W. C., Gill, V. J., Tuazon, C. U., Gelmann, E. P., Lane, H. C., Longfield, R., Overturf, G., Macher, A. M., Fauci, A. S., Parrillo, J. E., Bennett, J. E., and Masur, H. (1985). Cryptococcosis in the acquired immunodeficiency syndrome. *Ann. Intern. Med.* *103*:533-538.
64. Adams, R. D. and Victor, M. (1981). *Principles of Neurology*, 2nd ed. New York, McGraw-Hill, pp. 475-506.
65. Thompson, R. A. (1974). Clinical features of central nervous system fungus infection. In *Infectious Diseases of the Central Nervous System. Adv. Neurol. 6*: 93-100.
66. Armstrong, D., Gold, J. W. M., Dryjanski, J., Whimbey, E., Polsky, B., Hawkins, K. C., Brown, A. E., Bernard, E., and Kiehn, T. E. (1985). Treatment of infections in patients with the acquired immunodeficiency syndrome. *Ann. Intern. Med.* *103*:738-743.
67. Pitlik, S. D., Rios, L., Hersh, E. M., Bolivar, R., and Mansell, P. A. (1984). Polymicrobial brain abscess in a homosexual man with Kaposi's sarcoma. *South. Med. J.* *77*:271-272.

68. Wetli, C. V., Weiss, S. D., Cleary, T. J., and Gyori, E. (1984). Fungal cerebritis from intravenous drug abuse. *J. Forensic Sci. 29*:260-268.
69. Einstein, H. E. (1974). Coccidioidomycosis of the central nervous system. In *Infectious Diseases of the Central Nervous System. Adv. Neurol. 6*:101-105.
70. Zealer, D. S. and Winn, W. A. (1967). The neurosurgical approach in the treatment of coccidioidal meningitis. Report of 10 cases. In *Coccidioidomycosis.* (Allejo, L., ed.). Tuscon, University of Arizona Press, pp. 43-53.
71. Post, J. D., Jursunoglu, K. S. J., Hensley, G. T., Chan, J. C., Moskowitz, L. B., and Hoffman, T. A. (1985). Cranial CT in acquired immunodeficiency syndrome: Spectrum of diseases and optimal contrast enhancement technique. *Am. J. Neurol. Radiol. 145*:929-940.
72. Micozzi, M. S. and Wetli, C. V. (1985). Intravenous amphetamine abuse, primary cerebral mucormycosis and acquired immunodeficiency. *J. Forensic Sci. 30*:504-510.
73. Bishburg, E., Sunderam, G., Reichman, L. B., and Kapila, R. (1986). Central nervous system tuberculosis with the acquired immunodeficiency syndrome and its related complex. *Ann. Intern. Med. 105*:210-213.
74. Zakowski, P., Fligiel, S., Berlino, G. W., and Johnson, B. L. (1982). Disseminated *Mycobacterium avium-intracellulare* in homosexual men dying of acquired immunodeficiency syndrome. *JAMA 248*:2980-2982.
75. Hawkins, C., Gold, J. M., Whimberg, E. et al. (1986). *Mycobacterium avium* complex infections in patients with AIDS. *Ann. Intern. Med. 105*:184-188.
76. Sharer, L. R. and Kapila, R. (1985). Neuropathologic observations in acquired immunodeficiency syndrome (AIDS). *Acta Neuropathol. 66*:188-198.
77. Berger, J. R., Moskowitz, L., Fischl, M., and Kelley, R. E. (1984). The neurologic complicatioins of AIDS; frequently the initial manifestation. *Neurology 34*(supp. 1):134-135.
78. Berry, C. D., Hooton, T. M., Collier, A. C., Lukehart, S. A. (1987). Neurologic relapse after benzathine penicillin therapy for secondary syphilis in a patient with HIV infection. *N. Engl. J. Med. 316*:1587-1589.
79. Levy, R. M., Bredesen, D. E., and Rosenblum, M. L. (1988). Opportunistic central nervous system pathology in patients with AIDS. *Ann. Neurol. 23*(suppl): S7-S12.
80. Rosenblum, M. L., Levy, R. M., Bredesen, D. E., So, Y. T., Wara, W., and Ziegler, J. (1988). Primary central nervous system lymphomas in patients with AIDS. *Ann. Neurol. 23* (suppl):S13-S16.
81. Hollander, H., Golden, J., Mendelson, T., and Cortland, D. (1985). Extrapyramidal symptoms in AIDS patients given low-dose metaclopramide or chlorpromazine. *Lancet 2*:1186.
82. Bates, S., McKeever, P., Masur, H., Levens, D., Macher, A., Armstrong, G., and Magrath, I. T. (1985). Myelopathy following intrathecal chemotherapy in a patient with extensive Burkitt's lymphoma and altered immune status. *Am. J. Med. 78*:697-702.
83. Gold, J. W. M., Leyland-Jones, B., Urmacher, C., and Armstrong, D. (1984). Pulmonary and neurologic complications of treatment with FIAC (2'fluoro-5-

iodo-aracytosine) in patients with acquired immune deficiency syndrome (AIDS). *AIDS Res. 1*:243-252.

84. Fischl, M. A., Pitchenik, A. E., and Spira, T. J. (1985). Tuberculous brain abscess and toxoplasma encephalitis in a patient with the acquired immunodeficiency syndrome. *JAMA 253*:3428-3430.

85. So, Y. T., Holtzman, D., and Olney, R. (in preparation). Electrophysiological abnormalities of the peripheral nervous system in patients with AIDS.

86. Janssen, R. S., Saykin, A. J., Kaplan, J. E. et al. (1987). Neurologic complications of lymphadenopathy syndrome associated human immunodeficiency virus infection. *Neurology 37*(Suppl 1):344.

87. Bredesen, D. E. et al. (1987). Peripheral nervous system dysfunction in acquired immunodeficiency syndrome. In *AIDS and the Nervous System*. (Rosemblum, M. L., Levy, R. M., and Bredesen, D. E., eds.). New York, Raven Press, pp. 64-78.

88. Lipkin, W. I., Parry, G., Kiprov, D. D., and Abrams, D. (1985). Inflammatory neuropathy in homosexual men with lymphadenopathy. *Neurology 35*:1479-1483.

89. Miller, R. G., Parry, G., Lang, W. et al. (1985). AIDS-related inflammatory polyradiculoneurpathy: Prediction of response to plasma exchange with electrophysiologic testing. *Muscle Nerve 8*:626.

90. Mishra, B. B., Sommers, W., Koski, C. K., and Greenstein, J. I. (1985). Acute inflammatory demyelinating polyneuropathy in the acquired immune deficiency syndrome [Abstract]. *Ann. Neurol. 18*:131-132.

91. Cornblath, D. R., McArthur, J. C., Kennedy, P. G. E. et al. (1987). Inflammatory demyelinating peripheral neuropathies associated with HTLV-III infection. *Ann. Neurol. 21*:32-40.

92. Eidelberg, D., Sotrel, A., Vogel, H. et al. (1986). Progressive polyradiculopathy in acquired immune deficiency syndrome. *Neurology 36*:912-916.

93. Miller, R. G., Kiprov, D. D., Parry, G., Bredesen, D. E. (1988). Peripheral nervous system dysfunction in acquired immunodeficiency syndrome. In *AIDS and the Nervous System*. (Rosenblum, M. L., Levy, R. M., and Bredesen, D. E., eds.). New York, Raven Press, pp. 65-78.

94. Schmitt, F. A., Bigley, J. W., McKinnis, R., Logue, P. E., Evans, R. W., Drucker, J. L., and the AZT Collaborative Working Group. (1988). Neuropsychological outcome of zidovudine (AZT) treatment of patients with AIDS and AIDS-related complex. *N. Engl. J. Med. 319*:1573-1578.

95. Levy, R.M., Rosenbloom, S., and Perret, L. (1986). Neuroradiologic findings in the acquired immunodeficiency syndrome: A report of 200 cases. *Am. J. Radiol. 7*: 833-839.

7
Cutaneous Infections in Patients with Human Immunodeficiency Virus Infection

Clay J. Cockerell* and **Alvin E. Friedman-Kien**   *New York University Medical Center, New York, New York*

In many patients with human immunodeficiency virus (HIV) infection, cutaneous infections may be the first manifestation of immunodeficiency. The spectrum of dermatologic manifestations ranges from widespread fulminant mucocutaneous eruptions to very subtle localized skin lesions that often go unnoticed. Physicians must be familiar with the varied and unusual mucocutaneous infections that may occur in HIV-infected individuals. Quick recognition of the significance of the mucocutaneous manifestations of these opportunistic infections will permit early diagnosis and treatment. The HIV-infected patients may develop mucocutaneous infections caused by viruses, bacteria, fungi, or protozoa.

VIRAL INFECTIONS

Cytomegalovirus

Cytomegalovirus is a common pathogen in immunosuppressed patients. The most common manifestations of cytomegalovirus infection are predominantly systemic (see Chap. 11). However, the skin and mucosal surfaces may be involved. Thrombocytopenia is a common feature of cytomegalovirus

---

*Current affiliation: University of Texas Southwestern Medical Center, Dallas, Texas

infection, and petechiae and purpura may occur as well. A generalized morbilliform skin eruption involving the trunk and extremities is frequently associated with cytomegalovirus infection, whereas vesicular or bullous eruptions
are seen rarely (1). Hyperpigmented, indurated cutaneous plaques have been
reported occasionally as heralding disseminated cytomegalovirus infection
(2). One case of a generalized bullous toxic epidermal necrolysislike eruption in association with cytomegalovirus hepatitis in a patient with acquired
immunodeficiency syndrome (AIDS) has been reported (3). Persistent, severe perianal cytomegalovirus ulcerations that resemble those seen with anogenital herpes simplex infection have been reported in patients with AIDS
(4). Unlike herpes simplex infections, the perianal ulcers caused by cytomegalovirus do not respond to full doses of intravenous or oral acyclovir. In our
experience, these persistent perianal ulcers are associated with intractable
cytomegalovirus proctocolitis, and they are likely to represent contiguous
spread of gastrointestinal infection to the skin. Because it is not possible to
distinguish herpes simplex virus from cytomegalovirus in other agents by
clinical examination, virus culture, perhaps coupled with pathologic examination of biopsy specimens, is essential to confirm the etiology of persistent
perianal ulcerations in the AIDS patient. In some patients with ulcerative lesions of the mouth, anus, or around the nose, cytomegalovirus infection
may coexist with herpes simplex virus or with mycobacteria (6). Treatment
with the investigational nucleoside analogue, ganciclovir, may produce at
least temporary healing. Further details of treatment of cytomegalovirus
infections are provided in Chapter 11.

Varicella-Zoster

Zoster, also known as "shingles," results from reactivation of latent varicella-zoster virus infection in the trigeminal or dorsal root ganglia of patients
with previous varicella (chickenpox) infection. It is usually manifested by
the sudden occurrence of painful clusters of vesicles or an erythematous base
("dew drops on a rose petal"), in a localized neurodermatomal distribution.
Pain may precede the eruption by a few days, occasionally creating a diagnostic dilemma. In HIV-infected patients, initially well-localized infection
may spread to involve contiguous dermatomes, or it may become generalized with widely disseminated vesicles appearing at sites distant from the
original dermatome. In some cases of widely disseminated zoster, life-threatening systemic infection occurs with viremia and involvement of the central
nervous system, lungs, and other viscera. In addition, zoster infections in
HIV-infected patients tend to be severe and leave disfiguring residual scars
more often than is usually found in other patients; however, the prevalence
of residual postzoster neuralgia does not appear to be higher in AIDS pa-

tients, despite the greater frequency and severity of the acute zoster infection seen in these individuals. In a few HIV-infected patients, recurrent episodes of zoster have been observed. The occurrence of zoster in a patient from a risk group for developing AIDS should alert the physician to the possibility of other AIDS-related diseases (7). For details of diagnosis and treatment of zoster, see Chapter 10.

Herpes Simplex

Patients with HIV-infection, as well as those with other disorders of immunodeficiency, may have recurrent severe mucocutaneous herpes simplex virus infections. These infections are characterized by large, ulcerative lesions, often with satellite lesions, that run a protracted course. Untreated, localized anogenital herpetic eruptions, frequently observed especially in the HIV-infected immunocompromised host, may last for several weeks to months. These may result in extensive and painful perianal ulcerations that tend to coalesce. On occasion, these ulcers may become superinfected with bacteria or yeasts.

Treatment with acyclovir (oral or intravenous) will usually result in slow clearing of the herpetic lesions, but as they often recur when therapy is stopped, chronic suppressive therapy is frequently required. Occasional patients may develop acyclovir-resistant herpes simplex, which will not respond to acyclovir (Erlich et al., NEJM in press, 1989). Rarely a localized herpes simplex infection may become disseminated in patients with AIDS; then, the skin may be widely studded with discrete individual vesicular or ulcerated lesions as well as clusters of erythematous papules, vesicles, and ulcers. Such patients usually have high fevers and may develop visceral organ involvement and meningitis requiring hospitalization.

Patients with chronic, persistent perianal ulcers often require analgesics, stool softeners, and special hygienic attention to maintain the cleanliness of the infected area. These severe herpetic infections are best treated with large doses of intravenous acyclovir for 7 to 14 days. In patients with frequent recurrences of mucocutaneous herpes simplex infections, long-term prophylaxis with oral acyclovir (200 mg three times a day, or 400 mg twice a day) may be beneficial to lessen the frequency of recurrent outbreaks. Our experience is that many patients require this.

Molluscum Contagiosum

Molluscum contagiosum is a common viral infection of the skin caused by a poorly characterized human poxvirus. The infection is spread by close or intimate contact and by autoinoculation to distant areas of the skin of infected individuals. The eruptions resulting from molluscum contagiosum are characterized by multiple pearly, waxy papular lesions, 1 to 4 mm in diameter, which often have a central crusted umbilication [(Fig. 1) see Plate I, facing page 150]. In HIV-infected individuals the lesions of molluscum contagiosum are often more widely disseminated, more numerous, and usually larger than those seen in healthy patients. The large lesions, sometimes referred to as "giant" mollusca, can reach 1 cm in diameter. Molluscum lesions may be confused with basal cell carcinomas or keratoacanthomas.

In normal subjects, the lesions of molluscum contagiosum usually respond well to simple curettage or cryosurgery; however, the lesions found in AIDS patients are often refractory to standard treatment. Nevertheless, the usual methods of treatment are employed, but they may have to be repeated on multiple occasions.

Human Papillomavirus

Warts are a chronic, proliferative cutaneous infection caused by the human papillomavirus. They are spread by intimate contact. Extensive eruption of many types of warts, including flat warts, verrucae vulgares, condylomata acuminata [(Fig. 2) see Plate I, facing page 150], and plantar warts, are seen in HIV-infected patients. The sudden occurrence of disseminated warts in an individual in an AIDS risk group should alert the physician to look for possible HIV infection. Warts in HIV-infected patients tend to occur in the same areas as in healthy adults, but are found in greater numbers and are often considerably larger; they are also more resistant to conventional therapeutic modalities (F. Judson, personal communication). Clinically, the warts may be of several different morphologic varieities, including extensive flat or plane warts and filiform-shaped that are frequently found in the bearded area of the face and exuberant, often cauliflowerlike tumors of condylomata accuminata, especially involving the anogenital region. Multiple and often large hyperkeratotic common warts are most often seen on the hands, especially around the periungual regions. Multiple, sometimes large mosaic clusters of plantar warts have been observed in these immunosuppressed patients as well. Treatment usually consists of application of 40% salicylic acid plasters and paring of the lesions, but in this immunocompromised population, response to therapy is even less gratifying than in the immunocompetent. There are no data concerning the specific subtype of human papillomavirus that is associated with warts in these patients.

BACTERIAL INFECTIONS

Abcesses, Furunculosis, Impetigo, and Folliculitis

Infections caused by common bacterial pathogens, such as staphylococci, as well as those caused by more virulent bacteria, can cause localized, widely disseminated, and sometimes systemic life-threatening illnesses in HIV-infected patients. Bacterial folliculitis in the AIDS patient may present with acneiform eruptions consisting of erythematous papules and pustules widely distributed over the trunk, extremities, and the face. Bacterial cultures of such lesions have been found to not only grow "diphtheroids," but *Staphylococcus aureus* and *Streptoccocus pneumoniae* as well. In some cases, gram-negative organisms such as *Proteus* species have been isolated from these lesions. Like many of the other infectious diseases encountered in the patient with AIDS, folliculitis is often refractory to the standard doses of usual antibiotic therapy in the HIV-infected individual.

Folliculitis may progress to form localized abscesses, furuncles, and even multiloculated carbuncles. Occasionally, cellulitis may supervene. Whereas such skin infections in an immunocompetent individual might be managed as an outpatient with oral antibiotic therapy, such as erythromycin, dicloxacillin, or cephalosporin, the patient with AIDS may require hospitalization for intravenous treatment with penicillinase-resistant penicillin or cephalosporins, because the risk of systemic spread of the infection is much greater if the condition becomes more severe.

Clinically, one may not be able to distinguish pyogenic infection caused by *S. aureus* from one caused by a mycobacterium, candida, or unusual fungi. Delays in accurate diagnosis can be detrimental for the patient; hence, warn the clinical microbiology laboratory that unusual pathogens may be recovered.

A peculiar generalized acneiform, follicular, and papular eruption often associated with severe pruritus that clinically resembles urticarial papules surrounding a central pustule has been seen with increasing frequency among HIV-infected individuals. Interestingly, biopsy specimens of these pustular lesions are histologically distinguished by having numerous eosinophils within the infundubula of hair follicles (8). The nature and significance of this unique eruption in the HIV-infected, immunosuppressed patient is not yet understood. The symptoms of this rash respond to topical acne medications, with antihistamines to control the hivelike pruritic component; more recently, therapy with ultraviolet treatment has been shown to relieve pruritus and cause partial resolution of the process (9).

Impetigo is frequently seen among HIV-infected patients. This cutaneous infection is most often caused by group A streptococci [(Fig. 3) see Plate I, facing page 150] or *S. aureus*. Impetigo in children is seen predominantly on the face; however, in HIV-infected individuals, impetigo is seen more often in the axillary, inguinal, and other intertriginous areas. The infection usually begins with the development of multiple painful red macules and papules that rapidly develop into a blistering eruption with multiple superficial clusters of small vesicles and large flaccid bullae. These easily rupture, resulting in large shallow ulcerations that ooze serous or purulent fluid, forming characteristic honey-colored crusts overlying the erosions. In the untreated patient, satellite and distant vesicular and bullous skin lesions often continue to develop. Usually, impetigo responds most readily to systemic, oral antibiotic treatment such as penicillin or cephalosporin. However, in the patient with AIDS, the therapeutic responses may be delayed and high doses of medication, such as cephalexin (Keflex) 2 g/day, for longer periods may be required to resolve the infection.

In HIV-infected patients, cutaneous herpes simplex infections commonly become superinfected, resembling impetigo, and complicating diagnosis and treatment.

Mycobacteria

Patients with AIDS who have systemic mycobacterial infections (usually *Mycobacterium tuberculosis* or *M. avium* complex) may rarely develop cutaneous lesions. These lesions appear as small dome-shaped reddish papules and pustules that resemble folliculitis [(Fig. 4) see Plate I, facing page 150 (10)]. A diagnosis of mycobacterial infection can be rapidly made by microscopic examination of smears of the purulent fluid, or histologic examination of biopsy tissue sections stained for acid-fast bacilli. A microscopic diagnosis should always be confirmed by laboratory culture. These laboratory studies should be performed on any patient with AIDS who has developed unusual and suspicious cutaneous lesions. Reactivation of long-standing quiescent or latent *M. tuberculosis* is not uncommon in an individual who becomes immunodeficient. Of four AIDS patients (all intravenous drug users), seen at NYU Medical Center with disseminated mycobacterial infection with cutaneous involvement, three had *M. tuberculosis* and one had *M. avium* complex. All patients with pustular lesions of the skin were believed to be secondary to a disseminated spread of infection from a reactivated preexisting pulmonary foci of tubercular infection.

FUNGAL INFECTIONS

Superficial Fungal Infections

Many species of common superficial fungi may cause severe local and generalized cutaneous and, occasionally, systemic infections in the HIV-infected patient. Such infections may fail to respond to topical or systemic antifungal agents. Widespread dermatophytosis, especially that caused by *Trichophyton rubrum*, involving the palms, soles, nails, and intertriginous areas have been observed as an early sign of immunodeficiency in some HIV-infected individuals. In some patients, even systemic treatment with griseofulvin (500 mg p.o. b.i.d.) or ketoconazole (200 mg b.i.d.) in combination with topical antifungal medications such as econazole cream has not eradicated these severe and generalized fungal infections.

Candida albicans infection involving the oral mucosa (thrush), is one of the recognized early signs of immunodeficiency in HIV-infected patients; it occasionally progresses to cause esophagitis (see Chap. 8). *Candida albicans* may also infect the nails and surrounding tissue, resulting in hyperkeratosis and nail deformity, as well as an inflammatory paronychial infection that is often observed in HIV-infected individuals. Treatment consists of trimming the nails and application of topical antifungal solutions and creams such as clotrimazole. Ketoconazole, 200 mg p.o. b.i.d., may eventually be required.

Cryptococcus neoformans

Cutaneous lesions of systemic cryptococcal infection are rare. They appear as single or multiple disseminated pink to purple, indurated plaques and nodular lesions of the skin, varying in size from a few millimeters to a centimeter in diameter. Superficial erosion and crusting of cryptococcal lesions may be found. The cutaneous eruptions of cryptococcosis in AIDS patients may present as widespread, dome-shaped, and sometimes slightly umbilicated papules that may bear a striking resemblance to the benign, often disseminated lesions of molluscum contagiosum (11). Biopsy with microscopic examination and fungal culture will make the diagnosis. Occasionally, the AIDS patient may have simultaneous infections with both fungi and the molluscum contagiosum virus, which may cause confusion and delay the exact diagnosis because the individual skin lesions may be clinically indistinguishable. Cryptococcal skin lesions are found only in the setting of disseminated cryptococcal infection, and they respond to systemic antifungal chemotherapy (see Chap. 15).

Histoplasma capsulatum

Cutaneous eruptions are rare in disseminated histoplasmosis, even in patients with AIDS. Patients with early cutaneous lesions of histoplasmosis may not be acutely ill or have any evidence of systemic infection. The localized widespread skin lesions of histoplasmosis may mimic scattered reddish acneiform papules [(Fig. 5) see Plate II, after page 150 (12,13)]. Cutaneous histoplasmosis can be diagnosed with certainty by histopathologic examination and culture of biopsy specimens (see Chap. 16). In AIDS patients, histoplasmosis is most frequently due to reactivation of a prior infection; patients are often not aware of the prior infection, because histoplasmosis occurring in healthy individuals is often a mild subclinical pulmonary infection that is usually undiagnosed.

REFERENCES

1. Linn, C. S., Pinha, P. D., Krishnan, M. N. et al. (1981). Cytomegalic inclusion disease of the skin. *Arch. Dermatol. 117*:282.

2. Feldman, P. S., Walker, A. N., and Baker, R. (1982). Cutaneous lesions herald-ing disseminated cytomegalovirus infection. *J. Am. Acad. Dermatol.* 7:545.
3. Muehler-Stamou, A., Sen, H. J., and Emodi, G. (1974). Epidermolysis in a case of severe cytomegalovirus infection. *Br. Med. J.* 3:609.
4. Minars, N., Silverman, J. F., Escobar, N. R. et al. (1977). Fatal cytomegalic in-clusion disease: Associated skin manifestations in a renal transplant patient. *Arch. Dermatol.* 113:1569.
5. Chachoua, A., Dieterich, D., Krasinski, K., Greene, J., Laubenstein, L., Wernz, J., Buhles, W., and Koretz, S. (1987). 9-(1,3-dihydroxy-2-propoxymethyl) gua-nine (ganciclovir) in the treatment of cytomegalovirus gastrointestinal disease with the acquired immunodeficiency syndrome. *Ann. Intern. Med.* 107:133-136.
6. Kwan, T. H. and Kaufman, H. W. (1986). Acid fact bacilli with cytomegalo-virus and herpes virus inclusions in the skin of an AIDS patient. *Am. J. Clin. Pathol.* 85:236.
7. Friedman-Kien, A. E., LaFleur, F. L., Gendler, E. C., Hennessey, N. P. et al. (1986). Herpes zoster: A possible early clinical sign for development of acquired immunodeficiency syndrome in high risk individuals. *J. Am. Acad. Dermatol.* 14:1023.
8. Soeprono, F. F. and Schinella, R. A. (1986). Eosinophilic pustular folliculitis in patients with acquired immunodeficiency syndrome. *J. Am. Acad. Dermatol.* 14:1020.
10. Brown, F. S., Anderson, R. H., and Burnett, J. W. (1982). Cutaneous tubercu-losis. *J. Am. Acad. Dermatol.* 6:101.
11. Klein, R. S., Harris, C. A., Small, C. B. et al. (1984). Oral candidiadis in high risk patients as the initial manifestation of the acquired immunodeficiency syn-drome. *N. Engl. J. Med.* 311:354.
12. Rico, N. J. and Penneys, N. S. (1985). Cutaneous cryptococcosis resembling molluscum contagiosum in a patient with AIDS. *Arch. Dermatol.* 121:901.
13. Hazelhurst, J. A. and Vismer, H. F. (1985). Histoplasmosis presenting with un-usual skin lesions in acquired immunodeficiency syndrome (AIDS). *Br. J. Der-matol.* 113:345.

8
Oral Manifestations of Human Immunodeficiency Virus Infection

Deborah Greenspan and John S. Greenspan *University of California, San Francisco, California*

Oral manifestations of the acquired immunodeficiency syndrome (AIDS) and AIDS-related complex (ARC) were described in the very first reports of these syndromes. There is growing evidence that several otherwise relatively innocuous oral opportunistic infections, occurring in human immunodeficiency virus (HIV)-infected patients are indicators of marked immunosuppression and may predict the ultimate development of AIDS. The mouth has long been recognized as the site of residence of an extremely varied and complex microbial flora with marked potential to probe the host defenses and produce disease when those defenses are in the least compromised. Examples include the frequent and troublesome expressions of fungal, bacterial, and viral infection in patients with primary immunodeficiency, immunosuppressed graft recipients, and patients receiving immunosuppressive chemotherapy for malignancy (1). The prevalence and incidence of oral lesions seen in association with the AIDS epidemic has again drawn attention to the importance of this group of diseases (2-5).

Oral examination is an important part of any physical examination, and nowhere is this more important than in suspected HIV infection. All mucosal surfaces should be assessed using a mouth mirror, examination gloves, gauze squares for tongue extension and, of course, an adequate light source, which can be provided by a penlight held by an assistant if a better light source is not available. Any oral lesion should be subjected to further investigation with techniques such as smears, cultures, and a biopsy.

FUNGAL AND BACTERIAL LESIONS

Oral candidiasis was included in the first descriptions of AIDS and has been reported as occurring in about 75% of both ARC and AIDS patients (6). In one study, as many as 59% of the people in the high-risk groups with oral candidiasis developed AIDS (7). A study of 10 patients with AIDS and oral candidiasis, by Tavitian and co-workers, showed that all of the patients also had esophageal candidiasis (8). This has not been confirmed by others. Oral candidiasis in association with HIV infection may be predictive of the subsequent development of AIDS (9). However, many of the early studies of oral candidiasis in AIDS patients probably included undiagnosed cases of hairy leukoplakia. *Candida albicans* is frequently part of the normal oral flora and is the species most frequently found in oral candidal infections (10). Other species are sometimes found but produce similar-appearing oral lesions. Oral candidiasis associated with HIV infection may have several different appearances. These include pseudomembranous candidiasis, atrophic candidiasis, and angular cheilitis. Pseudomembranous candidiasis, sometimes called thrush, is characterized by the presence of creamy plaques on the oral mucosa [(Fig. 1) see Plate II, after page 150]. These white plaques can be removed, often revealing a bleeding surface. The atrophic form of candidiasis appears as a red lesion that may be found on the hard and soft palate and dorsal surface of the tongue [(Fig. 2) see Plate II, after page 150]. When candidiasis affects the dorsal surface of the tongue, patchy depapillated areas appear. Angular cheilitis may appear as cracking, fissuring, ulceration, or erythema at the corner of the mouth and may be seen either alone or in conjunction with the intraoral lesions. The prevalence of oral candidiasis in HIV infection is high, but exact numbers are not yet available. The relative frequency of the three types is also unknown. In association with HIV infection, oral candidiasis may persist for months if untreated. The diagnosis of oral candidiasis may be made from smears that are examined by potassium hydroxide suspension or by Gram stain showing hyphae and blastospores. Culture of the organism is unnecessary unless speciation is desired.

Little is known of the pathogenesis of HIV-associated oral candidiasis. Treatment involves the use of systemic or topical antifungal drugs. Topical therapy should be tried first and systemic therapy reserved for treatment failures. Ketoconazole (Nizoral) is a systemic antifungal imidazole, which is effective in the dose of one or two 200 mg tablets taken once daily with food. Oral topical medications include clotrimazole (Mycelex) oral troche 10 mg tablets, one tablet dissolved slowly in the mouth five times a day, nystatin vaginal tablets, 100,000 units, one tablet dissolved slowly in the mouth three times a day, or nystatin oral pastilles 200,000 units, one or two tablets dissolved in the mouth five times a day. The flavor and texture of the topical medications vary and patient preference should be considered when prescribing. A nystatin-triamcinolone (Mycolog) cream or other topical antifungal agents, such as clotrimazole or Ketoconazole creams, may be a useful adjunct in the treatment of angular cheilitis.

A number of other opportunistic infections have been found that cause oral lesions in HIV-infected individuals. They include infections with *Mycobacterium avium-intracellulare* complex and *Histoplasma* (11,12). These have been isolated case reports and no information is currently available on their prevalence.

VIRUS-ASSOCIATED LESIONS

Several viruses may reactivate, producing lesions in the mouth. These include the herpes group viruses and papillomaviruses. Human papillomaviruses (HPV) cause warts, including oral papillomas, condylomata, and focal epithelial hyperplasia (13). In particular, papillomavirus types 6, 11, 16, and 18 are associated with lesions of the mucous membrane and skin of the anogenital region, some of which have a high propensity to become malignant. Focal epithelial hyperplasia is associated with HPV type 13, which is uniquely associated with the oral mucosa. Papillomavirus types 2 and 4 have been identified in oral warts, and HPV 2 has been recently associated with carcinoma of the tongue. Immunosuppressed individuals show an increased tendency to develop skin warts, whereas anogenital warts occur as a sexually transmitted disease in male homosexuals and in heterosexual individuals of both sexes (14). Many cases of oral warts of varying clinical appearance have been seen in HIV-infected individuals [(Fig. 3) see Plate III, after page 150]. Some warts have a raised cauliflowerlike appearance, whereas others are well circumscribed, have a flat surface, and almost disappear when the mucosa is stretched. Some of the flat warts may be confused with small fibromas, and the diagnosis is made from a biopsy and histopathologic examination. The histologic appearance may show multiple fingerlike projections covered by hyperkeratotic epithelium with a prominent granular layer, or blunt projections covered by parakeratotic epithelium or solitary areas of focal acanthosis (focal epithelial hyperplasia). Some koilocytosis may be seen. Identification of the virus type is performed either by Southern blot analysis or by in situ hybridization. Surprisingly, both new and unusual types of papillomaviruses have been found in oral warts from HIV-infected individuals, including HPV types 7, 13, and a recently described new type, HPV 32 (Greenspan, D. et al., in press). The warts can be quite troublesome, with multiple lesions occurring throughout the oral cavity, and they frequently recur after surgical removal, whether laser, cryosurgery, or knife is used.

Herpes simplex can frequently produce recurrent painful episodes of ulceration, intraorally and circumorally. Lesions most commonly occur on the vermilion border, and occasionally the adjoining facial skin may be involved. Intraorally, lesions may appear on the palate or the gingival margin. The patient may report small vesicles, which erupt to form ulcers. Diagnosis can be made by virus culture, by cytologic smears showing characteristic viral giant cells (Tzanck preparation), or by detection of viral antigens using monoclonal antibodies. Intraoral ulceration can be a difficult diagnostic problem in patients with HIV infection. Recurrent herpes simplex produces vesicles and ulcers that occur on the keratinized mucosa, such as the hard palate or the attached gingiva. The ulcers usually heal within 10 days, but in association with HIV infection, resolution of the lesions may take longer. In some cases of delayed healing, oral acyclovir (200 mg orally five times a day) may be useful.

Herpes zoster caused by varicella-zoster virus, another member of the herpes group, can cause oral ulceration and pain. The prodomal symptoms may mimic dental pain. The vesicles and ulcers may occur intraorally, before the appearance of skin lesions. All mucosal surfaces may be involved, including the vermillion border. The lesions, however, are always unilateral. Treatment of herpes zoster requires higher doses of acyclovir, up to 800 mg five times daily to be effective.

Cytomegalovirus has been described in association with oral ulcers in a single case report (15).

Chapter 11 contains more detail.

Oral hairy leukoplakia (HL) is a white lesion of the oral mucosa, which is found predominantly on the lateral margins of the tongue. The condition was first seen in San Francisco in 1981 in a group of homosexual men (16). Over 300 cases have now been observed in San Francisco, and HL has been seen in different parts of the United States and in many areas of the world including Europe, South America, and Africa (17).

Oral hairy leukoplakia appears on the lateral margin of the tongue, either bilaterally or unilaterally and sometimes on the buccal or labial mucosa and floor of the mouth, palate, and oropharynx. It has been seen in these locations without coexistent tongue lesions in only a few cases. Hairy leukoplakia is white and does not rub off [(Fig. 4) see Plate III, after page 150]. The surface may be smooth, corrugated, or markedly prolific with projections giving a "hairy" appearance. The corrugations tend to run vertically along the lateral margin of the tongue. Hairy leukoplakia may extend onto the ventral surface of the tongue, where it may appear flat, and also onto the dorsal surface of the tongue, where it appears "hairy" [(Fig. 5) see Plate III, after page 150]. Microscopically, there are characteristic appearances with folds or "hairs," hyperparakeratosis, acanthosis, vacuolation of prickle cells, and little if any subepithelial inflammation (Fig. 6).

Hairy leukoplakia is probably a virally induced lesion. Immunocytochemical data support the presence of papillomavirus antigen in HL lesions (16) although human papillomavirus (HPV) DNA has not been identified by Southern blot or in situ hybridization (Greenspan, J. S., et al., unpublished observations). Ultrastructural findings are conflicting, with one study describing the "papillomavirus-like particles" (18) and two other studies not showing them (19,20).

Epstein-Barr virus (EBV) is readily demonstrated in HL (Fig. 7). Anticomplement immunofluorescence with human reference sera containing antibodies to the EBV capsid antigen, produced distinctive nuclear staining,

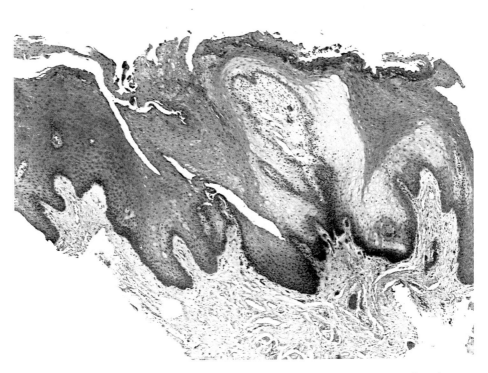

FIGURE 6 Histology of HL showing hyperkeratosis, acanthosis, and "ballooning cells."

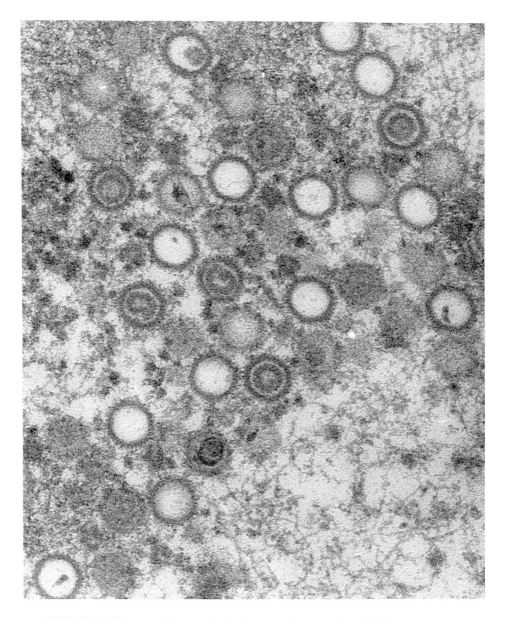

FIGURE 7   Electron micrograph showing Epstein-Barr virus in HL.

whereas Southern blot hybridization with probes for EBV, revealed the presence of the entire EBV genome (18). Intraepithelial Langerhans cells are reduced or absent in the HL lesion, and this decrease correlates with the presence of viral antigens (21). Virtually all patients with hairy leukoplakia are infected with HIV. Patients with HL have a similar clinical and laboratory profile to those with asymptomatic HIV infection and ARC. However, a recent study showed that patients with HL have a high risk of progression to AIDS. Forty-three of 143 patients with HL developed AIDS after a mean follow-up of 16 months (range 1 to 31 months). Seventy-four percent of the patients with HL developed *Pneumocystis carinii* pneumonia as their first manifestation of AIDS, as opposed to 55% in the general San Francisco AIDS population (22).

Originally, HL was reported only in the mouths of homosexual men. Recently, HL has been described in other risk groups (23,24). The lesion is usually asymptomatic, and treatment may not be indicated. However, patients with HL are often concerned about the appearance of the lesion, and also there may be soreness associated with coexisting candidal infection. Eliminating candida with antifungal therapy may reduce the symptoms, but no drug is known to eliminate the lesion permanently. Friedman-Kien noted that HL disappeared in patients who received high-dose acyclovir for herpes zoster (25). Resnick et al., have shown a similar effect (26). Preliminary trials with the experimental drug desciclovir, an analogue given orally that produces blood levels equivalent to intravenous acyclovir, showed temporary elimination or almost complete resolution in the clinical extent of the lesion. However, the lesions recurred from 1 to 4 months after desciclovir was stopped (27).

Hairy leukoplakia is a remarkable lesion because it is unique to HIV-infected people, having never been seen before the AIDS epidemic. It is a significant clinical marker of HIV infection, and may be one of the early changes associated with infection.

OTHER LESIONS

Recurrent aphthous ulcers (RAU) are a common oral lesion. The cause of RAU is unknown but hormonal factors, food allergy, stress, and viral factors have been implicated. A role for cellular immune dysfunction in the pathogenesis has been suggested (28). Preliminary reports suggest that there may be a recurrence of RAU in association with HIV infection. These lesions may occur in people with a history of RAU and also in those who have never had episodes of oral ulceration. The ulcers occur on the nonkeratinized mucosa and are usually painful. The lesions usually have the typical appearance of RAU, appearing as well-circumscribed ulcers with an erythematous margin. Sometimes, the ulcers persist and may become large with irregular margins and are locally quite destructive. These ulcers are usually of acute onset and heal in the course of 10 days to 2 weeks. Sometimes RAU, particularly of the major type, may persist for a month or longer. In association with HIV infection, the ulcers may last for long periods, and outbreaks may occur frequently. Some patients complain that they are never without an ulcer. Perhaps the local and systemic host defects in HIV infection are the cause of RAU in this group of patients. Diagnosis may be made from the clinical appearance, but in persistent lesions, a biopsy should be performed to rule out other causes. Differential diagnosis of RAU should include squamous cell carcinoma, trauma, vesiculoerosive disease, HSV, and syphilis. Treatment may include analgesics, such as viscous lidocaine (Xylocaine) used as an oral rinse and topical steroids, such as fluocinonide (Lidex) ointment mixed with 50% Orobase, applied topically several times daily.

Salivary gland enlargement has been reported in some HIV-infected adult and pediatric patients (29). The etiology is unknown and both parotid and submandibular gland involvement has been seen. Histologic examination of minor labial salivary glands reveal changes similar to those seen in Sjögren's syndrome (Greenspan, J. S. et al., unpublished observation). The ensuing changes of salivary function with reduced flow rates can be a significant problem, leading to increased dental caries. Symptomatic relief can sometimes be obtained with the use of salivary stimulants such as sugarless mints. Oral care should include the use of daily fluoride rinsing.

GINGIVITIS AND PERIODONTAL DISEASE

Even in health, the gingival crevice contains a diverse microflora (30). Many HIV-infected individuals show a tendency to develop severe gingival inflammation and progressive destructive periodontal disease (31-33). The gingivitis resembles acute necrotizing ulcerative gingivitis (ANUG), but it is prolonged and severe. The gingiva appear bright red and swollen with ulcers at the tips of the interdental papillae. Pain is often severe and halitosis is common. The HIV-associated periodontitis presents a rapid and progressive destruction of the supporting tissues, periodontal ligament, and alveolar bone, with loosening of and even exfoliation of teeth [(Fig. 8) see Plate III, after this page]. Plaque cultures show that a mixed flora is present, which has yet to be studied in detail. The pathogenesis of these lesions is also poorly understood. In particular, no information is yet available on the relative contributions to tissue damage made by microbial products and by the host response to infection, notably polymorphonuclear cells, macrophages, lymphocytes, and humoral factors.

PLATE I

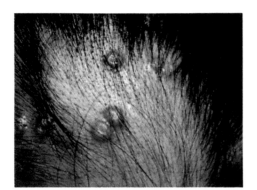

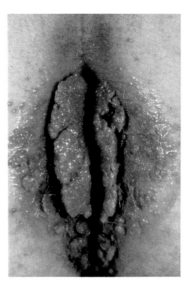

FIGURE 7.1 Molluscum contagiosum. Numerous large, waxy, umbilicated papules and nodules that have coalesced are characteristic of molluscum contagiosum infection in patients with AIDS. Treatment of such lesions may result in scarring.

FIGURE 7.2 Severe, exophytic perianal condyloma in a patient with AIDS.

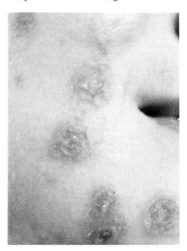

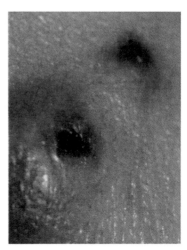

FIGURE 7.3 Severe impetigo, caused by group A streptococcus, in a patient with AIDS.

FIGURE 7.4 Papular cutaneous lesions secondary to *M. tuberculosis.* Nondescript cutaneous papules, sometimes ulcerated, may be caused by many infectious agents in patients with AIDS.

PLATE II

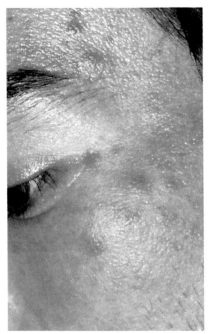

FIGURE 7.5 Papular skin lesions caused by *H. capsulatum*.

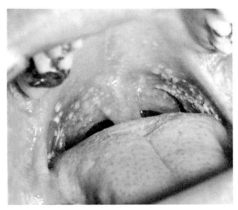

FIGURE 8.1 Pseudomembraneous candidiasis. Creamy white patches on erythematous mucosa.

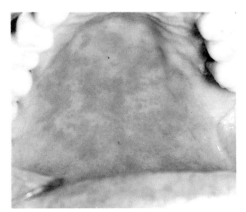

FIGURE 8.2 Atrophic candidiasis appearing as palatal erythema.

PLATE III

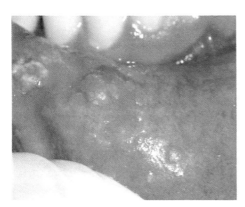

FIGURE 8.3. Wart on labial mucosa.

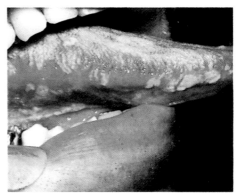

FIGURE 8.4 Hairy leukoplakia appearing as corrugations on the lateral margin of the tongue.

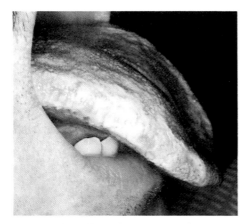

FIGURE 8.5 Extensive HL occurring on the dorsal surface of the tongue.

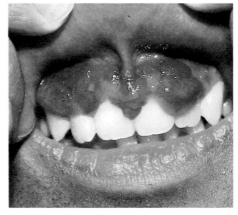

FIGURE 8.8 HIV-associated periodontal disease showing extensive destruction of the gingival tissue.

PLATE IV

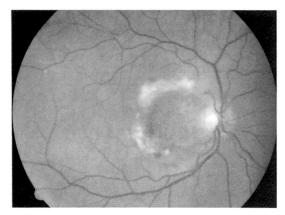

FIGURE 11.1   Typical appearance of cytomegalovirus retinitis. Fluffy, white retinal opacification is
associated with small hemorrhages. The lesions follow the distribution of the posterior vascular arcades
(courtesy Dr. James J. O'Donnell).

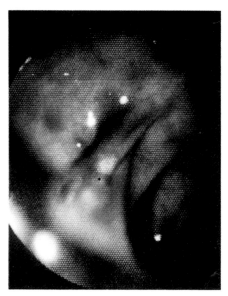

FIGURE 11.2   Typical appearance of cytomegalovirus colitis (courtesy of Dr. John
Cello).

REFERENCES

1. Greenspan, J. S. (1983). Infections and non-neoplastic diseases of the oral mucosa. *J. Oral. Pathol. 12*:139.
2. Greenspan, D. and Silverman, S., Jr. (1987). Oral lesions of HIV infection. *California Dent. Assoc. J. 15*:28.
3. Greenspan, D., Greenspan, J. S., Pindborg, J. J., and Schiodt, M. (1986). *AIDS and the Dental Team.* Copenhagen, Munksgaard.
4. Reichart, P. A., Pohle, D.-D., and Gelderblom, H. (1985). Oral manifestations of AIDS. *Dtsch. Z. Mund. Kiefererheilkd. Gesichtschir. 9*:167.
5. Reichart, P. A. et al. (1987). AIDS and the oral cavity. The HIV-infection: Virology, etiology, origin, immunology, precautions and clinical observations in 110 patients. *Int. J. Oral Maxillofac. Surg. 16*:129.
6. Pindborg, J. J. et al. (1986). Suggestion for a classification of oral candidiasis in patients with AIDS, ARC, and serum antibodies for LAV/HTLV-III. *J. Dent. Res. 65*:765.
7. Klein, R. S., Harris, C. A., Small, C. R. et al. (1984). Oral candidiasis in high-risk patients as the initial manifestation of the acquired immunodeficiency syndrome. *N. Engl. J. Med. 311*:354.
8. Tavitian, A., Raufman, J. P., and Rosenthal, L. E. (1986). Oral candidiasis as a marker for esophageal candidiasis in the acquired immunodeficiency syndrome. *Ann. Intern. Med. 104*:54.
9. Chandrasekar, P. H. and Molinari, J. A. (1985). Oral candidiasis: Forerunner of acquired immunodeficiency syndrome (AIDS). *Oral Surg. 60*:532.
10. Epstein, J. B., Truelove, E. L., and Izutzu, K. T. (1984). Oral candidiasis: Pathogenesis and host defense. *Rev. Infect. Dis. 6*:96.
11. Volpe, F., Schimmer, A., and Barr, C. (1985). Oral manifestations of disseminated *Mycobacterium avium intracellulare* in a patient with AIDS. *Oral Surg. 5*:567.
12. Fowler, C. B., Nelson, J. R., and Smith, B. R. (1986). A case of acquired immunodeficiency syndrome presented as a palatal perforation: Report of a case and review of the literature. Presented at 40th Meeting of American Association of Oral Pathology, Toronto, Canada.
13. Scully, C., Prime, S., and Maitland, N. (1985). Papillomaviruses: Their possible role in oral disease. *Oral Surg. 60*:166.
14. Owen, W. F. (1980). Sexually transmitted disease and traumatic problems in homosexual men. *Ann. Intern. Med. 92*:805.
15. Kanas, R. J., Jensen, J. L., Abrams, A. M. et al. (1987). Oral mucosal cytomegalovirus as a manifestation of the acquired immunodeficiency syndrome. *Oral Surg. 64*:153.
16. Greenspan, D., Greenspan, J. S., Conant, M. et al. (1984). Oral "hairy" leucoplakia in male homosexuals: Evidence of association with papillomaviruses and a herpes-group virus. *Lancet 2*:831.
17. Schiodt, M. and Pindborg, J. J. (1987). AIDS and the oral cavity. Epidemiology and clinical oral manifestations of human immune deficiency virus infection: A review. *Int. J. Oral Maxillofac. Surg. 16*:1.

18. Greenspan, J. S., Greenspan, D., Lennette, E. T. et al. (1985). Replication of Epstein-Barr virus within the epithelial cells of oral "hairy" leukoplakia, an AIDS-associated lesion. *N. Engl. J. Med. 313*:1564.

19. Belton, C. M. and Eversole, L. R. (1986). Oral "hairy" leukoplakia: Ultrastructural features. *J. Oral Pathol. 15*:493-439.

20. Kanas, R. J., Abrams, A. M., Jensen, J. L., Wuerker, R. B., and Handlers, J. P. (1988). Oral hairy leukoplakia: Ultrastructural observations. *Oral Surg. Oral Med. Oral Pathol. 65*:333-338.

21. Daniels, T. E., Greenspan, D., Greenspan, J. S. et al. (1987). Absence of Langerhans cells in oral hairy leukoplakia, an AIDS-associated lesion. *J. Invest. Dermatol. 89*:178.

22. Greenspan, D., Greenspan, J. S., Hearst, N. et al. (1987). Relation of oral hairy leukoplakia to infection with the human immunodeficiency virus and the risk of developing AIDS. *J. Infect. Dis. 155*:475.

23. Greenspan, D., Hollander, H., Friedman-Kien, A., Freese, U. K., and Greenspan, J. S. (1986). Oral hairy leukoplakia in two women, a haemophiliac and a transfusion recipient [Letter]. *Lancet 2*:978.

24. Greenspan, J. S., Mastrucci, M. T., Leggott, P. J. Freese, U. K., De Souza, Y. G., Scott, G. B., and Greenspan, D. (1988). Hairy leukoplakia in a child [Letter]. *AIDS 2*:143.

25. Friedman-Kien, A. E. (1986). Viral origin of hairy leukoplakia [Letter]. *Lancet 2*:694.

26. Resnick, L., Herbst, J. S., Ablashi, D. V., Atherton, S., Frank, B., Rosen, L., and Horwitz, S. N. (1988). Regression of oral hairy leukoplakia after orally administered acyclovir therapy. *JAMA 259*:384-388.

27. Greenspan, D., Greenspan, J. S., Chapman, S. et al. (1987). Efficacy of BWA515U in treatment of EBV infection in hairy leukoplakia [Abstract]. III International Conference of AIDS, Washington, D.C.

28. Greenspan, J. S., Gadol, N., Olson, J. A. et al. (1985). Lymphocyte function in recurrent aphthous ulceration. *J. Oral Pathol. 8*:592.

29. Ammann, A. J. (1985). The acquired immunodeficiency syndrome in infants and children. *Ann. Internal. Med. 103*:734.

30. Slots, J. (1979). Subgingival microflora and periodontal disease. *J. Clin. Periodontol. 6*:351.

31. Winkler, J. R. and Murray, P. A. (1987). Periodontal disease: A potential intraoral expression of AIDS may be rapidly progressive periodontitis. *Can. Dent. Assoc. J. 13*:20.

32. Winkler, J. R., Grassi, M., and Murray, P. A. (1987). Periodontal disease in HIV-infected male homosexuals [Abstract]. III International Conference on AIDS, Washington, D.C.

33. Murray, P. A., Grive, W. G., and Winkler, J. R. (1987). The humoral immune response in HIV-associated periodontitis [Abstract]. III International Conference on AIDS, Washington, D.C.

9
Pediatric Human Immunodeficiency Virus Infection

Peggy S. Weintrub   *University of California, San Francisco, California*

Gwendolyn B. Scott   *University of Miami School of Medicine, Miami, Florida*

EPIDEMIOLOGY

The number of pediatric patients with acquired immunodeficiency syndrome (AIDS) is currently doubling every year. The total reported cases in individuals under 13 years old was 292 by June 1986 and 512 by June 1987. These figures represent only a small fraction of the total number of symptomatic human immunodeficiency virus (HIV)-infected children, because their clinical findings do not fulfill the strict criteria for pediatric AIDS as defined by the Centers for Disease Control (CDC; 1). There are also an unknown number of asymptomatic seropositive children who are at risk for developing clinical disease.

Children can acquire HIV infection by several routes: (a) perinatally, from an infected mother; (b) from blood or blood products, including nonheat-treated factor VIII or IX concentrates; (c) sexual abuse or teenage sexual activity; or (d) intravenous drug use. At present, almost all of these HIV infections are perinatally transmitted, representing approximately 80% of the pediatric AIDS cases nationally. Blood transfusions or factor concentrates are responsible for 12% and 5% of the cases, respectively. In a small percentage of cases, the mode of transmission is either sexual, drug related, or undetermined because available histories are inadequate (2).

In the instances of perinatal transmission of HIV, the mother's risk factors or behaviors include intravenous drug abuse, blood transfusions, or women with sexual partners at risk (bisexual, drug abusing, transfused). Women from countries where heterosexual transmission is common are also at risk. Intravenous drug-abusing parents account for over 70% of the cases. Perinatal AIDS occurs more commonly in blacks (approximately 60% of cases) and Hispanics (25%) (2).

Most cases of pediatric AIDS have been reported from New York, New Jersey, and Florida. California has reported only small numbers of pediatric cases, relative to the large numbers of adult patients in the area (2). This is presumably related to the smaller numbers of intravenous drug abusers and the relatively lower prevalence of HIV infection among drug users (15-20%) on the West Coast.

Widespread use of HIV antibody assays for screening transfused blood and the new heat-treated factor concentrates will decrease the proportion of cases related to blood products. Unfortunately, however, with increasing heterosexual transmission and the high prevalence of infection in intravenous drug users, the number of infected women, and with this, the total number of infected children is expected to increase.

MATERNAL TRANSMISSION

Maternal infection is the most common source of infection in children, yet the risk and the exact route of transmission are not known. Estimates of the incidence of infection in infants of seropositive women range from 35% to 70% (3,4). In one study of women who had already delivered a child with AIDS or ARC, 12 subsequent pregnancies resulted in four clinically affected infants. This was reported before antibody testing was available and, hence, may underestimate the risk of transmission (4). Rubinstein noted an infection rate of approximately 35% in HIV seropositive primiparas, but a rate of 66% in women who already had one affected child (5). Larger numbers of HIV antibody-positive women need to be followed prospectively to accurately assess the risk of transmission to infants. The factors that determine which infants will become infected are not known; both maternal and fetal factors may play a role. Studies in twins have shown nonidentical twins who are both infected, as well as monozygotic twins who are discordant for HIV infection (6). Many women who have asymptomatic HIV infection during pregnancy deliver infected infants. Some mothers are unaware that they are infected with HIV until AIDS or ARC is diagnosed in an offspring. Scott et al. found that 15 of 16 mothers were asymptomatic at the time of delivery of their first HIV-infected infant (4). In addition, seropositive women frequently transmit infection to more than one infant. (This is not true of some congenital infections such as toxoplasmosis or cytomegalovirus, in which, with rare exceptions, only a primary infection during pregnancy leads to a symptomatic infection in the fetus.)

HIV infection may be transmitted from mother to infant in utero, intrapertum, or postnatally. Some data implicate intrauterine and postnatal transmission, but their relative contributions and the role of intrapartum transmission need further evaluation.

Cases of pediatric HIV infection from maternal-to-infant transmission frequently have symptoms within the first few months of life, although transfusion and sexually transmitted cases often have incubation periods of several years. The shorter incubation time in infants suggests that infection occurred in utero, affecting the immune system while it is relatively immature. More concrete evidence of intrauterine infection is the detection of HIV in abortus tissue of a 20-week fetus (7). Virus was grown from both lymphoid and brain tissue. It is not known how frequently virus can be found in the fetus or at what time during gestation HIV is most likely to cross the plancenta. The final piece of evidence suggesting in utero transmission is the embryopathy that has been described by Marion et al. (8). The features of this dysmorphic syndrome include microcephaly, growth failure, hypertelorism, a prominent boxlike forehead, a flattened nasal bridge, obliquity of the eyes, long palpebral fissures with blue sclera, a short nose with a flattened columella, a triangular philtrum, and patulous lips with a prominent vermillion border. The same authors have recently noted a correlation between the severity of the dysmorphism and the age at diagnosis of immunodeficiency. There is some controversy about the existence of this embryopathy because it has been seen only in a few centers involved in the care of children with AIDS.

It is not known if HIV can be transmitted during delivery. Infants have developed AIDS after both vaginal and cesarean deliveries, although intrauterine infection could not be excluded. The virus is present in blood as well as in cervical secretions, so infants could be exposed to HIV with either type of delivery (9). One retrospective report tested the infants of 12 seropositive women. Of the seven infants delivered vaginally, three were seropositive, and none of the five born by cesarean section were antibody-positive (10). Preliminary retrospective data from New York shows that cesarean delivery offers no protection from HIV infection (11). The retrospective nature of these studies, the small numbers investigated, and the limited information regarding these mother-infant pairs precludes drawing any conclusions at this time. Until more information is available, the mode of delivery of an antibody-positive woman should be determined by the usual obstetric criteria.

Breast milk may also be a vehicle for transmission of HIV. The virus is known to be lymphotropic and breast milk has abundant lymphocytes. The virus has been grown from cell-free breast milk of three healthy seropositive women, although it is not known how frequently virus is found in the milk of HIV-infected mothers (12). One case report strongly implicates breast milk as the likely route of infection (13). The parents of the child were not known to be in any risk group; the mother was transfused in the postpartum period with blood from a donor who subsequently developed AIDS. The child was breastfed for 6 weeks. When the diagnosis was made in the blood donor, the mother and 17-month old child were tested and found to be seropositive.

CLINICAL FEATURES

The typical case of pediatric HIV infection is a child born to a mother at risk, who develops recurrent bacterial infections, thrush, failure to thrive, lymphadenopathy, and hepatosplenomegaly within the first year of life. Most children die within 2 years. A number of features of AIDS in children are distinct from those seen in the adult population. We will describe the

TABLE 1 Common Clinical Manifestations of Pediatric HIV Infection

Recurrent bacterial infections
  S. pneumoniae
  H. influenzae
  S. aureus
  enteric gram-negative rods
Acute pneumonitis (PCP)
Chronic pneumonitis
  Lymphoid interstitial pneumonitis (LIP)
  Pulmonary lymphoid hyperplasia (PLH)
  Desquamative interstitial pneumonitis (DIP)
Oral thrush
Diarrhea
Lymphadenopathy
Hepatosplenomegaly
Failure to thrive
Developmental delay
Encephalopathy
Parotitis

signs and symptoms with emphasis on the aspects that are unique to pediatric AIDS. The most common clinical manifestations are listed in Table 1.

Recurrent Bacterial Infections

In adults with HIV infection scattered reports have noted severe infections with bacteria including *Salmonella* spp. and *Haemophilus influenzae* type B; however, they are a relatively minor component of the total spectrum of disease. In contrast, in children with pediatric HIV infection, recurrent bacterial infections are often the presenting symptom and are a major cause of morbidity and mortality. The types of bacterial infections seen are similar to those in patients with hypogammaglobulinemia. Infections with the encapsulated organisms, *Streptococcus pneumoniae, H. influenazae* type B, and enteric gram-negative rods, are common and can cause chronic or recurrent otitis media, pneumonia, mastoiditis, lymphadenitis, bacteremia, and meningitis (14). Malignant external otitis, a disease usually seen in older patients, has also been noted. The *Staphylococcus* is an important pathogen in HIV infected children; it can be particularly troublesome as the cause of skin infections, particularly in children with concomitant eczema. Salmonella infections are often quite severe, as in adults with prolonged gastroenteritis or bacteremia, and frequent relapses may occur.

Pulmonary Manifestations

The spectrum of pulmonary disease in children is also somewhat different from that seen in adults. *Pneumocystis carinii* pneumonia (PCP) is the most commonly diagnosed pulmonary infection in pediatric AIDS. Numerous cases of children with interstitial pneumonitis have been observed who upon open-lung biopsy have negative bacterial, viral, and fungal cultures, and negative stains for PCP. In these patients, lymphoid interstitial pneumonitis (LIP), pulmonary lymphoid hyperplasia (PLH), and desquamative interstitial penumonitis (DIP) have been seen. Lymphoid interstitial pneumonitis is characterized histologically by diffuse infiltration of the alveolar septa and peribronchiolar areas by lymphocytes, plasma cells with Russell bodies, plasmacytoid lymphocytes, and immunoblasts. Histologic sections from lung biopsies of patients with PLH reveal nodules containing lymphocytes and plasma cells; the larger ones often contain a germinal center and a thick-walled venule. Nodules tend to surround bronchiolar epithelium (15). Biopsy specimens of DIP show large intra-alveolar collections of mononuclear cells and cuboidal metaplasia of the alveolar lining epithelium (15). Alveolar septal lymphoplasmacytic infiltrates and fibrosis were present. These symptoms occur frequently in pediatric AIDS and, rarely, in adults. A typical chest radiograph of LIP is shown in Figure 1.

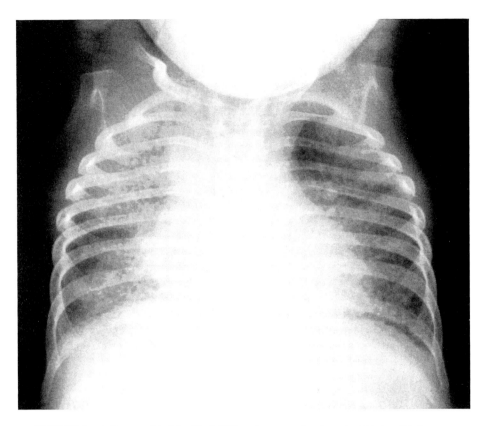

FIGURE 1 A 2-year-old girl with AIDS and progressive lymphoid interstitial pneumonitis. The lungs are hyperinflated with diffuse 1 to 2-mm reticulonodular densities with coalescence at both bases.

Rubinstein et al. have described the clinical, radiologic, and histologic characteristics of patients with PLH and compared them with patients with PCP (16). Children with PLH have cough but only rarely fever, tachypnea, or auscultatory findings. Extrapulmonary manifestations in this group include clubbing, generalized lymphadenopathy, and salivary gland enlargement, not seen in patients with PCP. The chest radiographs of children with PLH show a diffuse nodular pattern and widening of the superior mediastinum and hilum. The prognosis for children with this pulmonary complex is better than for those with PCP; DIP is seen less commonly. The few cases reported had a clinical picture different from LIP or PLH, without lymphadenopathy and with a poorer prognosis.

No pathogen has been consistently isolated from the lungs of patients with LIP or PLH, although there is some evidence to suggest that Epstein-Barr virus (EBV) may play a role in these entities. Patients with PLH and LIP frequently have persistently elevated EBV viral capsule antigen (VCA) IgA and IgM anti-EA titers. DNA hybridization studies have shown EBV-specific DNA in four of five lung biopsies from patients with PLH and in 8 of 10 patients with LIP; in contrast, EBV DNA was not found in specimens from patients with PCP or cytomegalovirus (CMV) infection (17). The association between LIP/PLH and EBV does not prove causality but is an intriguing possibility requiring further evaluation. Some centers treat patients with progressive LIP with steroids. Preliminary results are encouraging, but no controlled data are available (Scott, G. B., unpublished observation).

Parotitis

An additional, unique feature of HIV infection in children is the development of parotitis. The parotid involvement can be either acute, associated with pain, fever, and rapid enlargement, or chronic with slow, progressive, painless growth. Patients with the latter form may develop dry mouth and increased dental caries, as seen in patients with Sjögren's syndrome. The etiology is unknown. It is more common in patients who also have pulmonary lymphoid hyperplasia and, therefore, it has been postulated that EBV may be responsible.

Opportunistic Infections

The opportunistic infections seen in children are similar to those found in adults with AIDS. The most common are PCP, disseminated cytomegalovirus, *M. avium* complex, cryptosporidium, candida, and the herpes viruses. Toxoplasmosis of the CNS, an infection commonly found in most adult series, has been reported in only one case of pediatric AIDS (18). This low occurrence rate is easily explained if one remembers that CNS involvement is usually secondary to reactivation of latent infection, and most children will not have experienced primary infection.

Malignancies

Malignancies are reported in children with AIDS, although not as commonly as in adults. Kaposi's sarcoma, seen in a large proportion of homosexual AIDS patients, is rare in children. It has been postulated that a cofactor necessary for the development of this tumor may not be as common in the pediatric population. Lymphomas, including those involving the CNS, are also rarely seen in children.

Developmental Abnormalities and Central Nervous System Disease

Developmental and neurologic abnormalities can be a prominent part of the clinical spectrum of HIV infection in children (19). In addition, the effects of maternal drug use on the fetus, prematurity, multiple illness requiring hospitalization, and the often chaotic social environment in which many of these children live, may all compound the effects of HIV on the developing nervous system. The brain may be infected in utero, for HIV has been grown from fetal brain tissue (7). Postnatally, the most common neurologic manifestation is an encephalopathy that can be static or progressive. The progressive form is characterized by acquired microcephaly, loss of developmental milestones, progressive motor dysfunction, and generalized weakness with pyramidal tract signs. Pseudobulbar palsy, ataxia, extrapyramidal rigidity, and myoclonus have also been seen. Seizures are usually seen during a concomitant febrile illness. Developmental assessments have shown greater deficits in motor function and expressive speech than in receptive speech or cognitive skills. Deterioration of CNS symptoms is often coincident with deterioration of immune function.

Evaluation of cerebrospinal fluid (CSF) is more likely to show abnormalities in those with progressive encephalopathy. The presence of anti-HVI antibody in the CSF, which indicates active brain infection, has been documented in children. Computed tomography (CT) of the head has shown cerebral atrophy and enlargement of the ventricles, which correlates with the microcephaly. An additional interesting finding, seen only in children, is clacification of the basal ganglia and the periventricular white matter (19). Neuropathologic findings include low brain weight on gross examination and the presence of inflammatory cell infiltrates, including multinucleated giant cells, most prominent in the basal ganglia and brain stem, but also found throughout the gray and white matter. The small- and medium-sized vessels of the basal ganglia are often calcified. Examination of the white matter may show reactive astrocytosis or myelin pallor or both. As in adults, HIV-specific DNA has been demonstrated within brain tissue (20). In children dying with HIV infection, opportunistic CNS infections are infrequent, and it appears that the encephalopathy is most likely to be secondary to HIV infection (21).

Hematologic Manifestations

Hematologic manifestations of HIV infection in children include thrombocytopenia, anemia, and neutropenia. These conditions may accompany AIDS or may be an early manifestation of HIV in a seropositive child. Saulsbury reported three seropositive infants less than 1 year of age with thrombocytopenia; all had abundant bone marrow megakaryocytes and two of the three had elevated platelet-associated IgG levels, suggesting antibody-mediated platelet destruction (22). All of these patients were treated with prednisone and had a clinical response. We have also seen several HIV-infected infants of seropositive mothers with an asymptomatic neutropenia (absolute neutrophil counts between 500 and 1000). A few children have presented with a severe hemolytic anemia, requiring hospitalization; these patients also responded to prednisone (unpublished observation).

Other Manifestations

A number of other less common, but important, features of HIV infection include renal disease, presenting as nephrotic syndrome, cardiomyopathy, and hepatitis (23,24).

Overall, mortality in pediatric AIDS is high. The duration of survival is closely linked to the age of diagnosis. Children with a diagnosis of AIDS at less than 1 year of age have a median survival of 4 months; those whose diagnosis is made after 1 year of age survive an average of 22 months (25).

IMMUNOLOGY

Laboratory investigations of children with pediatric HIV infection have shown a variety of defects. As in other aspects of this infection in children, the abnormalities differ to some extent from those seen in older patients. Both T- and B-cell abnormalities are well described and correlate with the spectrum of clinical manifestations (Table 2).

In adults with AIDS, lymphopenia and a low ratio of T-helper/T-suppressor cells is an almost universal finding. Some children have similar findings. In contrast, despite clinical evidence of severe T-cell dysfunction, other children may have normal absolute lymphocyte counts, normal percentages of T cells and T-cell subsets, and normal nonspecific mitogen responses (24). Skin test anergy is common. Blanche and associates found that the response

---

TABLE 2 Immunologic Abnormalities in Pediatric HIV Infection

± Lymphopenia[a]
± Decreased helper/suppressor ratio[a]
± Decreased mitogen response[a]
Decreased T-cell response to antigen
Skin test anergy
Hypergammaglobulinemia (occasional panhypogammaglobulinemia)
Poor primary and secondary antibody response

[a]More common in advanced disease.

to antigens, rather than mitogens, was the most sensitive indicator of T-cell dysfunction in children. Prognosis also correlated with the ability to respond in the antigen-induced proliferation assay (26). Late in the course of the disease, T-cell numbers and responses to mitogens deteriorate and are similar to values seen in adults. Physicians taking care of children at risk should know that opportunistic infections can develop in children with normal laboratory values of T-cell numbers and function.

Evidence of B-cell dysfunction, manifested by recurrent bacterial infections, is seen early in symptomatic children. Pediatric patients with HIV infection, similarly to their adult counterparts, have increased B-cell numbers, polyclonal B-cell activation, and hypergammaglobulinemia. Immunoglobulin A, IgM, and IgG may reach adult levels by the time an infected child is 6 to 12 months of age. Occasionally, panhypogammaglobulinemia is seen. Although most patients with HIV infection make large quantities of antibodies, they have a poor response to new antigenic challenge. Bernstein et al. immunized six HIV-infected children with bacteriophage ϕX174, pneumococcal vaccine, and tetanus toxoid. They found decreased primary and secondary antibody responses in all patients; in five of six patients, the expected switch from IgM to IgG did not occur (27). This indicates an abnormal response to both T-cell-dependent and T-cell-independent antigens. Response to bacterial toxoids has been measured in 17 previously immunized HIV seropositive children. Protective antibody was seen in only 9 of 15 and 3 of 17 children to tetanus and diphtheria toxoids, respectively (28). Some children had a cell-mediated response to toxoid, despite low antibody levels. This lack of response to new antigens may explain the clinical difference in the number of bacterial infections in adults and children. Because of the polyclonal B cell activation, HIV-infected adult patients may make antibody against the numerous antigens or pathogens that they have previously encountered. By contrast, in children who are infected with HIV early in life, the past antibody repertoire is limited and the response to new antigens is poor, resulting in more clinical consequences of B-cell dysfunction.

DIAGNOSIS

A number of factors complicate the diagnosis of HIV infection in children, particularly those cases resulting from vertical transmission. The first is the necessity to distinguish symptomatic HIV infection from the various congenital immunodeficiencies. The clinical symptoms and time of presentation of pediatric HIV infection may be quite similar to those seen in severe combined immunodeficiency syndrome, Nezelof's syndrome, Wiskott-Aldrich syndrome, or agammaglobulinemia. In a child with symptoms of any of these disorders, it is important to evaluate risk behaviors of the parents that may subsequently lead to perinatal HIV transmission.

An additional diagnostic difficulty stems from the transport of maternal IgG across the placenta. If tested soon after delivery, all infants of seropositive mothers should be seropositive. Maternal IgG antibody may persist until the child is 15 months of age. Sequential antibody testing needs to be performed to determine whether the antibody is of maternal origin or is produced endogenously. Immunoglobulin M is not transported across the placenta, but there is now no reliable assay for anti-HIV IgM. In addition, it is not known whether or not infants infected in utero or perinatally will mount an IgM response.

In one mother-infant pair, true infection of the infant was proved by demonstrating the presence of HIV in peripheral blood lymphocytes by in situ hybridization (29). In a second pair, antibody was shown to be produced, by the infant, with Western blot techniques. Mother and baby were seropositive when tested by enzyme-linked immunosorbent assay (ELISA). Sequential western blot testing of the infant's sera showed the development of new antibody (not previously present) at 4 months of age (30). Other currently experimental tools, with potential to distinguish infants with passive antibody from those who are infected, are viral culture, HIV antigen detection, and IgG subclasses against HIV (31).

A negative antibody test result may also occur in young children at risk. These children, who are usually symptomatic, may have either positive cultures of HIV from peripheral blood mononuclear cells or the presence of HIV antigen in serum (32). As in adults, some children also lose the antibody to some HIV components when they are terminally ill, resulting in a negative ELISA. Therefore, in a high-risk situation, antibody testing alone may not be adequate to rule out HIV infection. The reason why some children do not make HIV antibody is unknown; it has been postulated that an in utero infection could lead to tolerance to HIV.

The following are general guidelines for evaluating an infant or child at risk (Fig. 2). Initial screening should include an ELISA or immunofluorescent antibody (IFA) HIV-test, and all positive results should be confirmed by a Western blot analysis.

In children over 15 months of age, a confirmed positive test result can be considered evidence of endogenous antibody production and, therefore, indicative of infection. In this same age group, a healthy, seronegative child does not need further testing.

In a child under 15 months old, a positive test may represent passive antibody; additional testing needs to be done to determine if the child is truly infected. When available, culture or p24 antigen testing may be diagnostically

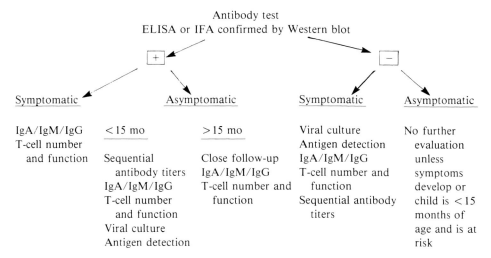

FIGURE 2   Evaluation of children at risk.

useful, if positive (negative results do not rule out infection). Quantitative immunoglobulins may be useful in these circumstances, because levels that are markedly elevated for age are consistent, although not diagnostic, of true infection. In asymptomatic, seropositive children, under 15 months of age, without other laboratory evidence of HIV infection, sequential antibody testing should be performed until the child is 15 months old, to determine if the antibody is passively acquired or endogenously produced.

Children at risk who are symptomatic, but seronegative, should have laboratory evaluation of both T- and B-cell function and, if possible, viral culture or antigen detection. Antibody testing should also be performed 3 to 6 months later to look for a later seroconversion.

MANAGEMENT AND THERAPY

Acute infections, routine or opportunistic, need prompt diagnosis and aggressive treatment. However, there are many unanswered questions concerning optimal ongoing management of both asymptomatic seropositive children and those with ARC or AIDS.

The first issue encountered is care of the infant of a high-risk mother in the immediate newborn period. Pediatricians must be encouraged to take a detailed maternal history, including a sexual and drug-use history. Occasionally, women who engage in high-risk behaviors know their HIV antibody status at delivery but, more commonly, this information is not available. Clearly, voluntary antibody testing of the mother and child must be encouraged to provide appropriate medical care. We have found that when the implications for the child are explained to the family, the vast majority of parents are willing to be tested. If the mother is in a high-risk group, in a geographic area where there is a high prevalence of AIDS, and she refuses testing for herself and her infant, it is safest to assume that the infant may be infected. Infants who are seropositive at birth may be infected with HIV or may have only passively acquired antibody. Until the status of such children can be more accurately determined, it appears prudent to care for these infants as if they are infected.

The management issues requiring special attention in the newborn period are breastfeeding, circumcision, and if needed, blood transfusions. Because of the known excretion of HIV in breast milk, and the case report indicating breast milk as the mode of transmission, in the United States it is recommended that an antibody-positive woman should not breastfeed her infant (33). Although this is easily accomplished in industrialized countries where safe formulas are readily available, in developing countries where prepared formulas may not be available and the water supply is often contaminated, the WHO has recommended breast feeding.

Some authorities have also recommended that circumcision be discouraged for the infants of antibody-positive women, although there have been no reports of complications of circumcision in this population. The basis for this recommendation is twofold: there is no clearcut medical reason to advocate this practice, and it provides a potential site for infection. It is difficult to be dogmatic about this precaution!

Some, but not all, centers taking care of seropositive children use blood products that are irradiated and are from CMV-seronegative blood donors. The rationale is to protect an HIV-seropositive, potentially immunodeficient infant from graft-versus-host disease and from CMV, which can cause severe disease in the compromised host.

Immunizations and Prophylaxis

Another major management issue in the HIV-infected child is how to administer childhood immunizations. There is general agreement that an HIV-seropositive child with clinical evidence of infection should not receive any live viral or bacterial vaccines, such as oral polio vaccine (OPV); measles, mumps, and rubella (MMR); or Bacille Calmette-Guerin (BCG). These children should be immunized according to the usual schedules with diphtheria, pertussis, and tetanus (DPT); inactivated polio vaccine (IPV) to replace OPV; and *H. influenzae* type B (HIB) vaccine. In addition, they should receive the pneumococcal vaccine at or after 2 years of age and inactivated influenza vaccine yearly (34). The use of IPV in this situation provides protection to the infant and prevents the possibility that other household members with HIV infection will be exposed to fecally excreted vaccine strain polio. This vaccine should also be used for seronegative children who are close contacts of seropositive children.

Because these symptomatic children cannot be immunized against measles or varicella, they are at risk of developing severe complications from these infections. Therefore, they should receive passive prophylaxis after a known exposure to these pathogens. Immune globulin (IG) or varicella-zoster immune globulin (VZIG) can be used for measles and varicella, respectively. Many children with symptomatic disease will be receiving monthly gamma globulin (see later discussion); the need for additional passive prophylaxis after an exposure would depend on the interval since the last dose of intravenous therapy.

The care of the child with asymptomatic HIV infection is more controversial. The DPT, IPV, and HIB can be given routinely, as in symptomatic children. However, opinions differ about the risk of MMR administration in healthy seropositive children.

The Advisory Committee on Immunization Practices (ACIP) of the Centers for Disease Control recommends that these patients receive the MMR and that further experience needs to be monitored (34). The committee expressed several reasons to immunize these patients. First, a retrospective study of 63 seropositive infants who had received MMR revealed no serious or unusual adverse events (35). There is also evidence that the MMR provides some protection; 60% of pediatric AIDS or ARC patients given MMR before diagnosis had protective levels of measles antibodies 5 to 66 months after vaccination. Outbreaks of measles could occur in an area with a high prevalence of HIV seropositive unvaccinated children. Finally, recent reports from Africa have shown that measles may cause a devastating illness in unvaccinated HIV-seropositive children (36).

Still, there are theoretical risks in administering this live vaccine to potentially immunodeficient children. Although there have not yet been reports of adverse effects after MMR, few children have been studied. Recently, a healthy HIV seropositive army recruit was given the live, attenuated smallpox vaccine and subsequently developed disseminated vaccinia. This emphasizes the need for caution in the healthy seropositive population. The alternative to vaccination is passive prophylaxis after exposure.

There are convincing arguments for both administering and withholding the MMR in this population. Until more information is available, one must evaluate the risks and benefits and consider, according to geographic area and the patient's accessibility to medical care, what are the patient's risks of exposure to natural infection as well as the likelihood of his receiving prompt, passive prophylaxis. Most centers follow the ACIP recommendations.

There are two additional prophylactic measures that may benefit children with symptomatic HIV infection: trimethoprim/sulfamethoxasole (TMP/SMX) and intravenous gamma globulin. The use of TMP/SMX in children with malignancy is well established for prophylaxis against PCP. This disease has been reported in more than 50% of pediatric AIDS cases. Therefore, although no trials have been performed to prove its efficacy in HIV-infected children, it seems logical that those with evidence of impaired cellular immunity be treated with a prophylactic dose of TMP/SMX (5 mg/kg TMP: 20 mg/kg SMX) daily. It may also decrease the number of pyogenic bacterial infections in these children.

As previously noted, although hypergammaglobulinemia is common, children with HIV infection have recurrent bacterial infections because of their poor specific antibody responses. A number of centers caring for these patients have used empiric immunoglobulin (IG) therapy and noted clinical improvement. Rubinstein et al. evaluated 16 patients (11 infants and 6 adults) treated with biweekly IG and found a decrease in the number of bacterial infections (37). They also noted improvement in some immunologic parameters including a decrease in the isomorphic elevations of lactate dehydrogenase (LDH) levels, which suggests feedback inhibition of B-cell proliferation, and restoration of suppressor T-cell function as measured in an assay of pokeweed mitogen-driven IgG secretion. Although precise guidelines are not available for when and how to treat HIV-infected children with IG, it should be considered for patients with chronic or frequently recurring bacterial infections, regardless of whether they have ARC or AIDS. A prospective multicenter trial is now underway to evaluate the efficacy of IG in symptomatic and asymptomatic HIV-infected children.

There is currently no available licensed antiviral treatment for children with AIDS. A small number of infants have been treated with ribavirin without improvement (38). Zidovudine (AZT), recently approved for the treatment of adults, is not approved for use in children under 13 years of age. Clinical studies of AZT in children are currently underway.

In addition to the care of the seropositive or infected child, a number of other issues may need to be discussed with the families of these children. In many instances of perinatally acquired infection, an affected child is the index case in a family. Under these circumstances, the family should be counseled, and antibody testing encouraged for parents and siblings. It is important to counsel the parents about the risks for future pregnancies. Appropriate referrals can then be made for care of these individuals. It is also important to discuss modes of transmission and to assure family members that there is no transmission by casual contact. Guidelines should be discussed for contact with body secretions and blood. Caretakers should practice thorough hand-washing after exposure to body fluids, and gloves should be worn if open lesions are present on the caretaker's hand (39).

REFERENCES

1. CDC (1985). Revision of the case definition of acquired immunodeficiency syndrome for national reporting—United States. *MMWR 34*:373-375.
2. Rogers, M. F., Thomas, P. A., Starcher, E. T. et al. (1987). Acquired immunodeficiency syndrome in children: Report of the Centers for Disease Control National Surveillance, 1982 to 1985. *Pediatrics 79*:1008-1014.
3. Rubinstein, A. and Bernstein, L. (1986). The epidemiology of pediatric acquired immunodeficiency syndrome. *Clin. Immunol. Immunopathol. 40*:115-121.
4. Scott, G. B., Fischl, M. A., Klimas, N. et al. (1985). Mothers of infants with the acquired immunodeficiency syndrome. Evidence for both symptomatic and asymptomatic carriers. *JAMA 253*:363-366.
5. Rubinstein, A. (1986). Pediatric AIDS. *Curr. Prob. Pediatr. XVI*:365-408.
6. Menez-Bautista, R., Fikrig, S. M., Pahwa, S. et al. (1986). Monozygotic twins discordant for the acquired immunodeficiency syndrome. *Am. J. Dis. Child 140*:678-679.
7. Jovaisas, E., Koch, M. A., Schafer, A. et al. (1985). LAV/HTLV-III in 20-week fetus. *Lancet 2*:1129.
8. Marion, R. W., Wiznia, A. A., Hutcheon, G., and Rubinstein, A. (1986). Human T-cell lymphotropic virus type III (HTLV-III) embryopathy: A new dysmorphic syndrome associated with intrauterine HTLV-III infection. *Am. J. Dis. Child. 140*:638-640.
9. Wofsy, C. B., Cohen, J. B., Hauer, L. B. et al. (1986). Isolation of AIDS-associated retrovirus from genital secretions of women with antibodies to the virus. *Lancet 1*:527-529.
10. Chiodo, F., Ricchi, E., Costigliola, P. et al. (1986). Vertical transmission of HTLV-III. *Lancet 1*:739.
11. Thomas, P. A., O'Donnell, R. E., Guigli, P. et al. (1987). Gestational characteristics and mode of delivery of 98 children with AIDS in New York City. *Abstr. III Int. Conf. AIDS.* June 1987, Washington, D.C.
12. Thiry, L., Sprecher-Goldberger, S., Jonckheer, T. et al. (1985). Isolation of AIDS virus from cell-free breast milk of three healthy virus carriers. *Lancet 2*: 891-892.
13. Ziegler, J. B., Cooper, D. A., Johnson, R. O., and Gold, J. (1985). Postnatal transmission of AIDS-associated retrovirus from mother to infant. *Lancet 1*: 896-897.
14. Bernstein, L. J., Krieger, B. Z., Novick, B. et al. (1985). Bacterial infection in the acquired immunodeficiency syndrome of children. *Pediatr. Infect. Dis. 4*:472.

15. Joshi, V. V., Oleske, J. M., Minnefor, A. B. et al. (1985). Pathologic pulmonary findings in children with the acquired immunodeficiency syndrome: A study of ten cases. *Hum. Pathol. 16*:241-246.
16. Rubinstein, A., Morecki, R., Silverman, B. et al. (1986). Pulmonary disease in children with acquired immune deficiency syndrome and AIDS-related complex. *J. Pediatr. 108*:498-503.
17. Andiman, W. A., Eastman, R., Martin, K. et al. Opportunistic lymphoproliferations associated with Epstein-Barr viral DNA in infants and children with AIDS. *Lancet 2*:1390-1393.
18. Shanks, G. D., Redfield, R. R., and Fisher, G. W. (1987). Toxoplasma encephalitis in an infant with acquired immunodeficiency syndrome. *Pediatr. Infect. Dis. 6*:70-71.
19. Epstein, L. G., Sharer, L. R., Oleske, J. M. et al. (1986). Neurologic manifestations of human immunodeficiency virus infection in children. *Pediatrics 78*: 678-687.
20. Ragni, M. V., Urbach, A. H., Taylor, S. et al. (1987). Isolation of human immunodeficiency virus and detection of HIV DNA sequences in the brain of an ELISA antibody-negative child with acquired immune deficiency syndrome and progressive encephalopathy. *J. Pediatr. 110*:892-894.
21. Sharer, L. R., Epstein, L. G., Cho, E. S. et al. (1986). Pathologic features of AIDS encephalopathy in children: Evidence for LAV/HTLV-III infection of brain. *Hum. Pathol. 17*:271-284.
22. Saulsbury, F. T., Bayle, R. J., Wykoff, R. F., and Howard, T. H. (1986). Thrombocytopenia as the presenting manifestation of human T-lymphotropic virus type III infection in infants. *J. Pediatr. 109*:30-34.
23. Steinherz, L. J., Brockstein, J. A., and Robins, J. (19867). Cardiac involvement in congenital acquired immunodeficiency syndrome. *Am. J. Dis. Child. 140*: 1241-1244.
24. Pahwa, S., Kaplan, M., Firkrig, S. et al. (1986). Spectrum of human T cell lymphotropic virus type III infection in children: Recognition of symptomatic, asymptomatic and seronegative patients. *JAMA 255*:2299-2305.
25. Oxtoby, M. J., Rogers, M., and Thomas, P. (1987). National trends in perinatally acquired AIDS, United States. *Abstr. III Int. Conf. AIDS.* June 1987, Washington, D.C.
26. Blanche, S., Le Deist, F., Fischer, A. et al. (1986). Longitudinal study of 18 children with perinatal LAV-HTLV III infection: Attempt at prognostic evaluation. *J. Pediatr. 109*:965-170.
27. Bernstein, L. J., Ochs, H. D., Wedgwood, R. J. et al. (1985). Defective humoral immunity in pediatric acquired immune deficiency syndrome. *J. Pediatr. 107*: 352-357.
28. Borkowsky, W., Steele, C. J., and Grubman, S. (1987). Antibody responses to bacterial toxoids in children infected with human immunodeficiency virus. *J. Pediatr. 110*:563-566.
29. Harnish, D. G., Hammerberg, O., Walker, I. R. et al. (1987). Early detection of HIV infection in a newborn. *Lancet 1*:272-273.

30. Johnson, J. P. and Nair, P. (1987). Early diagnosis of HIV infection in the neonate. *Lancet 1*:273-274.
31. Pyun, K. H., Ochs, H. D., Dufford, M. T. W. et al. (1987). Perinatal infection with human immune deficiency virus: Specific antibody responses by the neonate. *N. Engl. J. Med. 317*:611-614.
32. Borkowsky, W., Krasinski, K., Paul, D. et al. (1987). Human immunodeficiency-virus infections in infants negative for anti-HIV by enzyme-linked immunoassay. *Lancet 1*:1168-1170.
33. CDC (1985). Recommendations for assisting in the prevention of perinatal transmission of human T-lymphotropic virus type III/lymphadenopathy associated virus and acquired immunodeficiency syndrome. *MMWR 34*:721-731.
34. CDC (1986). Recommendation of the Immunization Practices Advisory Committee (ACIP) immunization of children infected with human T-lymphotropic virus type III/lymphadenopathy virus. *MMWR 35*:595-606.
35. McLaughlin, M., Thomas, P., Rubinstein, A. et al. (1986). Use of live virus vaccines in children with HTLV-III/LAV infection: A retrospective survey. International Conference on AIDS, June 23-25, 1986, Paris.
36. Sension, M. G., Nzila, N., Duma, M. et al. (1987). Does concomitant HIV and measles infection in African children lead to increased morbidity and mortality? Presented at the III International Conference on AIDS, June 1987, Washington, D.C.
37. Rubinstein, A., Sicklick, M., Bernstein, L. et al. (1984). Treatment of AIDS with intravenous gammaglobulin [Abstract]. *Pediatr. Res. 18*:264.
38. Blanche, S., Fischer, A., and Le Deist, F. (1986). Ribavirin in HTLV III/LAV infection of infants. *Lancet 1*:863.
39. CDC (1985). Education and foster care of children infected with human T-lymphotropic virus type III/lymphadenopathy-associated virus. *MMWR 34*:521.

Part III
Viral Infections

10
Herpes Simplex and Varicella-Zoster Virus Infections in Acquired Immunodeficiency Syndrome

Kim S. Erlich* *University of California, San Francisco, California*

Herpes simplex virus types 1 and 2 (HSV-1, HSV-2) and varicella-zoster virus (VZV), the neurotropic herpesviruses, typically produce an acute infection of epithelial and nerve tissue and latent infection of nerve root ganglia. These viruses can cause disease in both the normal and immunocompromised host, and are responsible for substantial morbidity in patients with acquired immunodeficiency syndrome (AIDS). Primary infection with these pathogens is unusual in adults with AIDS, because previous infection with HSV and VZV is common before HIV infection. However, reactivated infection and recurrent disease is common in AIDS patients and often results in severe illness with extensive tissue destruction and prolonged virus shedding. Prompt recognition of infection with these viruses is important because early intervention with antiviral chemotherapy in AIDS patients decreases morbidity and likely reduces the risk of fatal complications.

EPIDEMIOLOGY

Herpes Simplex Virus

Herpes simplex virus types 1 and 2 are isolated frequently from orolabial and genital lesions, respectively, but both viruses are capable of infecting any

Present affiliation: Seton Medical Center, Daly City, California

anatomic site (1). Sexual practices that involve oral-genital contact likely increase the risk of developing genital HSV-1 and orolabial HSV-2 infection. Recurrence rates, however, depend on the HSV type and the anatomic site of initial infection. Orolabial recurrences are more likely to occur if the infecting virus was HSV-1, whereas genital recurrences are more likely to occur if the initial infection was due to HSV-2 (2).

Prevalence rates for HSV infection depend on the HSV type and the social and demographic characteristics of the population studied (1). The prevalence of HSV infection in AIDS patients equals or exceeds that of the general population; probably reflecting the common risk factors for transmission of both HSV and HIV (sexual contact). Serologic studies have revealed that >95% of homosexual men with AIDS have been previously infected with both HSV-1 and HSV-2 (3,4). Other AIDS subgroups, such as hemophiliacs and transfusion recipients, undoubtably have lower rates of previous infection.

Varicella-Zoster Virus

Primary VZV infection is often a childhood illness, with secondary attack rates exceeding 90% in susceptible household contacts (5). As with HSV, most adults with AIDS have been previously infected with VZV and are not susceptible to primary infection (3).

AIDS patients develop recurrent VZV infection (zoster) more frequently than age-matched immunocompetent hosts. A retrospective review of 300 AIDS patients with Kaposi's sarcoma revealed that 8% of patients had experienced at least one attack of zoster, an incidence seven times greater than expected in a population that age. Zoster is also noted to occur with a higher than expected frequency in human immunodeficiency virus (HIV)-infected individuals who appear otherwise healthy. Additionally, more than one episode of zoster is fairly common in HIV-infected patients but is unusual in the immunocompetent host (6-10).

PATHOGENESIS

Transmission of either HSV or VZV requires inoculation of infected droplets directly onto mucosal surfaces or broken epithelium. Direct human-to-human spread appears to be the only important method of transmission, as the virus is enveloped and requires a moist environment for survival; additionally, there are no known animal vectors.

Herpes simplex virus infection and replication occurs in epithelial cells at the site of initial virus inoculation, but signs and symptoms of illness do not occur for 2 to 12 days. During this incubation period virions apparently travel along sensory nerve fibers from the site of inoculation to reach the corresponding nerve root ganglia. The virus produces latent infection in 0.01% to 0.1% of the ganglionic cells in a poorly understood fashion (11). Centrifugal spread of virus then occurs along peripheral nerve fibers, with virus replication and mucocutaneous lesions developing at the epithelial surface.

Transmission of VZV to a susceptible host probably occurs by aerosolization of infected droplets and deposition onto the oropharyngeal mucosa of a susceptible host. Virus initially replicates in tonsillar and lymphoid tissue, and this is followed by a primary viremia and seeding of internal organs. A secondary viremia, occurring 10 to 14 days later, results in spread of virus to cutaneous and mucosal surfaces and the characteristic "chickenpox" exanthem. Successive crops of new skin lesions during primary VZV infection are typical and suggest that recurrent viremia is common (5). During this primary infection, VZV establishes a latent infection in dorsal nerve roots or in trigeminal ganglia.

The mechanisms by which latent infection and virus reactivation occur are poorly understood. During latent infection viral DNA can be demonstrated in ganglion cells, but complete virions are not produced (11). Many HSV recurrences occur spontaneously, but various external stimuli (such as febrile illnesses, local irritation, ultraviolet radiation, stress, and menstruation) stimulate virus reactivation and result in recurrent disease in some individuals. Reactivation of VZV may occur spontaneously or as a result of immunosuppression (6). Although most episodes of zoster in AIDS are confined within a dermatomal distribution, cutaneous or visceral dissemination also occurs (9).

The host immune system probably plays a critical role in the recovery from acute HSV and VZV infection. Immunocompromised individuals, including patients with AIDS, are susceptible to severe illnesses after primary HSV or VZV infection, and often suffer from frequent and severe recurrent infections (12,13). The precise immune defect(s) responsible for the increased susceptibility of AIDS patients to these infections is unknown. Early studies had suggested that depletion of T lymphocytes that express the CD4 surface antigen ("helper" T lymphocytes) was the immune defect primarily responsible for the increased susceptibility of AIDS patients to opportunistic infections. Subsequent studies have revealed, however, that numerous other immune defects (including abnormalities in macrophage function, natural killer cell activity, cytotoxic T-lymphocyte activity, and antibody production) are also induced by HIV infection (14). The role of these immune abnormalities in the pathogenesis of herpesvirus infections in AIDS is unknown, and remains under investigation.

CLINICAL PRESENTATION

Herpes Simplex Virus

Because most AIDS patients are infected with HSV before infection with HIV, recurrent herpes is a much more common problem than primary HSV infection in this population. Infection is often atypical, compared with that observed in the normal host, with the severity of the illness depending on several factors, including the site of infection, the degree of immunosuppression, and whether the episode represents initial/primary infection (i.e., no previous exposure to either HSV type), initial/nonprimary infection (i.e., previous exposure to the heterologous HSV type), or recurrent infection (Table 1).

The Centers for Disease Control (CDC) have recently revised the diagnostic criteria for AIDS to include chronic mucocutaneous HSV infection (15). Large ulcerative HSV lesions (without visceral or cutaneous dissemination) are a frequent occurrence in HIV-infected patients. An ulcerative HSV infection that is present for longer than 1 month in an individual with no other cause of underlying immunodeficiency or with laboratory evidence of HIV infection is diagnostic of AIDS (Table 2).

TABLE 1 Clinical Features of HSV Infection in AIDS Patients Compared with Immunocompetent Hosts

Immunocompetent hosts	AIDS patients
May be due to primary or recurrent infection	Usually caused by virus reactivation and recurrent infection
Spontaneous healing occurs in 3 to 4 weeks (primary infection) and 7 to 10 days (recurrent infection)	Healing of mucocutaneous lesions often markedly delayed; chronic ulcerative lesions common
Virus shedding ceases as lesions crust and heal	Prolonged virus shedding common
Usual good response to antiviral chemotherapy	Delayed response to antiviral chemotherapy is common
Recurrences usually occur only infrequently (but wide patient-to-patient variability exists)	Frequent relapses after discontinuation of antiviral chemotherapy
Selection of acyclovir-resistant mutants has not been described while receiving therapy	Occasional selection of acyclovir-resistant mutants while receiving therapy

TABLE 2   Characteristics of HSV Infection Diagnostic of AIDS*

HSV infection causing a mucocutaneous ulcer that persists longer than 1 month; or HSV bronchitis, pneumonitis, or esophagitis for any duration affecting a patient over 1 month of age,

      and

No other cause of immunodeficiency [such as high-dose steroid or cytotoxic therapy, Hodgkin's disease, non-Hodgkin's lymphoma (other than primary brain lymphoma), lymphocytic leukemia, multiple myeloma, angioimmunoblastic lymphadenopathy, other lymphoreticular cancer, or a congenital or acquired immunodeficiency syndrome unrelated to HIV infection],

      or

Laboratory evidence of HIV infection

*From the Centers for Disease Control criteria (15).

Orolabial Infection

Although orolabial HSV infection in adults is usually due to recurrent disease, primary orolabial HSV infection may occur in children with AIDS, because HIV infection is more likely to have occurred before the initial HSV exposure.

The incubation period of primary infection ranges between 2 and 12 days. Primary orolabial infection in the normal host may produce no symptoms, or may result in a severe gingivostomatitis (1,11,16). Immunocompromised patients are at increased risk to develop a severe clinical illness during primary HSV-1 infection, with a painful vesicular eruption occurring along the lip, tongue, pharynx, or buccal mucosa. These vesicles rapidly coalesce and rupture to form large ulcers covered by a whitish-yellow necrotic film (16,17). Fever, pharyngitis, and cervical lymphadenopathy are frequently present in adults, whereas infants may display poor feeding and persistent drooling.

Recurrences of HSV in AIDS may increase in frequency and become more severe as immunosuppression increases. Alternatively, patients may have only infrequent, mild recurrences throughout their disease (12,13). Prodromal symptoms, consisting of tingling or numbness at the site of the impending recurrence, may be present from 12 to 24 hr before the onset of recurrent infection.

In the normal host, orolabial herpes usually heals over 7 to 10 days. In AIDS patients, however, a prolonged illness with delayed healing of lesions is common. Chronic ulceration and persistant virus shedding may occur for several weeks if the patient is left untreated (17).

Genital Infection

Local signs and symptoms develop in most individuals with primary genital herpes (18). A 2 to 12 day incubation period is followed by the emergence of small papules. These lesions rapidly evolve into fluid-filled vesicles, and they are usually painful and tender to palpation. The vesicles ulcerate rapidly and, in the normal host, heal over 3 to 4 weeks by crusting and reepithelialization. Tender inguinal adenopathy is a common finding. Dysuria is often present, even if the urethra is not infected. Systemic symptoms, such as fever, headache, myalgias, malaise, and meningismus, are also common during the primary infection (18,19).

In the normal host, recurrent genital herpes typically results in a milder illness than does the primary infection, with fewer external lesions, a shorter duration of illness, and no systemic symptoms (18,19). In AIDS patients, however, the severity and duration of recurrent genital herpes may be increased. Prolonged new lesion formation, with continued tissue destruction, persistent virus shedding, and severe pain, is common. As immunosuppression increases, the frequency of genital recurrences may also increase (12, 20).

Other causes must always be considered in the differential diagnosis of genital ulceration. All patients with AIDS (especially sexually active homosexual males and prostitutes) with genital ulcers should undergo serologic testing and dark-field examination for syphilis. Other sexually transmitted diseases, including chancroid, lymphogranuloma venereum, and granuloma inguinal, should also be included in the differential diagnosis. Other rare causes of genital ulcers, such as amebic infection, have been observed. Noninfectious etiologies, including Behcet's syndrome, Crohn's disease, traumatic ulceration, scabies, folliculitis, atopic dermatitis, and fixed drug eruption, are more unusual, but they may occasionally be confused with genital herpes (21).

Anorectal Infection

Chronic perianal herpes was among the first reported opportunistic infections associated with AIDS and has subsequently been recognized as the most frequent cause of nongonococcal proctitis in sexually active homosexual men (22,23). Proctitis caused by HSV usually results from primary infection with type-2 virus, but may also occur due to primary HSV-1 infection and may recur. Severe anorectal pain, perianal ulcerations, constipation, tenesmus, and neurologic symptoms in the distribution of the sacral plexus (i.e., sacral rediculopathy, impotence, and neurogenic bladder) are typical of HSV proctitis and assist with its differentiation from proctitis from other causes (23). Anorectal or sigmoidoscopic examination may reveal a friable mucosa, diffuse ulcerations, and intact vesicular or pustular lesions (23).

Recurrent perianal HSV lesions without proctitis are also common in patients with AIDS. Local pain, tenderness, itching, and pain on defecation are prominent symptoms. Shallow ulcers in the perianal region are often visible on external examination, and ulcerative lesions may coalesce and extend along the gluteal crease to involve the area overlying the sacrum. Because these atypical lesions may be confused with pressure decubitus ulcers, all perianal ulcerations and anal fissures should be cultured for HSV to prevent misdiagnosis.

Esophagitis

Symptoms of HSV esophagitis typically include retrosternal pain and odynophagia. Dysphagia may be of acute onset or chronic, and may be severe enough to interfere with eating. Typical herpetic oropharyngeal lesions may be absent, and the clinical picture may be identical with candidal esophagitis. Radiographic contrast studies typically reveal a "cobblestone" appearance of the esophageal musoca, but this finding is also present with candidial esophagitis. Definitive diagnosis is made only by direct endoscopic visualization of the esophageal mucosa with virus culture and biopsies for histopathologic examination.

Encephalitis

Herpes simplex viral encephalitis occurs infrequently, but it is the most life-threatening complication of HSV infection in AIDS. Both HSV-1 and HSV-2 have been identified in brain tissue of AIDS patients, and simultaneous brain infection with HSV and cytomegalovirus (CMV) has been reported (24,25). In adults with AIDS, HSV encephalitis usually occurs as a complication of primary or reactivated orolabial infection. In neonates, however, the disease usually occurs as a result of primary infection at the time of birth (11).

The presentation of HSV encephalitis in AIDS may be highly atypical, compared with that in the normal host. AIDS patients may initially develop only subtle neurologic abnormalities, suggesting that host immune responses contribute to the clinical manifestations of encephalitis caused by HSV (24, 25). Headache, meningismus, and personality changes develop gradually as the infection progresses. Alternatively, however, some AIDS patients develop more typical findings of acute encephalitis, with fever, headache, nausea, lethargy, temporal lobe abnormalities, cranial nerve defects, and focal seizures. If left untreated, grand mal seizures, obtundation, coma, and death eventually ensue.

The diagnosis of HSV encephalitis may be extremely difficult, as other central nervous system infections (including HIV encephalopathy, and those caused by *Cryptococcus neoformans* and *Toxoplasma gondii*) may manifest in an identical clinical fashion. Cerebrospinal fluid (CSF) usually reveals nonspecific abnormalities, with elevated protein concentration, a lymphocytic pleocytosis, and negative virus cultures (26). Detection of antibody to HSV in CSF has potential as a useful diagnostic test in patients with HSV encephalitis, but it has not been evaluated specifically in patients with AIDS (27). Computed tomography scanning, radionuclide brain scan, or electroencephalography reveal nonspecific abnormalities, and are often helpful in identifying abnormal areas of brain for tissue sampling. Definitive diagnosis requires brain biopsy and recovery of virus or demonstration of viral antigens (26). The histopathologic abnormalities typically observed in normal hosts (hemorrhagic cortical necrosis and lymphocytic infiltration) may be absent in AIDS patients (24,25).

Varicella-Zoster Virus

Primary Infection: Varicella

Varicella in immunocompetent children is usually a benign illness. Adults and immunocompromised individuals, however, are at markedly increased risk to develop a serious illness following primary VZV infection. Virus dissemination to visceral organs occurs in up to one-third of immunocompetent adults with primary infection (5). Because of their immune abnormalities, AIDS patients are at increased risk to develop a protracted and potentially life-threatening illness after primary VZV infection (3).

The rash of primary varicella (chickenpox) develops between 10 and 23 days (mean of 14 days) from the time of virus inoculation. Many individuals develop prodromal symptoms (consisting of low-grade fevers, malaise, and myalgias) 1 to 2 days before onset of the skin rash. Lesions begin as small erythematous macules, and progress to papules and vesicles over 12 to 36 hr. The vesicles are often variable in size and shape, and are filled with straw-colored fluid containing infectious virus particles. The characteristic VZV lesion has been compared to a "dewdrop on a rose petal" because of the appearance of the fluid-filled vesicle resting on an erythematous base. The vesicles rapidly dry, umbilicate, crust, and undergo reepithelialization. New vesicles continue to form for several days, resulting in the presence of lesions in all stages of development (i.e., macules, fresh vesicles, umbilicated lesions, and crusts). In immunocompetent individuals, complete healing usually occurs within 7 to 10 days (5).

Recurrent Infection: Zoster

Unlike primary VZV infection, recurrent VZV infection (zoster) is common in patients with AIDS. The illness is often heralded by radicular pain and begins with a localized or segmented erythematous rash covering one to three dermatomes. Maculopapules develop in the dermatomal area and the patient often experiences increasing pain. The maculopapules progress to become fluid-filled vesicles, and contiguous vesicles may become confluent with true bullae formation. In many AIDS and ARC patients the lesions remain confined in a dermatomal distribution; eventually drying and healing by crusting and reepithelialization (7-10,28). Occasionally, however, widespread cutaneous or visceral dissemination occurs (29). Patients with extensive cutaneous dissemination may appear identical with individuals with primary varicella.

Reactivated infection involving the ophthalmic division of the trigeminal nerve results in infection of the cornea (zoster ophthalmicus). The presence of vesicles on the tip of the nose is often associated with involvement of the eye. Although healing without sequelae may occur, untreated patients may develop anterior uveitus, corneal scarring, and suffer from permanent visual loss (10,28).

Complications

Complications of VZV infection are common in immunocompromised patients and are a frequent cause of prolonged morbidity. Dissemination of virus to the lung, liver, and CNS has been associated with a mortality of 6% to 17% (6).

Varicella pneumonia may occur during primary VZV infection or during reactivated infection and visceral dissemination. Symptoms of varicella pneumonia are often quite variable; many patients develop only mild respiratory symptoms, whereas others develop severe and fatal hypoxemia resulting from respiratory failure. Radiographic abnormalities are usually out of proportion to the clinical findings, with diffuse nodular densities present on chest x-ray films with occasional pleural effusions.

Encephalitis is a rare complication of VZV infection, but may also occur in AIDS. In the normal host, the illness begins 3 to 8 days after the onset of varicella, or 1 to 2 weeks after the development of zoster. AIDS patients, however, have developed progressive VZV neurologic disease up to 3 months after an episode of localized zoster (29). Headache, vomiting, lethargy, and cerebellar findings (ataxia, tremors, dizziness) may be prominent physical findings. Diagnosis based on clinical criteria alone can be difficult because other central nervous system infections can present in a similar fashion.

Postherpetic neuralgia (local pain that persists long after resolution of the acute infection) is unusual in patients with AIDS. This complication is more common in elderly individuals, and most AIDS patients are less than 65 years of age.

LABORATORY DIAGNOSIS

Virus Culture

For diagnosis of an HSV infection in AIDS, virus isolation is the procedure of choice (Table 3). Virus culture is widely available and relatively rapid, with

TABLE 3 Laboratory Procedures for Diagnosis of HSV and VZV Infections

Procedure	HSV	VZV
Virus culture	Very sensitive (95-100%) Very specific (100%) Relatively rapid (1-5 d) Expensive ($30-100)	Good sensitivity (50-90%) Very specific (100%) Slow (7-14 d) Expensive ($30-100)
Antigen detection	Very sensitive (50-75%) Very specific Very rapid (usually 1 d) Not expensive ($10-25)	May be more sensitive than culture (75-90%) Very specific Very rapid (usually 1 d) Not expensive ($10-25)
Cytology	Insensitive (40-50%) Not specific Very rapid (hr)	Insensitive (40-50%) Not specific Very rapid (hr)
Serology	Usually not helpful during acute infection May be useful retrospectively	Usually not helpful during acute infection May be useful retrospectively

positive results usually available within 3 to 4 days (30). Fresh vesicles should be preferentially sampled for HSV and VZV culture because they have the highest concentrations of live virus (31). Cultures of unroofed vesicles and shallow ulcerations are also frequently positive, whereas crusted and dried lesions are usually negative (31).

Unlike HSV, a typical VZV infection may be associated with a negative virus culture. Virus cultures from the normal host are more likely to be falsely negative if obtained late in the course of VZV infection (32). However, AIDS patients may shed virus for prolonged periods, and virus culture may be a more sensitive diagnostic test in this group of patients. Growth of VZV in cell culture usually takes 10 days to 2 weeks, however, limiting the usefulness of virus culture in the rapid diagnosis of acute VZV infection (32).

Virus cultures from intact vesicles are obtained by gently unroofing the vesicle and swabbing the fluid and cellular debris with a cotton-tipped or Dacron applicator. Broken vesicles and ulcers are cultured in a similar manner by gently swabbing the base of the ulcerative lesion. Specimens can be inoculated directly into cell culture, but this is often an infeasible approach. The routine use of a viral transport medium in obtaining specimens allows for a delay of several hours from the time the specimen is obtained until it is inoculated into cell culture. If a viral transport medium is not available, material for culture can be kept moistened in a small amount of nonbacteriostatic sterile saline (30,31). Calcium alginate swabs (used routinely for the culture of *Neisseria gonorrhoeae*) should not be used for obtaining HSV or VZV cultures; they produce false-negative results by inactivating the viruses (33). Care should be taken to avoid introducing blood, stool, soap, alcohol, or iodine into the sample, because these substances may also inactivate the virus and are toxic to the cell culture. Specimens should be transported to the laboratory immediately, but they can be kept at 4°C (i.e., refrigerated or in an ice bath) in a buffered salt solution for up to 48 hr without a substantial drop in virus titer. Specimens for virus culture should not be frozen at −20°C, but can be stored at −70°C.

To culture for virus, specimens are inoculated into tubes containing cell monolayers capable of supporting virus growth. Tissue biopsies or autopsy samples are minced or homogenized before inoculation. Virus replication in the cell monolayer produces morphologic changes visible under light microscopy. These changes, referred to as cytopathic effects (CPE), begin with cytoplasmic granulation and progress to rounded, swollen, and refractile cells with occasional syncitial formation. Newer techniques have demonstrated that "modified culture" techniques (consisting of centrifuging clinical specimens directly onto cell monolayers followed by staining the monolayer with specific monoclonal antibodies) permits a more rapid diagnosis of HSV infection (34).

Antigen Detection

Identification of HSV antigens is routinely used in the identification of virus in cell culture displaying CPE, and is gaining wide use in the rapid diagnosis of HSV or VZV infection by application directly to clinical material. These techniques employ immunofluorescent or immunoperoxidase staining of cellular material, using virus-specific monoclonal antibodies, and achieve a high sensitivity and specificity compared with that of virus culture (31). The major advantage of this technique is that results are often available in less than 24 hr (see Table 3).

Specimens from mucocutaneous lesions are obtained by gently swabbing the base of an unroofed vesicle or ulcerative lesion with a cotton tipped applicator. The cells are then transferred to glass microscope slides by gentle rolling of the applicator tip along the slide (to preserve the cellular morphology) and are allowed to air dry. Unlike virus culture, vesicular fluid may not be suitable for antigen detection because the amount of exfoliated cellular material in vesicular fluid is usually small. Tissue biopsies and autopsy samples (e.g., brain) are trypsinized and the single-cell suspension is processed in an identical fashion. Several slides should be prepared for antigen detection because lesions caused by HSV-1, HSV-2, and VZV may appear similar. Additionally, antigen testing for all three viruses assures a negative laboratory control (30,32).

Cytology

Morphologic changes in HSV- or VZV-infected cells can be observed by examining stained cell or tissue preparations under light microscopy. Cytologic examination is rapid, inexpensive, and widely available, but the sensitivity is only 40% to 50%, compared with that of virus culture or antigen detection. Additionally, a positive result does not allow differentiation between HSV-1, HSV-2, and VZV (see Table 3).

To obtain specimens for cytologic examination, mucocutaneous lesions are gently scraped and the cells transferred onto glass microscope slides. The slides are stained with either Papanicolaou or Wright-Giemsa stain (Tzanck preparation) and examined under 40× magnification. Cells that have been recently infected display a slightly enlarged nucleus and thickened nuclear membrane. As infection progresses, cell fusion and multinuclear giant cells appear. Eosinophilic intranuclear (Cowdry type A) inclusion bodies are visible with Papanicolaou staining, but they are not observed with the Tzanck preparation (30,32).

Serology

Antibody to HSV can be detected by several techniques, including complement fixation, virus neutralization, enzyme-linked immunosorbent assay (ELISA), indirect hemagglutination, indirect immunofluorescence, and radioimmunoasssay. Serology, however, is rarely useful in the diagnosis and management of AIDS patients with acute HSV infection because antibody formation occurs late in the course of primary HSV infection and is usually unchanged during recurrent infection. Additionally, infection with one HSV type induces antibodies that cross-react with the heterologous HSV type (30).

The VZV antibody can be detected by the fluorescent antibody-membrane antigen (FAMA) test, ELISA, complement fixation, and anticomplement immunofluorescence. Serologic testing usually is not helpful in the diagnosis of VZV because the humoral response occurs late following primary or recurrent infection (see Table 3). However, a rise in antibody concentration may be diagnostic of a recent VZV infection, if paired sera are available. Immunity to primary VZV infection can be confirmed by demonstrating antibody by either FAMA or ELISA (32).

Treatment

Antiviral Chemotherapy

Acyclovir

The prompt administration of antiviral chemotherapy to AIDS patients with acute HSV or VZV infection reduces morbidity and minimizes the risk of fatal

TABLE 4   Dosage Adjustment of Intravenous Acyclovir
in Patients with Compromised Renal Function

Creatinine clearance (ml/min)	Percentage of standard dose[a]	Dosage interval (hr)
>50	100	8
25-50	100	12
10-25	100	24
0-10	50	24

[a]Usually 5 mg/kg for mucocutaneous HSV infections and 10
mg/kg for severe HSV infections and VZV infections.

complications. Acyclovir, the antiviral agent of choice for all HSV and VZV
infections in AIDS, can be administered orally (35-38), intravenously (39-
43), and topically (20,44). The optimal route of administration, dosage, and
duration of therapy depend on the infecting virus as well as the site and severity of the infection.

Acyclovir has a high therapeutic ratio because it undergoes selective activation (by phosphorylation) in HSV-infected cells. Acyclovir triphosphate,
the active antiviral, acts by selective inhibition of viral DNA polymerase
and termination of DNA chain synthesis. The drug is slightly more active
against HSV-1 than HSV-2, and is about 10 times more active against HSV
than VZV. Acyclovir distributes into all tissues, including the brain and
cerebrospinal fluid, and is cleared by renal mechanisms. The serum half-life
in patients with normal renal function is 2 to 3 hr, and the intravenous dose
should be adjusted in patients with impaired renal function (Table 4; 45).

Management of Herpes Simplex Virus Infection

Most AIDS patients with primary or recurrent mucocutaneous HSV infections are not ill enough to require hospitalization and can be treated as outpatients. Outpatient therapy should be initiated with oral acyclovir 200 mg
five times daily (Table 5). Therapy can be started while awaiting results of
virus culture (if the clinical suspicion is high) or when the diagnosis has been
confirmed by laboratory techniques (35).

Intravenous acyclovir should be reserved for patients with severe or extensive mucocutaneous HSV infection and for patients with virus dissemination,
visceral organ involvement (e.g., brain, esophagus, eye), or neurologic complications (atonic bladder, transverse myelitis; see Table 5). Additionally,
intravenous acyclovir should be used for individuals who require antiviral
chemotherapy but are unable to tolerate oral cyclovir because of nausea,
dysphagia, or protracted diarrhea. The dosage of intravenous acyclovir for

TABLE 5 Management of HSV Infections in AIDS

Clinical presentation	Modifying circumstances	Treatment
Primary mucocutaneous infection	None	Acyclovir 200 mg p.o. five times daily[a]
Primary mucocutaneous infection	Complications or dissemination[b]	Acyclovir 15 mg/kg per day IV[a,c]
Visceral organ infection	None	Acyclovir 30 mg/kg per day IV[d]
Recurrent mucocutaneous infection	None	Acyclovir 200 mg p.o. five times daily[a]
Recurrent mucocutaneous infection	Complications or dissemination[b]	Acyclovir 15 mg/kg per day IV[a,c]
Recurrent mucocutaneous infection (suppressive therapy)	Frequent and/or severe recurrences	Acyclovir 200 mg p.o. t.i.d. or 400 mg p.o. b.i.d.
Severe infection caused by acyclovir-resistant HSV	Thymidine-kinase-negative strain	Vidarabine 15 mg/kg per day IV[d] or foscarnet, 180 mg/kg/d IV

[a]Treatment should be continued until all external lesions have crusted or reepithelialized.
[b]Cutaneous dissemination, visceral dissemination, or neurologic involvement (atonic bladder, transverse myelitis, severe meningismus).
[c]If prolonged therapy is required after hospital discharge, oral acyclovir (200 mg five times daily) may be substituted.
[d]Intravenous therapy should be continued for a minimum of 10 days.

patients with mucocutaneous HSV infection and normal renal function is 15 mg/kg per day in three divided doses (41). Patients with life-threatening HSV infection (encephalitis, neonatal infection, disseminated infection) or visceral organ involvement (esophagitis, proctitis) should receive a higher dosage; usually 30 mg/kg per day in three divided doses (39,40). Treatment should last for a minimum of 10 days, but longer therapy may be necessary. The intravenous dosage should be adjusted in patients with impaired renal function (see Table 4). If prolonged therapy is required and the patient is ready for hospital discharge, oral acyclovir can be substituted for intravenous therapy.

Topical acyclovir is probably less effective than either oral or intravenous therapy, although comparative trials have not been performed. Topical acyclovir decreases the duration of virus shedding in compromised hosts with mucocutaneous HSV infection, but it does not reduce new lesion formation or the risk of dissemination (20,44). There appears to be no benefit to the combination of topical medication with oral or intravenous acyclovir (46).

Topical acyclovir should be reserved for patients with chronic ulcerative mucocutaneous HSV infection who are unable to tolerate oral medication (see Table 5).

Treatment with acyclovir should be continued until all mucocutaneous lesions have crusted or reepithelialized. The HSV lesions in AIDS patients may heal quite slowly, however, even with optimal antiviral chemotherapy. If healing of lesions does not occur while the patient is receiving acyclovir therapy, repeat virus cultures should be obtained, and the possibility of acyclovir-resistant HSV should be considered.

Because vidarabine (ara-A) is less effective than acyclovir in the treatment of HSV infections, it should be reserved only for patients with severe HSV infections caused by thymidine kinase-negative HSV mutants, which are acyclovir resistant (see later discussion) and for patients who require intravenous antiviral chemotherapy for severe HSV infection but are unable to tolerate acyclovir (39,40).

Suppressive Acyclovir Therapy for Herpes Simplex Virus Infection

Many AIDS patients suffer from frequently recurring HSV infection and develop new HSV recurrences shortly after antiviral chemotherapy is discontinued. Frequently recurring or chronic HSV infections can be managed with suppressive acyclovir (36-38). AIDS patients requiring suppressive therapy should receive oral acyclovir, 200 mg three times daily or 400 mg twice daily (see Table 5). Adjustment of the daily dosage can be attempted based on gastrointestinal tolerance to the drug and the overall clinical response. "Breakthrough recurrences" that develop while receiving suppressive acyclovir may be controlled by increasing the daily suppressive dosage, because these recurrences may not represent the emergence of acyclovir-resistant strains (47). Patients who demonstrate a good response to the initial oral regimen may attempt a reduction in the daily suppressive dosage. Although suppressive acyclovir therapy is approved by the Food and Drug Administration for no longer than 6 months, patients have been maintained on daily acyclovir for up to 4 years with no evidence of adverse reactions or cumulative toxicity. Individuals maintained on long-term suppressive therapy should be cautioned, however, that recurrences will likely develop after discontinuation of therapy, and that the first recurrence may be more severe than those previously experienced (36-38).

Acyclovir-Resistant Herpes Simplex Virus

The emergence of acyclovir-resistant HSV occurs infrequently and is usually due to selection of virus mutants that lack the enzyme thymidine kinase

[TK($-$) strains]. Most resistant strains have been obtained from immuno-suppressed patients treated with prolonged acyclovir therapy for severe mu-cocutaneous infections (48,49). The large number of virus in these patients probably offers an ideal setting for the selection of acyclovir-resistant iso-lates. Alternative mechanisms of resistance to acyclovir, including mutation of viral DNA polymerase and alteration of substrate specificity for thymi-dine kinase, occur less frequently in patients receiving this drug (50).

Resistance to acyclovir should be considered in all HSV-infected AIDS patients who fail to respond to acyclovir therapy, or who were previously well-controlled on acyclovir but who relapsed while maintained on therapy. Because the absorption of oral drug may be erratic, a trial of intravenous acyclovir may be attempted in patients who fail oral therapy. If resistance to acyclovir is suspected, virus isolates should be tested for in vitro suscepti-bility to the drug and for production of thymidine kinase. If acyclovir re-sistance is documented the drug should be discontinued. Serial virus cultures should be obtained, and the isolates should be tested for acyclovir suscepti-bility because susceptibility to acyclovir may return once the drug is with-drawn (48,49).

We have recovered acyclovir-resistant HSV from twelve AIDS patients with HSV infection (Erlich et al., in press). All of these patients had been treated previously with oral or intravenous acyclovir or both, and all patients pre-sented with chronic, localized mucocutaneous lesions. All of the HSV strains were highly resistant to acyclovir (ID_{50} = 7.1-91.4 μg/ml) and ganciclovir (ID_{50} = 425 μg/ml), but remained susceptible to vidarabine (ID_{50} = 1.9-23.5 μg/ml) and foscarnet (ID_{50} = 3.3-33.3 μg/ml).

Since vidarabine and foscarnet do not require viral thymidine kinase-in-duced phosphorylation for activity, these drugs should remain effective for TK($-$) acyclovir-resistant HSV. Because foscarnet remains investigational in the United States, AIDS patients with severe HSV infections due to TK($-$) strains should be treated with vidarabine 15 mg/kg per day for a minimum of 10 days (51). Herpes keratoconjunctivitis caused by TK($-$) acyclovir-resistant virus can also be managed with topical idoxuridine treatment.

Management of Varicella-Zoster Infection

In immunocompromised hosts with primary or recurrent VZV infection, acyclovir decreases the duration of virus shedding, the numbers of new le-sions, the incidence of dissemination, and the overall mortality (42,43). In view of these data, acyclovir treatment of all HIV-infected patients with VZV infection appears warranted. Management of severe primary or recurrent VZV infection in AIDS often requires intravenous acyclovir therapy, but many AIDS patients with uncomplicated, localized zoster are not ill enough

TABLE 6 Management of VZV Infections in AIDS

Clinical presentation	Modifying circumstances	Treatment
Primary infection (varicella)	None	Acyclovir 30 mg/kg per day IV[a] or acyclovir 600-800 mg p.o. five times daily[a,b]
Recurrent infection (zoster)	None	Acyclovir 30 mg/kg per day IV or acyclovir 600-800 mg p.o. five times daily[a,b]
Recurrent infection (zoster)	Cutaneous or visceral dissemination	Acyclovir 30 mg/kg per day IV[a,c]

[a]Treatment should be continued until all external lesions are crusted or reepithelialized.
[b]Oral acyclovir is not approved by FDA for this purpose.
[c]Treatment should be continued for at least 10 days.

to require hospitalization. The decision on whether or not to hospitalize an individual patient for intravenous antiviral chemotherapy must be based on several factors, including the severity of the infection, the immune status of the host, and whether visceral or cutaneous dissemination has occurred (Table 6).

AIDS patients with disseminated VZV infection—either cutaneous or visceral—should be hospitalized and treated with intravenous acyclovir 30 mg/kg a day in three divided doses (with dosage adjustment in renal failure; see Table 2). Treatment should be continued for at least 10 days or until all external lesions are crusted. Oral acyclovir in the standard dosage regimen (200 mg five times daily) does not result in serum drug levels adequate to inhibit VZV in tissue culture (45) and is not approved in the United States for the treatment of VZV infection. Higher dosages of oral acyclovir (600 to 800 mg five times daily) produce virustatic serum drug levels and is efficacious in the management of acute zoster (52). This regimen is costly, however, and may be poorly tolerated because of gastrointestinal side effects.

Although some studies have suggested that the use of steroids reduces the incidence of postherpetic neuralgia, other studies have failed to confirm an overall beneficial effect. Steroids should not be used in AIDS patients with zoster because postherpetic neuralgia is infrequent in this population, and the potential immunosuppressive effect of these drugs outweighs any possible benefits.

ACKNOWLEDGMENT

The author was supported by Public Health Service grant 5-T32-AI07234 from the National Institutes of Health.

REFERENCES

1. Nahmias, A. J. and Josey, W. E. (1982). Herpes simplex viruses 1 and 2. In *Viral Infections of Humans: Epidemiology and Control*, 2nd ed. (Evans, A., ed.). New York, Plenum Press, pp. 351-372.

2. Lafferty, W. E., Coombs, R. W., Benedetti, J., Critchlow, C., and Corey, L. (1987). Recurrences after oral and genital herpes simplex virus infection: Influence of site of infection and viral type. *N. Engl. J. Med. 316*:1444-1449.

3. Rogers, M. F., Morens, D. M., Stewart, J. A. et al. (1983). National case control study of Kaposi's sarcoma and *Pneumocystis carinii* pneumonia in homosexual men: Part 2, Laboratory results. *Ann. Intern. Med. 99*:151-158.

4. Nerurkar, L., Goedert, J., Wallen, W., Madden, D., and Sever, J. (1983). Study of antiviral antibodies in sera of homosexual men. *Fed. Proc. 42*:6109.

5. Weller, T. H. (1983). Varicella and herpes zoster: Changing concepts of the natural history, control, and importance of a not-so-benign virus (Parts 1 and 2). *N. Engl. J. Med. 309*:1362-1368, 1434-1440.

6. Dolin, R., Reichman, R. C., Mazur, M. H., and Whitley, R. J. (1978). Herpes zoster and varicella infections in immunosuppressed patients. *Ann. Intern. Med. 89*:375-388.

7. Cone, L. A. and Schiffman, M. A. (1984). Herpes zoster and the acquired immunodeficiency syndrome [Letter]. *Ann. Intern. Med. 100*:462.

8. Friedman-Kien, A. E., Lafleur, F. L., Gendler, E. et al. (1986). Herpes zoster: A possible early clinical sign for development of acquired immunodeficiency syndrome in high-risk individuals. *J. Am. Acad. Dermatol. 14*:1023-1028.

9. Verroust, F., Lemay, D., and Laurian, Y. (1987). High frequency of herpes zoster in young hemophiliacs [Letter]. *N. Engl. J. Med. 316*:166-167.

10. Sandor, E., Croxson, T. S., Millman, A., and Mildvan, D. (1984). Herpes zoster ophthalmicus in patients at risk for AIDS. *N. Engl. J. Med. 310*:1118-1119.

11. Corey, L. and Spear, P. G. (1986). Infections with herpes simplex viruses (Parts 1 and 2). *N. Engl. J. Med. 314*:686-91, 749-757.

12. Armstrong, D., Gold, J. W. M., Dryjanski, B. J. et al. (1985). Treatment of infections in patients with the acquired immunodeficiency syndrome. *Ann. Intern. Med. 103*:738-743.

13. Quinnan, G. V., Masur, H., Rook, A. H. et al. (1984). Herpes simplex infections in the acquired immune deficiency syndrome. *JAMA 252*:72-77.

14. Seligman, M., Pinching, A. J., Rosen, F. S. et al. (1987). Immunology of human immunodeficiency virus infection and the acquired immunodeficiency syndrome: An update. *Ann. Intern. Med. 107*:234-242.

15. CDC (1987). Revision of the CDC surveillance case definition for acquired immunodeficiency syndrome. *MMWR 36*(Suppl.):1S-15S.

16. Spruance, S. L., Overall, J. C., Kern, E. R. et al. (1977). The natural history of recurrent herpes simplex labialis: Implications for antiviral therapy. *N. Engl. J. Med. 297*:68-75.

17. Straus, S. E., Smith, H. A., Brickman, C., de Miranda, P., McClaren, C., and Keeney, R. E. (1982). Acyclovir for chronic mucocutaneous herpes simplex virus infection in immunosuppressed patients. *Ann. Intern. Med. 96*:270-277.

18. Corey, L., Adams, H. G., Brown, Z. A., and Holmes, K. K. (1983). Genital herpes simplex virus infections: Clinical manifestations, course, and complications. *Ann. Intern. Med. 98*:958-972.

19. Corey, L. and Holmes, K. K. (1983). Genital herpes simplex virus infections: Current concepts in diagnosis, therapy, and prevention. *Ann. Intern. Med. 98*: 973-983.

20. Whitley, R. J., Levin, M., Barton, N. et al. (1984). Infections caused by herpes simplex virus in the immunocompromised host: Natural history and topical acyclovir therapy. *J. Infect. Dis. 150*:323-329.

21. Chapel, T., Brown, W. J., Jeffries, C., and Stewart, J. A. (1978). The microbiological flora of penile ulcerations. *J. Infect. Dis. 137*:50-57.

22. Siegel, F. P., Lopez, C., Hammer, G. S. et al. (1981). Severe acquired immunodeficiency in male homosexuals, manifested by chronic perianal ulcerative herpes simplex lesions. *N. Engl. J. Med. 305*:1439-1444.

23. Goodell, S. E., Quinn, T. C., McKritchian, E., Schuffler, M. D., Holmes, K. K., and Corey, L. (1983). Herpes simplex proctitis in homosexual men: Clinical, sigmoidoscopic, and histopathologic features. *N. Engl. J. Med. 308*:868-871.

24. Dix, R. D., Waitzman, D. M., Follansbee, S. et al. (1985). Herpes simplex virus type 2 encephalitis in two homosexual men with persistent adenopathy. *Ann. Neurol. 17*:203-206.

25. Dix, R. D., Bredeson, D. E., Davis, R. L., and Mills, J. (1985). Herpesvirus neurologic diseases associated with AIDS: Recovery of viruses from CNS tissues, peripheral nerve and CSF. *Abstr. Int. Conf. AIDS.* Atlanta, Georgia, Abstr. M82.

26. Nahmias, A. J., Whitley, R. J., Visintine, A. N. et al. (1982). Herpes simplex virus type 2 encephalitis: Laboratory evaluations and their diagnostic significance. *J. Infect. Dis. 146*:829-836.

27. Kahlon, J., Chatterjee, S., Lakeman, F. D., Lee, F., Nahmias, A. J., and Whitley, R. J. (1987). Detection of antibodies to herpes simplex virus in the cerebrospinal fluid of patients with herpes simplex encephalitis. *J. Infect. Dis. 155*: 38-44.

28. Cole, E. L., Meisler, D. M., Calabrese, L. H. et al. (1984). Herpes zoster ophthalmicus and acquired immune deficiency syndrome. *Arch. Ophthalmol. 102*: 1027-1029.

29. Ryder, J. W., Croen, K., Kleinschmidt-DeMasters, B. K., Ostrove, J. M., Straus, S. E., and Cohn, D. L. (1986). Progressive encephalitis three months after resolution of cutaneous zoster in a patient with AIDS. *Ann. Neurol. 19*:182-188.

30. Drew, W. L. and Rawls, W. E. (1985). Herpes simplex viruses. In *Manual of Clinical Microbiology*, 4th ed. (Lennette, E. H., Balows, A., Hausler, W. J., and Shadomy, H. J., eds.). Washington, D.C., American Society for Microbiology, pp. 705-710.

31. Moseley, R. C., Corey, L., Benjamin, D. et al. (1981). Comparison of viral isolation, direct immunofluorescence, and indirect immunoperoxidase techniques for detection of genital herpes simplex virus infection. *J. Clin. Microbiol. 13*: 913-918.

32. Schmidt, N. J. (1985). Varicella-zoster virus. In *Manual of Clinical Microbiology*, 4th ed. (Lennette, E. H., Balows, A., Hausler, W. J., and Shadomy, H. J., eds.). Washington, D.C., American Society for Microbiology, pp. 720-727.
33. Crane, L. R., Gutterman, P. A., Chapel, T. et al. (1980). Incubation of swab materials with herpes simplex virus. *J. Infect. Dis. 141*:531.
34. Pruneda, R. C. and Almanza, I. (1987). Centrifugation-shell vial technique for rapid detection of herpes simplex virus cytopathic effect in Vero cells. *J. Clin. Microbiol. 25*:423-424.
35. Shepp, D. H., Newton, B. A., Dandliker, P. S., Flournoy, N., and Meyers, J. D. (1985). Oral acyclovir therapy for mucocutaneous herpes simplex virus infections in immunocompromised marrow transplant recipients. *Ann. Intern. Med. 102*:783-785.
36. Wade, J. C., Newton, B., Flournoy, N., and Meyers, J. D. (1984). Oral acyclovir for prevention of herpes simplex virus reactivation after marrow transplantation. *Ann. Intern. Med. 100*:823-828.
37. Straus, S. E., Seidlin, M., Takiff, H., Jacobs, D., Bowen, D., and Smith, H. A. (1984). Oral acyclovir to suppress recurring herpes simplex virus infections in immunodeficient patients. *Ann. Intern. Med. 100*:522-524.
38. Douglas, J. M., Critchlow, C., Benedetti, J. et al. (1984). Double blind study of oral acyclovir for suppression of recurrences of genital herpes simplex virus infection. *N. Engl. J. Med. 310*:1551-1556.
39. Skoldenberg, B., Alestig, K., Burman, L. et al. (1984). Acyclovir versus vidarabine in herpes simplex encephalitis. *Lancet 2*:707-711.
40. Whitley, R. J., Alford, C. A., Hirsch, M. S. et al. (1986). Vidarabine versus acyclovir therapy in herpes simplex encephalitis. *N. Engl. J. Med. 314*:144-149.
41. Wade, J. C., Newton, B., McLaren, C., Flournoy, N., Keeney, R. E., and Meyers, J. D. (1982). Intravenous acyclovir to treat mucocutaneous herpes simplex virus infection after marrow transplantation. *Ann. Intern. Med. 96*:265-269.
42. Balfour, H. H., Bean, B., Laskin, O. L. et al. (1983). Acyclovir halts progression of herpes zoster in immunocompromised patients. *N. Engl. J. Med. 308*:1448-1453.
43. Shepp, D. H., Dandliker, P. S., and Meyers, J. D. (1986). Treatment of varicella zoster virus infection in severely immunocompromised patients. *N. Engl. J. Med. 314*:208-212.
44. Corey, L., Nahmias, A. J., Guinan, M. E., Benedetti, J. K., Critchlow, C. W., and Holmes, K. K. (1982). A trial of topical acyclovir in genital herpes simplex virus infections. *N. Engl. J. Med. 306*:1313-1319.
45. Laskin, O. (1984). Acyclovir: Pharmacology and clinical experience. *Arch. Intern. Med. 144*:1241-1246.
46. Kinghorn, G. R., Abeywickreme, I., Jeavons, M. et al. (1986). Efficacy of combined treatment with oral and topical acyclovir in first episode genital herpes. *Genitourin. Med. 62*:186-188.
47. Nusinoff-Lehrman, S., Douglas, J. M., Corey, L., and Barry, D. W. (1986). Recurrent genital herpes and suppressive oral acyclovir therapy: Relation between clinical outcome and in-vitro sensitivity. *Ann. Intern. Med. 104*:786-790.

48. Crumpacker, C. S., Schnipper, L. E., Marlowe, S. I., Kowalsky, P. N., Hershey, B. J., and Levin, M. J. (1982). Resistance to antiviral drugs of herpes simplex virus isolated from a patient treated with acyclovir. *N. Engl. J. Med. 306*:343-346.

49. Schnipper, L. E., Crumpacker, C. S., Marlowe, S. I., Kowalsky, P. N., Hershey, B. J., and Levin, M. J. (1982). Drug resistant herpes simplex virus in vitro and after acyclovir treatment in an immunocompromised patient. *Am. J. Med. 73*: 387-392.

50. Sacks, S. L., Reece, D. E., Galloway, P., and Moquin, J. P. (1987). Acyclovir resistance in herpes simplex virus isolates from a patient with esophagitis: A thymidine kinase positive, foscarnet-resistant strain with response to intravenous foscarnet. *Abstr. 27th Intersci. Conf. Antimicrob. Agents Chemother.*, New York, 1987, (Abstr. 1155).

51. Whitley, R. J., Soong, S. J., Dolin, R. et al. (1977). Adenine arabinoside therapy of biopsy proved herpes simplex encephalitis: National Institute of Allergy and Infectious Diseases collaborative antiviral study. *N. Engl. J. Med. 297*:289-294.

52. McKendrick, M. W., McGill, J. I., White, J. E., and Wood, M. J. (1986). Oral acyclovir and herpes zoster. *Br. Med. J. 293*:1529-1532.

11
Cytomegalovirus Disease in Acquired Immunodeficiency Disease

Mark A. Jacobson *University of California and San\Francisco General Hospital, San Francisco, California*

Among the viral infections affecting patients with the acquired immunodeficiency syndrome (AIDS), cytomegalovirus (CMV) is the most common cause of life-threatening disease. Although prior CMV infection is found in 70% to 90% of the general population, serious disease caused by CMV is largely confined to neonates or immunocompromised hosts.

As with other human herpesvirus infections (herpes simplex, varicella-zoster, Epstein-Barr, and herpesvirus-6 viruses), a latent state follows primary CMV infection. Primary infection occurs in childhood or young adulthood in 30% to 50% of the population. In the latent state, CMV genomic material is present in host cells, but virions are absent (1). Reactivation can occur at any time after primary infection, resulting in renewed shedding of virus (1). This change from latency to reactivation is most likely to occur during an immunosuppressed state, but it may also occur spontaneously.

Asymptomatic reactivated CMV infection is commonly associated with human immunodeficiency virus (HIV) infection. Among HIV-infected homosexual men, more than half shed CMV in urine or semen (2). Ninety percent or more of patients with AIDS have had histopathologic evidence of CMV infection in autopsy series, and half or more AIDS patients may have CMV viremia (3-5).

Although reactivated CMV infection is very common in the HIV-infected population, serious end-organ CMV disease (e.g., retinitis, colitis, encephalitis) is considerably less frequent. Because of the overlap between CMV infection and serious CMV disease, prevalence data for CMV in AIDS must be interpreted carefully. According to San Francisco Public Health Department statistics, only 1.2% of AIDS cases have had serious CMV disease as their primary case-defining diagnosis (6). However, we have followed approximately 760 AIDS patients at San Francisco General Hospital during 1986. The prevalence of serious CMV retinitis or gastrointestinal disease in this population was 5.7% for retinitis and 2.2% for gastrointestinal disease (7). In a UCLA ophthalmologic autopsy series, 8 of 30 (27%) patients had evidence of CMV retinitis (8). Selection bias may have contributed to this high figure.

The prevalence of clinically evident CMV pneumonitis is difficult to estimate. Cytomegalovirus was recovered from lung tissue or bronchoalveolar lavage fluid at bronchoscopy in 43% of 221 AIDS patients in one series (9). However, a positive culture could indicate either colonization or invasive infection. Because CMV is usually isolated from bronchoscopy specimens in the presence of other opportunistic pathogens, the clinical significance of CMV isolation from the lung is unclear (10).

LABORATORY DIAGNOSIS

When the diagnosis of CMV disease is suspected, laboratory confirmation of CMV in the target organ is required. For retinitis, direct retinal biopsy is neither practical nor safe. Because the ophthalmologic findings in CMV retinitis are quite specific for CMV disease, laboratory confirmation of active systemic infection by recovering the virus from blood or urine is adequate. However, with all other forms of CMV end-organ disease, a biopsy specimen from the target organ should be taken to confirm active CMV infection.

The histopathologic lesions of CMV infection consist of enlarged cells containing characteristic intranuclear or paranuclear cytoplasmic inclusions. The presence of such lesions in endothelial, epithelial, or macrophage cells, with surrounding inflammatory cells, is almost certainly pathognomonic of CMV disease, and treatment may be initiated based on histologic results alone. However, in our experience, patients may have histopathologic changes typical of CMV, with positive cultures, without disease that requires treatment.

Cultures should be obtained before initiating therapy. This serves the purpose of confirming target-organ infection, and cultures of blood and urine can be followed to monitor the efficacy of therapy. See Chapter 21 for further details of culture technique.

The importance of obtaining virologic confirmation of CMV disease is emphasized by a recent report suggesting that some patients, in whom the

disease has been diagnosed as CMV colitis, may actually be infected by adenovirus (11).

CYTOMEGALOVIRUS RETINITIS

The onset of CMV retinitis is usually heralded by blurred vision, decreased
visual acuity, and visual field defects, almost always affecting one eye more
than the other (12,13). Pain is absent, and visual loss usually progresses over
time. Most AIDS-related CMV retinitis infections occur in patients that already carry a diagnosis of AIDS, usually on the basis of previously diagnosed *Pneumocystis carinii* pneumonia. In 1986, we treated 43 patients with
newly diagnosed CMV retinitis at San Francisco General Hospital. Over
90% of these patients already had an AIDS diagnosis (7).

By funduscopic examination, CMV retinitis is characterized by granular
white lesions that coalesce and spread with time (8,14-18). Typically there
are fluffy, white lesions, which are often associated with hemorrhage, and
follow a vascular pattern of distribution [(Fig. 1) see Plate IV, facing page
151 (12,16,19,20)]. Histopathologically, the characteristic appearance is of
full-thickness retinal necrosis and swollen retinal cells with intranuclear and
intracytoplasmic inclusions (8,17). Uveitis may be present, although usually
mild in comparison with the degree of retinal inflammation. With severe
retinal disease, diffuse vitreous inflammation may also occur, making it difficult to visualize the fundus.

The natural history of untreated CMV retinitis has been well described
for previous non-AIDS, immunocompromised patients. Among transplant
patients, reduction in immunosuppressive drug therapy is frequently followed
by spontaneous healing of retinitis, leaving an atrophic scar (16,20). However, in lymphoma patients, retinitis tends to progress and is associated with
substantial visual loss (16,20).

The largest series of AIDS patients followed with untreated CMV retinitis
was reported by Holland et al. (8). None of the eight patients described survived more than 6 weeks after retinitis was diagnosed. Acute inflammation
was more prominent than in previously described immunocompromised patients. These few anecdotal case reports suggest that untreated CMV retinitis
in AIDS is a relentlessly progressive disease, eventually leading to blindness.
Retinitis patients are also susceptible to retinal detachment. This complication often occurs during the healing stage, in areas of the retina thinned by
retinal necrosis (21).

The differential diagnosis of retinal lesions in AIDS includes cotton wool
spots (present in half of patients with AIDS), retinal hemorrhages, Roth
spots, choroidal granulomas, retinal periphlebitis, and central nervous sys-

TABLE 1   Diagnostic Criteria for AIDS-Related CMV Disease

Retinitis
  patches of fluffy white retinal opacification, often with associated hemorrhage
    and following a vascular distribution
  no other likely explanation for retinal findings
  recovery of CMV from any body site (optional)
  a clinical response to ganciclovir or foscarnet therapy (stabilization or decrease in
    retinal inflammation) may be confirmatory
Gastrointestinal disease
  symptoms referable to colitis (diarrhea with or without abdominal pain), esopha-
    gitis (dysphagia, substernal burning pain), or gastritis (epigastric pain)
  colonoscopy or endoscopy reveals focal or diffuse areas of erythema with mucosal
    edema and erosions
  biopsy of involved gastrointestinal mucosa reveals typical histopathologic changes
    of CMV infection and other stains and cultures are negative for pathogens
  a positive culture of the biopsy specimen later confirms the diagnosis
Pneumonitis
  hypoxemia
  chest x-ray film reveals diffuse infiltrates
  transbronchial or open-lung biopsy reveals typical histopathologic changes of CMV
    infection, and other stains and cultures are negative for pathogens
  a positive culture of the biopsy specimen later confirms the diagnosis

tem toxoplasmosis (8). Because experience is a requisite to differentiate between these entities fundoscopically, an ophthalmologist should always confirm the diagnosis of CMV retinitis.

The diagnosis of CMV retinitis is usually based on the criteria in Table 1
(12,19,21).

CYTOMEGALOVIRUS GASTROINTESTINAL DISEASE

Symptomatic CMV involvement of the gastrointestinal tract has been increasingly recognized in patients with AIDS. Most data about this clinical
entity come from individual case reports, in which clinical syndromes of
colitis, gastritis, and esophagitis have since been described along with histologic evidence of severe CMV vasculitis in these end organs (22-29). Cytomegalovirus has also been implicated as a primary gastrointestinal pathogen
in renal transplant patients who developed a syndrome of colonic ulceration
and lower gastrointestinal bleeding (30). We treated 17 AIDS patients with
CMV gastrointestinal disease in the last year at San Francisco General Hospital—11 with colitis, 4 with esophagitis, and 2 with gastritis (7). Five of 17

patients (29%) had CMV gastrointestinal disease as their primary AIDS-defining diagnosis. Among patients with CMV colitis, 100% presented with diarrhea (2 to 20 liquid stools per day) and 82% with abdominal pain. Abdominal pain was usually intermittent and cramplike, although occasionally continuous. Other investigators have reported hematochezia or perforation as complications of CMV colitis in AIDS patients (27,28,31,32).

In our experience, CMV gastrointestinal disease is a more severe systemic disease than CMV retinitis. The mean Karnofsky performance score at time of diagnosis was 70 for retinitis patients compared with 50 for gastrointestinal disease patients (7). Also, retinitis patients were more likely to become CMV culture-negative during therapy and to survive longer than patients with gastrointestinal disease (7).

Among patients with CMV colitis, colonoscopy usually reveals focal or diffuse areas of erythema, submucosal edema and hemorrhage (occasionally appearing as "thumbprints"), and mucosal erosions [(Fig. 2) see Plate IV, facing page 151 (29)]. Hemorrhage and mucosal ulcers 0.5 to 1 cm in diameter are also commonly observed. In most instances these changes occur distally in the colon, well within reach of the flexible 60-cm sigmoidoscope. The barium enema radiograph is abnormal in most patients, demonstrating a variety of diffuse, segmental, and focal colonic abnormalities (29). Colonic biopsy may reveal nonspecific inflammatory cells and colonic epithelial, connective tissue, and endothelial cells containing cytoplasmic and intranuclear inclusions. Histologic changes and positive viral cultures have been found in areas of normal-looking mucosa from patients suspected of CMV colitis. A characteristic histopathologic finding in CMV colitis is submucosal endothelial cells bearing CMV inclusions and associated with neutrophil infiltration of blood vessels and vascular occlusion (Fig. 3; 27). Without specific therapy, most patients have a prolonged, indolent, symptomatic course, and occasional patients suffer rapidly progressive disease leading to severe hemorrhagic colitis, colonic perforation, or peritonitis (29).

The differential diagnosis of CMV colitis includes *Campylobacter jejuni* infection, shigellosis, salmonellosis, *Mycobacterium-avium* complex disseminated infection, cryptosporidiosis, amebiasis, *Clostridium difficile* colitis, vasculitis, and idiopathic ulcerative colitis. The optimal diagnostic workup for a patient with AIDS or with AIDS-related complex (ARC), with persistent diarrhea, includes sending stool samples for routine bacterial culture, examination for ova and parasite, modified Kinyoun stain for cryptosporidia, and assay for *C. difficile* toxin. Stool may also be stained and cultured for mycobacteria; however, because of colonizing atypical mycobacteria, such tests may not be diagnostically reliable. If all of these tests are negative, a flexible sigmoidoscopy is indicated and should include a biopsy for histo-

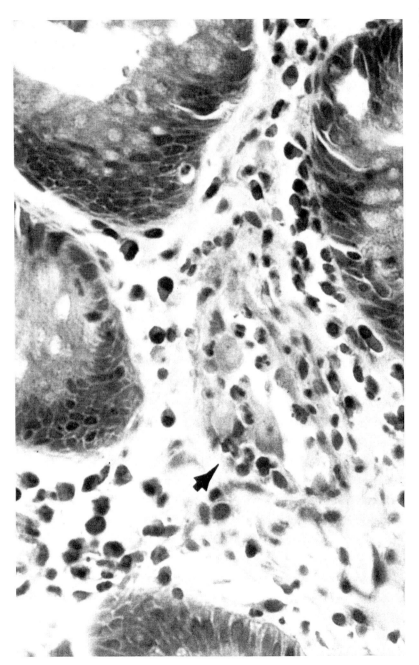

FIGURE 3 Photomicrograph of cytomegalovirus colitis demonstrating endothelial cells (arrow) with cytomegalovirus inclusions (courtesy of Dr. John Cello).

logic examination and viral culture as well as repeat bacterial cultures and special stains for ova and parasites.

The diagnosis of CMV colitis can be made only by a rectal or colonic biopsy specimen that demonstrates typical histopathology or growing CMV in cell culture. A positive CMV culture of the specimen can also later confirm the diagnosis. Stool and blood cultures for virus are of little use in the workup or diagnosis of CMV colitis.

Cytomegaloviral esophagitis or gastritis may appear as severe dysphagia, odynophagia, substernal or epigastric pain. In our experience at San Francisco General Hospital, esophagitis patients have severe dysphagia, odynophagia, and variable substernal chest pain, whereas gastritis patients have severe continuous epigastric pain (7). Endoscopy reveals large, shallow mucosal ulcers, erythema, and edema (23). Radiographic findings are nonspecific and include esophageal mucosal thickening, focal ulcers, and multiple small, filling defects, large rugal folds, and gastric ulcers. Esophageal or gastric biopsy specimens show the same histologic appearance as CMV colitis. As in CMV colitis, untreated patients tend to have protracted, progressive symptoms that may be complicated by perforation (22).

The differential diagnosis of CMV esophagogastritis includes candidal esophagitis, herpes simplex esophagitis, and reflux esophagitis. Differentiation is best made by endoscopy, with esophageal biopsies for viral culture (herpes simplex virus and CMV), and biopsy of inflamed mucosa for histologic studies and viral culture (herpes simplex virus, candida, and CMV).

In the AIDS or ARC patient who presents with dysphagia or epigastric pain, especially with oral thrush, an empiric trial of ketoconazole may be diagnostic for esophageal candidiasis. If dysphagia persists despite a course of ketoconazole, the patient should then undergo endoscopy to rule out CMV or herpes simplex esophagitis.

CYTOMEGALOVIRUS PNEUMONITIS

In retrospective autopsy series, CMV inclusions were observed in lungs of 90% or more of AIDS patients (3,4). These inclusions were frequently associated with focal or diffuse pneumonitis and often occurred in the absence of other pathogens, suggesting that CMV might be an important opportunistic pulmonary pathogen in AIDS; however, such studies do not establish a clear etiologic link between CMV lung infection and CMV pneumonitis.

In clinical reviews of AIDS patients with active, symptomatic pneumonitis, CMV is commonly demonstrated in bronchoscopy specimens by culture or characteristic cytopathic effect (8,10). Yet most of these patients have other coexistent opportunistic infections. Rarely, is CMV the only pulmonary pathogen isolated (10). The importance of CMV coexisting with other opportunistic pulmonary pathogens in AIDS is unclear. In one study, respiratory failure and death in *P. carinii* pneumonia were associated with the presence of coexistent CMV infection (4); however, in another, recovery of CMV from the lung had no prognostic value in predicting mortality or duration of hospitalization (33).

Thus, CMV pneumonitis is not a well-characterized syndrome in patients with AIDS. In the few well-documented cases of pneumonitis caused by CMV alone, fever, dyspnea, and nonproductive cough were reported (34). Interstitial, rather than alveolar, infiltrates were described from chest x-ray films. However, the clinical findings have ranged from asymptomatic to rapidly fatal pneumonia.

In our experience, CMV pneumonitis is almost always an incidental diagnosis, resulting from bronchoscopy performed in a patient with symptomatic interstitial lung disease in whom other pulmonary pathogens are present (M. A. Jacobson et al., unpublished data). The isolated presence of CMV in bronchoscopy specimens may or may not be associated with progressive clinical pneumonitis (M. A. Jacobson et al., unpublished data).

CYTOMEGALOVIRUS ENCEPHALITIS

Evidence of CMV involvement in the central nervous system has been described in up to 30% of AIDS patients (35,36). Pathologic findings have included microglial nodules, isolated inclusion-bearing cells, focal parenchymal necrosis, necrotizing ventriculoencephalitis, and necrotizing radiculomyelitis; yet no clear correlation of these findings with a clinical syndrome has emerged (36). As with CMV pneumonitis, coinfection with other opportunistic pathogens, as well as HIV itself, is commonly present so that a distinct encephalitis syndrome attributable to CMV is difficult to define. However, Post et al. (37) described six AIDS patients with a progressive syndrome of altered mental status, fever, and confusion, who, at autopsy, had intranuclear inclusions typical of CMV in the brain and no other evidence of opportunistic central nervous infection. Neither a computed tomography (CT) scan nor cerebrospinal fluid analysis showed specific findings that might have led to an antemortem diagnosis. A CMV polyradiculopathy syndrome associated with paralysis has also been recently described (38).

CYTOMEGALOVIRUS LIVER DISEASE

In autopsy series, up to 44% of AIDS patients have evidence of hepatic CMV infection (3,39). However, in an autopsy review correlating histologic findings to clinical data, hepatic inclusions were seen in only 5% of patients with CMV involvement of other organs, and those patients had mildly elevated alkaline phosphatase with normal bilirubin values (40). We have recently reviewed our cases of CMV retinitis, gastrointestinal disease, and viremia. A syndrome of markedly abnormal cholestatic liver function test values was noted in 20% (4 of 20) of patients with CMV retinitis versus 50% (8 of 16) of patients with CMV gastrointestinal disease (41). Among patients with no evidence of CMV end-organ disease, this cholestatic pattern was present in 40% of those with CMV viremia compared with 11% of those with negative viral blood cultures ($p = 0.02$) (41). This suggests that cholestasis may result directly from CMV hepatocellular or biliary injury.

Cytomegaloviral biliary pathology has been correlated to clinical disease in AIDS. AIDS patients with acalculous cholecystitis and CMV inclusions present in gallbladder epithelial cells have been described (42). Recently, a syndrome of papillary stenosis and sclerosing cholangitis was reported in AIDS patients. Both cryptosporidia and CMV have been implicated as causal agents (43). The patients described had tender hepatomegaly, markedly elevated alkaline phosphatase, mildly elevated transaminases, and normal bilirubin levels. Bacterial cholangitis has been a common secondary complication. Clinical improvement has resulted from endoscopic papillotomy in some cases.

CYTOMEGALOVIRUS ADRENALITIS

AIDS patients with symptomatic hypoadrenalism during life and adrenal necrosis with CMV inclusions at autopsy have been described (44). At San Francisco General Hospital, about one-third of AIDS patients with CMV retinitis or gastrointestinal disease have had abnormal adrenal function (45). The abnormal pattern most commonly seen has been a high baseline cortisol level, exceeding 17 μg/dl, with a subnormal incremental response to synthetic adrenocorticotropic hormone stimulation (M. A. Jacobson, unpublished data). Recent data show that some of the adrenal functional deficit observed in AIDS patients is due to central nervous system disease, i.e., decreased corticotropin-releasing factor (46). When CMV patients develop symptoms compatible with hypoadrenalism (e.g., postural hypotension, low-grade fever, or fatigue) it is appropriate to test for hypoadrenalism, even in the absence of hyperkalemia or hyponatremia.

THERAPY FOR CYTOMEGALOVIRUS DISEASE

Ganciclovir

Ganciclovir (9-[2-hydroxy-1-(hydroxymethyl)ethoxymethyl]guanine, DHPG, BW759U) is a nucleoside analolgue of thymidine that inhibits viral DNA synthesis and exhibits in vitro activity against all human herpesviruses. Although structurally similar to acyclovir, ganciclovir's greater activity towards CMV appears to be due to this drug's more efficient phosphorylation in CMV-infected cells (47). The ED_{50} (minimum dose required to reduce CMV plaque formation by 50%) of ganciclovir for most strains of human CMV has been reported to range from 1 to 6.4 μmol (48,49). Most CMV isolates do not become resistant to ganciclovir during therapy with this drug (50).

The pharmacokinetics of ganciclovir in humans are remarkable for the drug's complete lack of metabolism (99% renal excretion), mean serum steady-state half-life of 3.3 hr, poor oral bioavailability, and adequate penetration into cerebrospinal fluid (51-53). In adults with normal renal function who receive a typical induction course of 2.5 mg/kg of intravenous ganciclovir every 8 hr, peak and trough steady-state plasma levels average 18 to 24 μmol and 1 to 2 μmol, respectively, with cerebrospinal fluid levels of 2.0 to 2.7 μmol (51).

Ganciclovir therapy for serious end-organ CMV disease is usually administered in two phases. Initially, there is an induction phase consisting of 2.5 mg ganciclovir per kilogram body weight given intravenously every 8 hr or 5 mg/kg given every 12 hr over 10 to 14 days (21,34,54,55). Because clinical and virologic relapse often has occurred after the induction course, most patients receive long-term maintenance ganciclovir therapy after the induction phase (21,34,54,55). This second, maintenance phase is usually administered as a single daily dose of ganciclovir (5 to 7.5 mg/kg) given 5 to 7 days per week. Ganciclovir dosage should be reduced if the estimated creatinine clearance is less than 50 ml/min, and it probably should not be administered to patients whose creatinine clearance is less than 10 ml/min.

Ganciclovir treatment is commonly limited by dose-related, reversible neutropenia. A decrease in absolute neutrophil count by 50% from baseline or to less than 1000/μL has been reported in up to 68% of patients receiving this drug (34,56). Neutropenia severe enough to require dosage adjustment (< 800 neutrophils per microliter) occurred in 31% of patients receiving maintenance ganciclovir at San Francisco General Hospital (7). However, in our experience, absolute neutrophil counts as low as 800 are well tolerated, although occasional cases of life-threatening bacteremia (especially in patients with central intravenous indwelling catheters) have occurred)7). In patients who develop serious neutropenia (less than 500 cells/μL) during ganciclovir therapy, we temporarily discontinue the drug until the absolute neutrophil count is greater than 800 cells/μL. Ganciclovir is then reinstituted at full dose (if induction therapy) or with a 30% to 50% dose reduction (if maintenance therapy).

We noted thrombocytopenia requiring dose reduction in 5% (2 of 44) patients (7). Anemia, though commonly associated with ganciclovir therapy, did not bear a direct relationship to ganciclovir dosage and may have been a result of underlying disease (7). Rare adverse reactions that have been reported to occur in association with ganciclovir include disorientation, psychosis, hepatitis, anorexia, nausea, rash, and eosinophilia. As the pH of ganciclovir solution is about 10.5, pain or phlebitis at the infusion site is common with peripheral intravenous infusions (45).

At doses equivalent to those used to treat humans, the drug has caused azoospermia in all animal species tested (45). Human data regarding testicular toxicity are not yet available.

In uncontrolled, prospective trials, ganciclovir induction therapy has been reported to stabilize or improve CMV retinitis in 80% or more of AIDS patients treated (19,21,24,54,56). This has been paralleled by a decreased recovery of CMV from blood and urine during therapy. With cessation of therapy, retinitis has frequently progressed concomitant with virologic relapse. There have been no placebo-controlled comparative studies of ganciclovir induction therapy for retinitis. Considering the historical data on untreated CMV retinitis in AIDS and the stabilization described in most patients treated with ganciclovir, placebo-controlled studies of ganciclovir are no longer ethical for immediately sight-threatening disease.

At San Francisco General Hospital, we recently completed a controlled trial of ganciclovir maintenance therapy (7). Sixteen AIDS patients with CMV retinitis, who all received a 10-day course of ganciclovir induction therapy, either began daily ganciclovir maintenance therapy (5 mg/kg given 5 days/week) immediately following induction or had further therapy deferred until there was evidence of retinitis progression. Median time to retinitis progression was 54 days for the immediate maintenance group versus 19 days for the deferred maintenance group ($p = 0.01$, log rank test). Among all retinitis patients treated at San Francisco General Hospital in 1986, only 9% of viral cultures obtained while patients received maintenance ganciclovir were positive for CMV compared with 35% of those obtained off maintenance therapy ($p = 0.01$, Fisher exact test) (7).

Ganciclovir therapy delays, but does not halt, the progression of CMV retinitis, and suppresses, but does not eradicate, CMV shedding in patients with AIDS. Hence, some form of lifelong maintenance regimen is requisite to prevent blindness in these patients. Studies of other routes of ganciclovir therapy (oral, intravitreal) have been undertaken in an attempt to minimize toxicity or improve convenience of administration. Orally administered ganciclovir might be a possible alternative for maintenance therapy (53). Four patients given repeated oral ganciclovir doses, 20 mg/kg, at 6-hr intervals demonstrated no evidence of drug intolerance and achieved mean steady-state peak and trough plasma ganciclovir levels of 2.96 μmol and 1.05 μmol. With this oral regimen, the mean drug peak exceeded the ED_{50} for most CMV isolates (51,53). Intravitreal administration of ganciclovir has been described in a few cases without apparent retinal toxicity or systemic drug absorption (57). The long elimination half-life of intravitreal ganciclovir ($<$ 13 hr) is compatible with an intermittent maintenance regimen (57).

Ganciclovir has also been shown to be effective treatment for CMV colitis, esophagitis, and gastritis. Dieterich et al. (58) reported that well over half of 65 patients with CMV gastrointestinal disease had a clinical response to ganciclovir induction therapy, defined as resolution of dysphagia or dyspepsia, 50% decrease in diarrhea, or 50% decrease in ulcer size. Relapse was common following induction, and most patients required maintenance therapy. At SFGH, we have followed 17 patients with CMV gastrointestinal disease (7). Sixty-three percent of colitis patients and 67% of esophagitis/gastritis patients had resolution of abdominal pain, and 73% of colitis patients totally resolved diarrhea with induction ganciclovir. Maintenance therapy was associated with control of diarrhea but not of pain.

There are very few data on ganciclovir efficacy for CMV pneumonitis in AIDS. Masur et al. (34) described an AIDS patient with progressive diffuse pulmonary infiltrates, hypoxemia, and lung histology consistent with CMV pneumonitis, in the absence of other causes of pneumonia. The patient's pneumonitis resolved after 10 days of ganciclovir. He remained stable for 2 months on thrice-weekly ganciclovir maintenance therapy, relapsing after maintenance ganciclovir was discontinued. In a multicenter study, seven patients with CMV pneumonitis were treated with ganciclovir (19). Four died before induction was completed, and the other three died of pulmonary failure within 7 weeks.

At San Francisco General Hospital, we currently consider ganciclovir therapy for CMV pneumonitis only if a transbronchial biopsy reveals interstitial inflammation and cytopathic changes characteristic of CMV, in the absence of other pulmonary pathogens. We have treated only three patients in four years (M. Jacobson, unpublished data).

Foscarnet

Foscarnet (trisodium phosphonoformate, PFA) is a pyrophosphate analogue that inhibits replication of all human herpesviruses and HIV at concentrations well below those achievable in human plasma (59,60). The drug has a half-life of 0.7 to 3.6 hr, is excreted by the kidneys without metabolic conversion, and has poor penetration of cerebrospinal fluid (59). Foscarnet has a very long terminal half-life (months) in bone and cartilage (59). Continuous intravenous infusion of foscarnet, 112 mg/kg a day, can achieve average steady-state plasma levels of approximately 100 μg/ml, equalling or exceeding the ED_{50} for CMV isolates (61,62). In an ongoing phase 1 study of intermittent intravenous foscarnet, we have observed that 60 mg/kg of foscarnet, given over 2 hr and repeated every 8 hr results in similar average steady-state levels (M. A. Jacobson et al., unpublished data).

Reversible nephrotoxicity, characteristically appearing as a rise in serum creatinine concentration without azotemia, is the most frequent adverse effect observed with foscarnet therapy (62,63). Hypercalcemia, hypocalcemia, hyperphosphatemia, mild anemia, reversible tremor, seizures, irritability, and superficial thrombophlebitis at the infusion site have also been reported during foscarnet administration (62,63). Bone, tooth, and cartilage histologic changes have been described in animal studies (Astra Lakemedel AB, unpublished data). The significance of these findings are unknown. Unlike ganciclovir, myelosuppression is not reported as an adverse effect of foscarnet.

Over 100 bone marrow and renal transplant patients have received foscarnet for CMV pneumonitis in Europe and Canada. A 50% to 100% clinical and virologic response has been reported in these patients (61-64). Only a prospective, randomized trial comparing ganciclovir to foscarnet therapy will determine the relative efficacy and risk/benefit of each drug as therapy for acute CMV disease.

Other Therapy

Acyclovir inhibits CMV replication in concentrations achievable with high-dose intravenous therapy (40 to 117 μmol; 50). High-dose prophylactic, intravenous acyclovir appeared to be of value in preventing CMV pneumonia in bone marrow transplant patients (65); however, studies in patients with HIV-related disease have not been done.

Desciclovir (6-deoxyacyclovir) is an investigational derivative of acyclovir that is converted in vivo to acyclovir (66). Because of the drug's high oral bioavailability, administration of desciclovir by mouth results in plasma acyclovir levels that are equivalent to those achieved with intravenous acyclovir (66). In the future, desciclovir may be of value in maintenance therapy for CMV disease.

Several 2'-deoxypurine nucleosides and pyrrolo-[2,3-d]pyrimidine nucleosides have shown in vitro activity versus CMV. These compounds also may be evaluated in future trials (67,68).

LONG-TERM OUTCOME IN AIDS-RELATED CYTOMEGALOVIRUS DISEASE

In assessing long-term visual outcome, we noted that 15 (65%) of 23 retinitis patients followed for a mean 4.3 months after induction had a corrected visual acuity of 20/30 or better in at least one eye at the time last examined; only one was legally blind (7).

One retrospective study comparing nine untreated patients with CMV disease to 18 ganciclovir-treated patients showed survival to be prolonged from a median of 2 months to 5 months (69). However, the diagnosis was made in the untreated patients several years before that in the treated patients; and no data on comparative survival post-*P. carinii* pneumonia were reported. Dieterich et al. (58) reported a significant survival advantage post-CMV diagnosis and post-*P. carinii* pneumonia diagnosis in patients who received maintenance ganciclovir (8 to 10 months) versus patients who did not receive maintenance therapy (4 to 8 months); however, comparability of the two groups' clinical characteristics was not reported (58). We observed no difference in survival between patients who were given immediate versus deferred maintenance ganciclovir therapy; however, few patients went longer than 1 month without therapy (7). Among our CMV retinitis patients, survival was a median 5.4 months from the time of CMV diagnosis and 11.5 months from the time of *P. carinii* pneumonia diagnosis. For patients with gastrointestinal CMV disease, survival from the time of CMV diagnosis (4.5 months) did not differ significantly from retinitis patients, but survival post-*P. carinii* pneumonia (7.0 months) was significantly shorter ($p < 0.05$) (7).

REFERENCES

1. Jordan, M. C. (1983). Latent infection and the elusive cytomegalovirus. *J. Infect. Dis.* 5:205-215.
2. Mintz, L., Drew, W. L., Miner, R. C., and Braff, E. H. (1983). Cytomegalovirus infections in homosexual men: An epidemiologic study. *Ann. Intern. Med.* 98: 326-329.
3. Reichert, C. M., O'Leary, T. J., Levens, D. L., Simrell, C. R., and Macher, A. M. (1983). Autopsy pathology in the acquired immune deficiency syndrome. *Am. J. Pathol.* 12:357-82.
4. Pass, H. I., Potter, D. A., Machen, A. M. et al. (1984). Thoracic manifestations of the acquired immunodeficiency syndrome. *J. Thorac. Cardiovasc. Surg.* 88:654-658.
5. Quinnan, G. V., Jr., Masur, H., Rook, A. H., Armstrong, G., Frederick, W. R., Epstein, J. et al. (1984). Herpes virus infections in the acquired immune deficiency syndrome. *JAMA* 252:72-77.
6. San Francisco Health Department (1987). AIDS Monthly Surveillance Report, January 31.

7. Jacobson, M. A., O'Donnell, J. J., Porteous, D., Feigal, D., and Mills, J. (1988). Retinal and gastrointestinal disease due to cytomegalovirus in patients with the acquired immunodeficiency syndrome. *Quart. J. Med. 67*:473-486.

8. Holland, G. N., Pepose, J. S., Petiti, T. H., Gottlieb, M. S., Yee, R. D., and Foos, R. Y. (1983). Acquired immune deficiency syndrome: Ocular manifestations. *Ophthalmology 90*:859-873.

9. Broaddus, C., Dake, M. D., Stulbarg, M. S., Golden, J., and Hopewell, P. (1985). Bronchoalveolar lavage and transbronchial biopsy for the diagnosis of pulmonary infection in AIDS. *Ann. Intern. Med. 102*:747-752.

10. Murray, J. F., Felton, C. P., Garay, S. M. et al. (1984). Pulmonary complications of the acquired immunodeficiency syndrome: Report of a National Heart, Lung and Blood Institute Workshop. *N. Engl. J. Med. 310*:1682-1688.

11. Parkin, J., Tyms, S., Roberts, A., Burnell, R., Jeffries, D., and Pinching, A. (1987). "Cytomegalovirus" colitis: Can it be caused by adenovirus? *Abstr. III Int. Conf. AIDS.* Washington, D.C., Abstr. TH8.3.

12. Palestine, A. G., Stevens, G., Lane, H. C. et al. (1986). Treatment of cytomegalovirus retinitis with dihydroxypropoxymethylguanine. *Am. J. Ophthalmol. 101*: 95-101.

13. Felsenstein, D., D'Amico, D. J., Hirsch, M. S. et al. (1985). Treatment of cytomegalovirus retinitis with 9-(2-hydroxy-1-(hydroxymethyl)ethoxymethyl)guanine. *Ann. Intern. Med. 103*:377-380.

14. Aaberg, T. M., Cesarz, T. J., and Rytel, M. W. (1972). Correlation of virology and clinical course of cytomegalovirus retinitis. *Am. J. Ophthalmol. 74*:407.

15. Murray, H., Knox, D., Green, W., and Susel, R. (1977). Cytomegalovirus retinitis in adults. *Am. J. Med. 65*:574.

16. Egbert, P., Pollard, R., Gallagher, J., and Merigan, T. C. (1980). Cytomegalovirus retinitis in immunosuppressed hosts: II. Ocular manifestations. *Ann. Intern. Med. 93*:664-670.

17. Holland, G. N., Gottlieb, M. S., and Yee, R. D. (1982). Ocular disorders associated with a new severe acquired cellular immunodeficiency syndrome. *Am. J. Ophthalmol. 93*:393-402.

18. Freidman, A. H., Orellana, J., Freeman, W. R. et al. (1983). Cytomegalovirus retinitis: A manifestation of the acquired immune deficiency syndrome. *Br. J. Ophthalmol. 67*:372-380.

19. Collaborative DHPG Treatment Study Group (1986). Treatment of serious cytomegalovirus infections with 9-(1,3-dihydroxy-2-propoxymethyl)guanine in patients with AIDS and other immunodeficiencies. *N. Engl. J. Med. 314*:801-805.

20. Pollard, R. B., Egbert, P. R., Gallagher, J. G., and Merigan, T. C. (1980). Cytomegalovirus retinitis in immunosuppressed hosts: I. Natural history and effects of treatment with adenine arabinoside. *Ann. Intern. Med. 93*:655-664.

21. Holland, G. N., Sakamoto, M. J., Hardy, D. et al. (1986). treatment of cytomegalovirus retinopathy in patients with acquired immunodeficiency syndrome: Use of the experimental drug 9-[2-hydroxy-1-(hydroxymethyl)ethoxymethyl]guanine. *Arch. Ophthalmol. 104*:1794-1800.

22. Freedman, P. G., Weiner, B. C., and Balthazar, E. J. (1985). Cytomegalovirus esophagastritis in a patient with AIDS. *Am. J. Gastroenterol. 80*:434-437.
23. Balthazar, E. J., Megibow, A. J., and Hulnick, D. H. (1985). Cytomeaglovirus esophagitis and gastritis in AIDS. *Am. J. Radiol. 144*:1201-1204.
24. St. Onge, G. and Bezahier, G. H. (1982). Giant esophageal ulcer associated with cytomegalovirus. *Gastroenterology 83*:127-150.
25. Knapp, A. B., Horst, D. A., Elipoulos, G. et al. (1983). Widespread cytomegalovirus gastroenterocolitis in a patient with acquired immunodeficiency syndrome. *Gastroenterology 85*:1399-1402.
26. Gertler, S. L., Pressman, J., Price, P., Brozinsky, S., and Miyai, K. (1983). Gastrointestinal cytomegalovirus infection in a homosexual man with severe acquired immunodeficiency syndrome. *Gastroenterology 85*:1403-1406.
27. Meiselman, M. S., Cello, J. S., and Margareten, W. (1985). Cytomegalovirus colitis. *Gastroenterology 88*:171-175.
28. Frank, D. and Ratent, R. F. (1984). Intestinal perforation associated with cytomegalovirus infection in patients with acquired immunodeficiency syndrome. *Am. J. Gastroenterol. 79*:201-205.
29. Frager, H. H., Frager, J. D., Wolf, E. L. et al. (1986). Cytomegalovirus colitis in acquired immune deficiency syndrome: Radiologic spectrum. *Gastrointest. Radiol. 11*:241-246.
30. Foucar, E., Mukai, K., Foucar, K., Sutherland, D. E., and Van Buren, C. T. (1981). Colonic ulceration in lethal cytomegalovirus infection. *Am. J. Clin. Pathol. 76*:788-801.
31. Balthazer, E. J., Megobow, A. J., Fazzini, E., Opulencia, J., and Seigal, I. (1985). Cytomegalovirus colitis in AIDS: Radiographic findings in 11 patients. *Radiology 155*:585-589.
32. Fernandes, B., Brunton, J., and Koven, I. (1986). Ileal perforation due to cytomegaloviral enteritis. *Can. J. Surg. 29*:453-456.
33. Brodie, H. R., Broaddus, C., Blumenfield, W., Hopewell, P., Mos, A., and Mills, J. (1985). Is cytomegalovirus a cause of lung disease in patients with AIDS? *Clin. Res. 33*:396A.
34. Masur, H., Lane, H. C., Palestine, A. et al. (1986). Effect of 9-(1,3-dihydroxy-2-proposymethyl)guanine on serious cytomegalovirus disease in eight immunosuppressed homosexual men. *Ann. Intern. Med. 104*:41-44.
35. Snider, W. D., Simpson, D. M., and Nielson, S. (1983). Neurological complications of acquired immune deficiency syndrome. *Ann. Neurol. 14*:403-418.
36. Morgello, S., Cho, E. S., Nielsen, S., Devinsky, O., and Petito, C. K. (1987). Cytomegalovirus encephalitis in patients with the acquired immunodeficiency syndrome: An autopsy study of 30 cases and a review of the literature. *Hum. Pathol. 18*:289-297.
37. Post, M. J. D., Hensley, G. T., Moskowitz, L. B., and Fischl, M. (1986). Cytomegalic inclusion virus encephalitis in patients with AIDS: CT, clinical and pathologic correlation. *AJR 146*:1229-1234.
38. Behar, R., Wiley, C., and McCutchan, J. A. (1987). Cytomegalovirus polyradiculopathy in acquired immune deficiency syndrome. *Neurology 37*:557-561.

39. Guzda, L. A., Luna, M. A., Smith, J. L. et al. (1984). Acquired immunodeficiency syndrome: Postmortem findings. *Am. J. Clin. Pathol. 81*:549-557.
40. Glasgow, B. J., Ardens, K., and Layfield, L. J. (1985). Clinical and pathologic findings of the liver in the acquired immunodeficiency syndrome. *Am. J. Clin. Pathol. 83*:582-588.
41. Jacobson, M. A., Cello, J. P., and Sande, M. A. (1988). Cholestasis and disseminated cytomegalovirus disease in patients with the acquired immune deficiency syndrome. *Amer. J. Med. 84*:218-224.
42. Kavin, J., Jones, R. B., Chowdwy, L. et al. (1986). Acalculous cholecystitis and cytomegalovirus infection in the acquired immunodeficiency syndrome. *Ann. Intern. Med. 104*:53-54.
43. Schnediderman, D. J., Cello, J. P., and Laing, F. C. (1987). Papillary stenosis and sclerosing cholangitis in patients with the acquired immunodeficiency syndrome. *Ann. Intern. Med. 106*:546-550.
44. Greene, L. W., Cole, W., Greene, L. B. et al. (1984). Adrenal insufficiency as a complication of the acquired immunodeficiency syndrome. *Ann. Intern. Med. 101*:497-498.
45. Mills, J. (1986). 9-(1,3-Dihydroxy-2-propoxymethyl)guanine (DHPG) for treatment of cytomegalovirus infections. In *Antiviral Chemotherapy: New Directions for Clinical Application and Research*, (Mills, J. and Corey, L., eds.). New York, American Elsevier, p. 199.
46. Membrano, L., Irony, I., Dere, W., Klein, R., Biglieri, E., and Cobb, E. (1987). Adrenocortical function in acquired immune deficiency syndrome. *J. Clin. Endocrinol. Metab. 65*:482-487.
47. Freitas, V. R., Smee, D. F., Chernow, M., Boehmer, R., and Matthews, T. R. (1985). Activity of 9-(1,3-dihydroxy-2-propoxymethyl)guanine compared with that of acyclovir against human, monkey and rodent cytomegalovirus. *Antimicrob. Agents Chemother. 28*:240-245.
48. Field, A. K., Davies, M. E., De Witt, C. et al. (1983). 9-[2-hydroxy-1-(hydroxymethyl)ethoxymethyl]guanine: A selective inhibitor of herpes group virus replication. *Proc. Natl. Acad. Sci. USA 80*:4139-4143.
49. Tocci, M. J., Livelli, T., Perry, H. C., Crumpacker, C. S., and Field, A. K. (1984). Effect of the nucleoside analogue 2′-NDG on cytomegalovirus replication. *Antimicrob. Agents Chemother. 25*:247-252.
50. Elion, G. B. (1986). History, mechanism of action, spectrum and selectivity of nucleoside analogs. In *Antiviral Chemotherapy: New Directions for Clinical Application and Research.* (Mills, J. and Corey, L., eds.). New York, American Elsevier, p. 127.
51. Fletcher, C., Sawchuck, R., Chinnock, B. et al. (1985). Human pharmacokinetics of 9-[2-hydroxy-1-(hydroxymethyl)ethoxymethyl]guanine. *Program Abstr. 25th Intersci. Conf. Antimicrob. Agents Chemother.* Minneapolis, Minn., Abstr. 127.
52. Laskin, O. L., Stahl-Bayliss, C., Kalman, C. et al. (1985). Multidose pharmacokinetics of 9-[2-hydroxy-1-(hydroxymethyl)ethoxymethyl]guanine. *Program Abstr. 25th Intersci. Conf. Antimicrob. Agents Chemother.*, Minneapolis, Minn., Abstr. 443.

53. Jacobson, M. A., De Miranda, P., Cederberg, D. M. et al. (1987). Oral ganciclovir: Human pharmacokinetics and toleration. *Antimicrob. Agents Chemother. 31*:1251-1254.

54. Laskin, O. L., Stahl-Bayliss, C. M., Kalman, C. M., and Rosecan, L. R. (1987). Use of ganciclovir to treat serious cytomegalovirus infections in patients with AIDS. *J. Infect. Dis. 155*:323-327.

55. Jacobson, M. A., O'Donnell, J. J., Brodie, H. R., O'Donnell, J. J., Wofsy, C., and Mills, J. (1988). Randomized prospective trial of ganciclovir maintenance therapy for cytomegalovirus retinitis. *J. Med. Virol. 25*:339-349.

56. Cederberg, D., Laskin, O. L., Mills, J. et al. (1986). Efficacy and safety of 9-[2-hydroxy-1-(hydroxymethyl)ethoxymethyl]guanine (BW759U) in AIDS patients with cytomegalovirus retinitis. *Program Abstr. 26th Intersci. Conf. Antimicrob. Agents Chemother.* New Orleans, La., Abstr. 565.

57. Henry, K., Cantrill, H., Fletcher, C., Chinnock, B. J., and Balfour, H. H. (1987). Use of intravenous ganciclovir (dihydroxypropoxymethylguanine) for cytomegalovirus retinitis in a patient with AIDS. *Am. J. Opthalmol. 103*:17-23.

58. Dieterich, D., Lafleur, F., Chachoua, A., and Warrell, C. (1987). Successful therapy of cytomegalovirus infections in patients with acquired immunodeficiency syndrome with ganciclovir. *Proc. III Int. Conf. AIDS.* Washington, D.C., Abstr. TH4.5.

59. Oberg, B. (1983). Antiviral effects of phosphononformate. *Pharmacotherapy 19*:387-415.

60. Vogt, M. W., Chou, T. C., Hartshorn, K. L. et al. (1987). Synergism and antagonism in vitro among various antiviral drugs in the treatment of HIV infections. *Proc. III Int. Conf. AIDS.* Washington, D.C., Abstr. TP30.

61. Akeeson-Johansson, A., Lernestedt, J. O., Rigden, O., Lonnqvist, B., and Wahren, B. (1986). Sensitivity of cytomegalovirus to intravenous foscarnet treatment. *Bone Marrow Transplant. 1*:215-220.

62. Ringdon, O., Lonnqvist, B., Paulin, T. et al. (1986). Pharmacokinetics, safety and preliminary clinical experiences using foscarnet for the treatment of cytomegalovirus infections in bone marrow and renal transplant recipients. *J. Antimicrob. Chemother. 17*:373-387.

63. Klintmalm, G., Lonnqvist, B., Oberg, B. et al. (1985). Intravenous foscarnet for the treatment of severe cytomegalovirus infection in allograft recipients. *Scand. J. Infect. Dis. 17*:157-163.

64. Walmsley, S., Chew, E., Fanning, M. M. et al. (1986). Treatment of cytomegalovirus retinitis with trisodium phosphonoformate. *Program Abstr. 26th Intersci. Conf. Antimicrob. Agents Chemother.* New Orleans, La, Abstr. 568.

65. Meyers, J. D., Reed, E. C., Shepp, D. H. et al. (1986). Prevention of cytomegalovirus infection after marrow transplant with high-dose intravenous acyclovir. *Program Abstr. 26th Intersci. Conf. Antimicrob. Agents Chemother.* New Orleans, La., Abstr. 732.

66. Selby, P., Slake, S., Mbidde, E. K. et al. (1984). Amino(hydroxyethoxymethyl)purine: A new well-absorbed prodrug of acyclovir. *Lancet 2*:1428-1430.

67. Turk, S. R., Townsend, L. B., Genzlinger, G. N., Cook, P. D., Shipman, C., and Drach, J. C. (1986). Inhibition of human cytomegalovirus by pyrrolo-(2,3-*d*)-pyrimidine nucleosides. *Program Abstr. 26th Intersci. Conf. Antimicrob. Agents Chemother.*, New Orleans, La, Abstr. 570.
68. Murray, B. K., Burns, N. J., McKernan, P. A., Robins, R. K., and North, J. A. (1985). Structure-activity relationship of certain 2'-deoxypurine nucleoside analogs against human cytomegalovirus. *Program Abstr. 25th Intersci. Conf. Antimicrob. Agents Chemother.* Minneapolis, Minn., Abstr. 123.
69. Kotler, D. P., Culpepper-Morgan, J. A., Tierney, A. R., and Klein, E. B. (1986). Treatment of disseminated cytomegalovirus infection with 9-(1,3-dihydroxy-2-propoxymethyl)guanine: Evidence of prolonged survival in patients with the acquired immunodeficiency syndrome. *AIDS Res.* 4:299-307.

12
Epstein-Barr and Other Viral Infections

Mark A. Jacobson *University of California and San Francisco General Hospital, San Francisco, California*

EPSTEIN-BARR VIRUS INFECTION

Epistein-Barr virus (EBV) is a highly prevalent, endemic human herpesvirus with a unique tropism for oral epithelial cells and B lymphocytes. More than 80% of the adult population in the United States, and a higher percentage of Asian and African populations, have serologic evidence of prior EBV infection. Like other herpesviruses, EBV regularly establishes latent infection in the host.

Humoral and cellular immunity to EBV is augmented in the majority of human immunodeficiency virus (HIV)-infected patients, compared with healthy HIV-negative controls (1-6). There is evidence that EBV may play an important role in the immunologic dysfunction that characterized HIV infection (6,7). In addition, opportunistic EBV infection may be directly involved in three HIV-associated syndromes: high-grade lymphoma, lymphoid interstitial pneumonitis, and hairy leukoplakia (8-10).

Role of Epstein-Barr Virus in HIV-Associated Syndromes

Non-Hodgkin's B-Cell Lymphoma

High- and intermediate-grade B-cell lymphomas, including Burkitt's lymphoma, have been increasingly recognized as a complication of HIV infection (11). Considerable epidemiologic and molecular biologic data suggest that some B-cell lymphomas occurring in immunocompromised hosts are associated with the presence of cytoplasmic circularized EBV genome and the possible integration of EBV DNA sequences into the host genome (12, 13). Not surprisingly, there are now reports of undifferentiated lymphomas occurring in acquired immunodeficiency syndrome (AIDS) patients which contain EBV DNA (8,9) and display chromosomal translocations characteristic of Burkitt's lymphoma (14,15).

Lymphoid Interstitial Pneumonitis

Many children with AIDS have developed a chronic diffuse interstitial pneumonitis with a characteristic follicular lymphocytic infiltrate (lymphocytic interstitial pneumonitis, LIP; 16). Andiman et al. (17) demonstrated EBV DNA in 8 of 10 lung biopsies from children with AIDS and LIP. Ten of 11 children with AIDS and LIP had IgG EBV viral capsid antigen titers greater or equal to 1:320, 8 of 11 had EBV early antigen titers greater or equal to 1:80, and only 2 of 11 had EBV nuclear antigen titers greater or equal to 1:40,960. This is the same serologic pattern described in the X-linked lymphoproliferative syndrome that is also characterized by uncontrolled EBV infection (18). Among children with AIDS without pathologic evidence of LIP on lung biopsy, only two of four had such high IgG viral capsid antigen or early antigen titers (17).

Hairy Leukoplakia

Hairy leukoplakia (HL) is a form of leukoplakia that occurs in patients with AIDS-related complex (ARC) or AIDS. It is typically an asymptomatic 2-mm to 3-cm raised lesion with a corrugated surface, most commonly located on the lateral aspect of the tongue. Epidemiologic data suggests that the presence of HL in an ARC patient is highly predictive of future progression to AIDS (19). Both human papillomavirus and EBV DNA have been demonstrated within epithelial cells of HL lesions (10). The EBV viral capsid antigen has also been detected in HL biopsies, suggesting that EBV actively replicates in these lesions. The response of these lesions to high-dose acyclovir also substantiates the etiologic role of EBV (20,21).

Laboratory Diagnosis

Because direct culture for EBV is insensitive and technically difficult, evidence of EBV infection is generally obtained by indirect means. The tests described in the following are not recommended as routine diagnostic tests for HIV-infected patients because they are mainly used as research methods, and the information gained generally will not alter prognosis or therapy.

Peripheral Blood Mononuclear Cell Transformation

Peripheral B lymphocytes latently infected with EBV in vivo produce immortal (transformed) cell lines when cultured in the absence of suppressor or cytotoxic T cells (22,23). The frequency of such transformed cells can be used as a measurement of the number of circulating EBV-infected B cells (23). This technique usually involves separation of peripheral blood mononuclear cells (PBMCs) by Ficoll-Hypaque centrifugation, followed by removal of T lymphocytes by rosetting with sheep erythrocytes, and culturing the remaining B cells for at least 4 weeks (4,5). Healthy controls without active EBV infection have approximately 0.1 spontaneously transforming cells per million PBMC (4,23). As compared with healthy controls, patients with AIDS or ARC have markedly increased numbers of transformed PCMCs similar to those observed in acute infectious mononucleosis (2-6).

Oropharyngeal Epstein-Barr Virus Excretion

The EBV shed from oropharyngeal epithelial cells and present in these secretions can be detected by transformation of human cord blood lymphocytes inoculated with throat washings (24). AIDS and ARC patients, as well as infectious mononucleosis patients, appear to have significantly increased oropharyngeal EBV excretion compared with healthy controls (2,3).

Direct Detection of EBV DNA

Hybridization of DNA is the most direct method of demonstrating the presence of EBV in tissue. DNA extracted from the specimen is fixed to nitrocellulose filters (25). Single-stranded, radioactively labeled EBV DNA probes are then used to detect, by specific hybridization, homologous DNA sequences in the filter (26). This method has been used to demonstrate EBV DNA in tissue specimens from ARC and AIDS patients with HL, LIP, and undifferentiated non-Hodgkin's lymphoma (8-10).

Epstein-Barr Virus Serology

Primary EBV infection (i.e., infectious mononucleosis) is characterized by development of serum IgM and IgG antibody responses to the EBV viral capsid antigen (VCA) and an IgG response to the EBV early antigen (EA; 27) (see Table 1). Whereas the IgM VCA and IgG EA response usually persists for only a few months (27), the IgG VCA response virtually always persists throughout life (27). Antibodies to EBV nuclear antigen (EBNA) develop weeks to months after primary infection and generally also persist for life (27). The immunocompetent adult with remote primary infection typically has EBNA antibodies and low titers of IgG antibody to VCA. Immunoglobulin M VCA and antibodies to EA are usually absent.

Certain classes of immunocompromised patients, including bone marrow transplant and ataxia telangiectasia patients, have been noted to have a pattern of increased EA and IgG VCA titers, which may be associated with a fatal lymphoproliferative disorder (18,28-30). Many of these patients have also had low or absent EBNA titers, thought to represent a T-cell deficiency

TABLE 1 Epstein-Barr Virus Serologic Patterns

	Serum antibody titers to EBV antigens		
	IgG VCA	EA	EBNA
Primary EBV infection	High	High	Absent
Immunocompetent, remote EBV infection	Low	Low or absent	Moderate
Ataxia telangiectasia, BMT	High	High	Low or absent
HIV infection	Low-high	Low-high	Moderate

Abbreviations: EBV, Epstein-Barr virus; VCA, viral capsid antigen; EA, early antigen; EBNA, Epstein-Barr nuclear antigen; BMT, bone marrow transplant; HIV, human immunodeficiency virus.

in controlling EBV activity (27). Recently, it has been proposed that EBV reactivation is a cause of a chronic fatigue syndrome in otherwise immuno-competent persons (27); however, therapeutic trials with acyclovir have not been confirmatory (69).

Rinaldo et al. (1), and Sumya et al. (3), both noted significantly higher titers of IgG VCA in healthy HIV-seropositive, gay men with lymphadeno-pathy syndrome (LAS) and patients with AIDS compared with healthy sero-negative controls. However, Chang et al. (4) reported similar antibody pro-files for gay men with LAS and healthy controls (4). Three studies (1,4,31) showed no significant difference between EA titers in HIV-infected and non-infected groups, whereas one study (3) reported a two to fourfold increased titer in an HIV infected group. Two studies reporting EBNA titers (3,4) noted no significant difference in HIV-infected and noninfected groups. Although these studies show a trend toward a serologic pattern similar to that asso-ciated with lymphoproliferative EBV disease, the data are too contradictory to draw any conclusion. In addition, higher than normal titers of antibodies to other viral antigens (e.g., CMV) have been noted in AIDS patients.

Role of Epstein-Barr Virus in HIV-Associated Immune Dysfunction

Although the role of EBV in the natural history of HIV disease is controver-sial, there can be little doubt that EBV reactivation frequently occurs in HIV-infected patients. As mentioned in the previous section, most AIDS and ARC patients have an enhanced antibody response to EBV antigens, an increased shedding of EBV in oropharyngeal secretions, and increased peripheral B-lymphocyte transformation, when compared with healthy adults. These find-ings are similar to those seen in individuals with primary EBV infection.

Several lines of evidence now suggest that EBV reactivation may be a co-factor in the immune dysfunction that occurs in HIV disease. Birx et al. (6)

cultured EBV-stimulated peripheral B lymphocytes from 17 AIDS or ARC patients and 18 normal controls. The EBV-stimulated immunoglobulin production was reduced by 80% in the presence of autologous T cells in healthy controls but markedly increased in the AIDS/ARC group. This suggests that AIDS and ARC patients have a profound defect in T-cell regulation of EBV infection. Blumberg et al. (7) demonstrated that HIV disrupted immune control of latent EBV infection by its cytopathic effect in the T4 lymphocyte and that this effect could be reversed in vitro by adding recombinant interleukin-2. The EBV-specific cytotoxic T-cell activity was also decreased in HIV-infected patients compared with HIV-seronegative controls. Rinaldo et al. (1) reported a positive correlation between titers of antibody to HIV determinants and IgG titers to EBV VCA and EA. Two of three patients in this study who experienced seroconversion to HIV had a concurrent fourfold rise in IgG VCA titer.

These studies demonstrate that HIV infection is associated with reduction in the host immune mechanisms responsible for maintaining latent EBV in a quiescent state. The resulting EBV reactivation may have an additive or even synergistic immunosuppressive effect in HIV infection (32). Expression of the T-suppressor subset could be amplified by EBV reactivation (33). Also, the manifestations of B-cell activation in HIV infection (hypergammaglobulinemia, autoimmune phenomena, and follicular hyperplasia of lymph nodes) might be linked to deregulation of EBV infection (7).

It has been recently demonstrated that EBV genome-positive B lymphocytes can be infected by HIV even in the apparent absence of the CD4 molecule, which functions as the receptor for HIV (34). Epstein-Barr virus may code for or induce synthesis of other surface molecules that permit direct HIV infection of B lymphocytes.

Therapy

Acyclovir has been shown to inhibit EBV replication in vitro at concentrations of 10 to 25 μmol (35,36), in spite of the fact that EBV may lack the thymidine kinase enzyme necessary for optimal drug phosphorylation (37). This effect may be explained by the sensitivity of EBV DNA polymerase to small amounts of acyclovir phosphorylated by cellular kinases (38) or to the poorly-characterized EBV-specified thymidine kinase. In any event, antiviral therapy with acyclovir is feasible only for permissive EBV infection (24) in which active virus replication is occurring. Acyclovir has no effect on EBV in latently infected or transformed cells (39,40). Generally, oropharyngeal epithelial cells are permissively infected by EBV, whereas B lymphocytes usually undergo nonpermissive infection (30,41).

Results of acyclovir therapy for life-threatening EBV infection in several transplant and X-linked lymphoproliferative syndrome patients have been mixed (30). Failure of therapy may have been due to nonpermissive infection. A technique that discriminates between linear and circular EBV DNA may be useful in determining if patients with serious EBV infection are likely to benefit from acyclovir therapy (30).

Although generally asymptomatic, hairy leukoplakia would be predicted to respond to antiviral therapy because EBV infects oral epithelial cells in the permissive form. Four of six patients with HL undergoing tongue biopsy had linear EBV DNA detected in one study (10). Recent trials of desciclovir (a prodrug of acyclovir, metabolized in vivo to acyclovir) and oral acyclovir have demonstrated resolution of tongue lesions in 85% to 100% of patients treated (20,21). However, HL recurred when acyclovir was discontinued. Because HL lesions are usually asymptomatic and do not cause progressive, invasive disease, antiviral therapy cannot now be generally recommended for HL. There is also evidence of acyclovir efficacy in normal hosts with EBV-associated acute infectious mononucleosis (42).

PROGRESSIVE MULTIFOCAL LEUKOENCEPHALOPATHY

Progressive multifocal leukoencephalopathy (PML) is a rare demyelinating disease affecting immunocompromised hosts, particularly patients with hematologic malignancies or AIDS (see also Chap. 6; 43-47). Multiple progressive lesions in the cerebral white matter cause signs and symptoms that correlate with the site of pathologic involvement. The disease is caused by a papovavirus, specifically a polyoma virus of the JC type, infecting the central nervous system. No treatment is available.

Etiology

Serologic studies have shown that the JC virus infects most people by adolescence (48). These infections are inapparent, and the tissues supporting primary virus replication are unknown. However, shedding of JC virus in the urine of kidney transplant patients was accompanied by rising serum antibody titers, supporting the hypothesis that immunosuppression results in reactivation of virus, with an augmented antibody response (49).

The JC virus has been recovered from primary cultures of human fetal glial cells inoculated with homogenized PML brain tissue (50). More than 10^{10} viral particles can be present per gram of brain tissue (51). Papovavirus-like particles have also been detected in oligodendroglia nuclei of fresh brain autopsy material from PML patients (52).

Pathologic Findings

The JC types of polyoma virus appears to cause PML in both AIDS and non-AIDS patients. A JC nonstructural protein [large tumor (T) antigen] has been detected in both AIDS and non-AIDS-related PML cases (53). In one study, brain tissue samples from two AIDS patients appeared to be much more diffusely and more heavily infected with JC virus than those from three non-AIDS PML patients (53).

Pathologic findings of PML do not differ between AIDS and non-AIDS-related cases. The characteristic histologic appearance is multiple asymmetric discrete foci of demyelination, often forming large plaques, without preferential localization to any one region of the central nervous system (43). Oligodendrocytes with swollen nuclei containing intranuclear inclusions and giant astrocytes with pleomorphic nuclei are observed in most cases (43). Inflammatory cells are generally sparse or absent. With electron microscopy, typical papovaviruslike particles are seen within nuclei of oligodendrocytes located in foci of demyelination (52).

Clinical Presentation and Course

Progressive multifocal leukoencephalopathy is rare, even among patients with AIDS. In two large series of AIDS patients with neurologic complications, only 2% to 4% had PML (45,46). In many reported cases, PML has been an index diagnosis of AIDS (44); however, PML occurring after other AIDS-defining opportunistic infections is also well recognized (44,45).

Like non-AIDS patients with PML, patients with AIDS and PML present with mental status changes, blindness, aphasia, hemiparesis, ataxia, or other focal central nervous system deficits (44-46,54,55). Generally, headache, fever, and seizures are absent; these findings are helpful, but not always reliable, in differentiating between PML and central nervous system toxoplasmosis or cryptococcal meningitis, the two most important treatable opportunistic infections affecting the central nervous system in AIDS. Results from examination of cerebrospinal fluid are normal in PML, unless other central nervous system disease is also present, and electroencephalogram studies often show background slowing (55). In reported cases of PML in AIDS, initial focal deficits have progressed, either slowly or rapidly; and additional deficits have commonly occurred, often leading to quadriparesis and dementia. Generally, these patients have died within 1 to 6 months of diagnosis of PML (44,45,54). However, two patients with AIDS and PML have been reported to have recovered neurologic function spontaneously and to have survived 17 to 22 months (56). Brain biopsy revealed an uncharacteristic intense inflammatory response in the region where papovavirus was detected by electron microscopy.

Diagnosis

The diagnosis of PML is often suggested by computed tomography (CT) scans of the brain that demonstrate focal areas of diminished density or demyelination within the hemispheric or posterior fossa white matter (44-46). The lack of mass effect and absence of contrast enhancement distinguish these lesions from tumors, granulomas, and other infections (57).

Recent experience with magnetic resonance imaging (MRI) suggests that it is a more sensitive method than a CT scan for detecting diffuse central nervous system demyelination in AIDS patients. The MRI scans of AIDS patients with PML have been reported to reveal a characteristic pattern on T2-weighted images of multiple, discrete high-signal foci with ill-defined margins (in contrast with the sharply defined margins in central nervous system toxoplasmosis; 58). We have followed several AIDS patients with progressive neurologic deficits consistent with PML who initially had normal CT scans. Concurrent MRI scans demonstrated focal white matter zones with an abnormal increased signal characteristic of PML (M. A. Jacobson et al., unpublished data). The "CT-clinical dissociation" (an initial CT scan which is normal or reveals only subtle abnormalities at a time when the clinical symptoms and signs are far more prominent) noted by some authors (44) may also reflect the relative insensitivity of CT compared with MRI in detecting demyelination. In our experience, the neuroradiologic appearance of PML is usually sufficiently characteristic, especially in a patient without headache or fever, that open-brain biopsy is rarely necessary to confirm the diagnosis.

Brain biopsy may be an indicated in patients with atypical neuroradiologic findings, especially if the patient does not already have an AIDS diagnosis. In situ hybridization with a biotinylated JC virus probe has been recently described as a rapid, sensitive method of confirming PML in brain biopsy or autopsy material (59).

Therapy

Partial remission has been described in several cases of PML in non-AIDS patients treated with cytosine arabinoside (60,61). There are two case reports (44,45) of cytosine arabinoside therapy for AIDS patients with PML. Transient improvement occurred in one patient, and no detectable effect on outcome was noted in the other. To date, no other treatment modalities have been reported for PML in AIDS.

ADENOVIRUS INFECTION

Adenoviruses, like EBV and papovaviruses, are double-stranded DNA viruses with a propensity to establish persistent infection in humans. Adenoviruses may cause acute upper respiratory, ocular, or urinary tract infections in immunocompetent adults; however, most infections are asymptomatic.

Adenoviruses may persist in tonsillar lymphoid cells for long periods without causing disease (62). Recent studies have documented frequent isolation of an unusual adenovirus strain in the urine of AIDS patients (62,63).

Although invasive adenovirus infection has been correlated with disease in some transplant patients (63,64), there is, as yet, no evidence that adenovirus is an opportunistic pathogen in patients with AIDS. Adenovirus was isolated from 4.9% of bone marrow transplant patients, most commonly from the urine (62). A large proportion of these isolates belong to subgroup B, types 34 and 35, which have not been reported in immunocompetent community outbreaks (63). Hemorrhagic cystitis has been correlated with the presence of a positive urine culture in bone marrow transplant patients at the University of Washington (63). In addition, several patients with renal insufficiency or hepatic necrosis had an adenovirus cultured from the involved tissue as well as histologic evidence of viral inclusions (63). In three bone marrow transplant patients, adenovirus pneumonia contributed to death.

Adenovirus was reported in the urine of 10 patients with AIDS (65). Ten of 13 isolates were subgroup B, type 34 or 35, by hemagglutination; all 13 isolates had a restriction endonuclease pattern similar to types 34 and 35. This group of investigators (66) later compared serotypes of adenovirus isolates from AIDS and non-AIDS patients, from urine and other sites. Twenty urine isolates from AIDS patients were all type 34/35, whereas none of 36 non-AIDS patients were type 34/35. Adenoviruses persisted in the urine of AIDS patients for up to 12 months (66). However, only 2 of 10 AIDS patients with adenovirus in urine had detectable serum antibody to type 34/35 determinants (66). This same group reported a 20% prevalence of adenovirus in urine of AIDS patients (65). In our experience, adenovirus has also been isolated from urine of AIDS patients; however, the prevalence has been less than 5% (J. Rush and M. A. Jacobson, unpublished data).

The significance of finding adenovirus in the urine of AIDS patients is unknown. This asymptomatic shedding could result from endogenous reactivation of latent virus. However, the rarity of the 34/35 serotype in the general population argues against this hypothesis. Perhaps, patients with HIV infection become uniquely susceptible to colonization with this unusual serotype. Although the adenovirus infection appears to be a benign process in these patients, it may have some immunosuppressive or transforming potential yet to be described.

Recent evidence from one center suggests that the group D adenovirus may be an opportunistic pathogen in AIDS patients with colitis (67,68). Although adenovirus is occasionally isolated from colonic biopsies of patients with cytomegalovirus (CMV) colitis (J. Rush and M. A. Jacobson, unpublished data), a group at Saint Mary's Hospital in London (68) has observed nine AIDS colitis patients with colonic biopsy cultures that were negative for CMV and positive for adenovirus. Histologic sections showed a cytopathic effect similar to CMV, but electron microscopy revealed viral particles with a structure more characteristic of adenovirus. Confirmation studies of these data will be of interest, especially because adenovirus isolates from these patients have been relatively sensitive to genciclovir (ED_{50} 7-10 μmol) (67).

REFERENCES

1. Rinaldo, C. R., Kingsley, L. A., Lyter, D. W., Rabin, B. S., Atchison, R. W., Bodner, A. J., Weiss, S. H., and Sexinger, W. C. (1986). Association of HTLV-III with Epstein-Barr virus infection and abnormalities of T lymphocytes in homosexual men. *J. Infect. Dis. 154*:556-561.
2. Quinnan, G. V., Masur, H., Rook, A. H., Armstrong, G., Frederick, W. R., Epstein, J., Manischewitz, J. F., Macher, A. M., Jackson, L., Ames, J., Smith, H. A., Parker, M., Pearson, G. R., Parrillo, J., Mitchell, C., and Straus, S. E. (1984). Herpesvirus infections in the acquired immune deficiency syndrome. *JAMA 252*:72-77.
3. Sumaya, C. V., Boswell, R. N., Ench, Y., Kisner, D. L., Hersh, E. M., Rueben, J. M., and Mansell, P. W. A. (1986). Enhanced serological and virological findings of Epstein-Barr virus in patients with AIDS and AIDS-related complex. *J. Infect. Dis. 154*:864-870.
4. Chang, R. S., Thompson, H., and Pomerants, S. (1985). Epstein-Barr virus infections in homosexual men with chronic persistent generalized lymphadenopathy. *J. Infect. Dis. 151*:459-463.
5. Yarchoan, R., Redfield, R. R., and Broder, S. (1986). Mechanisms of B cell activation in patients with acquired immunodeficiency syndrome and related disorders. *J. Clin. Invest. 78*:439-447.
6. Birx, D. L., Redfield, R. R., and Tosato, G. (1986). Defective regulation of Epstein-Barr virus infection in patients with acquired immunodeficiency syndrome (AIDS) or AIDS-related disorders. *N. Engl. J. Med. 314*:874-879.
7. Blumberg, R. S., Paradis, T., Byington, R., Henle, W., Hirsch, M. S., and Schooley, R. T. (1987). Effects of human immunodeficiency virus on the cellular immune response to Epstein-Barr virus in homosexual men: Characterization of the cytotoxic response and lymphokine production. *J. Infect. Dis. 155*: 877-890.
8. Groopman, J. E., Sullivan, J. L., Mulder, C., Ginsburg, D., Orkin, S. H., O'Hara, C. J., Falchuk, K., Wong-Staal, F., and Gallo, R. C. (1986). Pathogenesis of a B cell lymphoma in a patient with AIDS. *Blood 67*:612-615.
9. Andiman, W. A., Martin, K., Rubinstein, A., Pahwa, S., Eastman, R., Katz, B. Z., Pitt, J., and Miller, G. (1985). Opportunistic lymphoproliferations associated with Epstein-Barr viral DNA in infants and children with AIDS. *Lancet 2*:1390-1393.
10. Greenspan, J. S., Greenspan, D., Lennette, E. T., Abrams, D. I., Conant, M. A., Petersen, V., and Freese, U. K. (1985). Replication of Epstein-Barr virus

within the epithelial cells of oral "hairy" leukoplakia, an AIDS-associated lesion. *N. Engl. J. Med. 313*:1564-1571.

11. Ziegler, J. L., Beckstead, J. A., Volberding, P. A., Abrams, D. I., Levine, A. M., Likes, R. J. et al. (1984). Non-Hodgkin's lymphoma in 90 homosexual men. *N. Engl. J. Med. 311*:565-570.

12. Sullivan, J. L., Medveczky, P., Forman, S. J., Baker, S. M., Monroe, J. E., and Mulder, C. (1984). Epstein-Barr virus induced lymphoproliferation. *N. Engl. J. Med. 311*:1163.

13. Cleary, M. L., Warnke, R., and Sklar, J. (1980). Monoclonality of lymphoproliferative lesions in cardiac-transplant recipients: Clonal analysis based on immunoglobulin-gene rearrangements. *N. Engl. J. Med. 302*:302.

14. Peterson, J. M., Tubbs, R. R., Savage, R. A. et al. (1985). Small noncleaved B cell Burkitt-like lymphoma with chromosome t (8;14) translocation and Epstein-Barr virus nuclear-associated antigen in a homosexual man with acquired immune deficiency syndrome. *Am. J. Med. 78*:141-148.

15. McGrath, I. T., Erikson, J., Whang-Peng, J. et al. (1983). Synthesis of kappa light chains by cell lines containing an 8;22 chromosomal translocation derived from a male homosexual with Burkitt's lymphoma. *Science 222*:1094-1098.

16. Scott, G. B., Buck, B. E., Leterman, J. G., Gloom, F. L., and Parks, W. P. (1984). Acquired immunodeficiency syndrome in infants. *N. Engl. J. Med. 310*:76-81.

17. Bar, R. S., Delor, C. J., Clausen, K. P., Hurtubise, P., Henle, W., and Heweston, J. F. (1974). Fatal infectious mononucleosis in a family. *N. Engl. J. Med. 290*:363-367.

18. Sullivan, J. L., Byron, K. S., Brewster, F. E., Baker, S. M., and Ochs, H. D. (1983). X-linked lymphoproliferative syndrome: Natural history of the immunodeficiency. *J. Clin. Invest. 71*:1765-1778.

19. Greenspan, D., Greenspan, J. S., Hearst, N. G., Li-Zhen Pan, Conant, M. A., Abrams, D. I., Hollander, H., and Levy, J. (1987). Relation of oral hairy leukoplakia to infection with human immune deficiency virus and the risk of developing AIDS. *J. Infect. Dis. 155*:475-481.

20. Resnick, L., Herbst, J., Ablashi, D. V., Salahuddin, S. Z., Frank, B., Atherton, S. et al. (1987). Regression of oral hairy leukoplakia with acyclovir. *Proc. III Int. Conf. AIDS.* Washington, D.C., Abstr. MP146.

21. Greenspan, D., Greenspan, J. S., De Souza, Y., Chapman, S. K., Lennette, E., and Petersen, V. (1987). Efficacy of BWA515 in treatment of EBV infection in hairy leukoplakia. *Proc. III Int. Conf. AIDS.* Washington, D.C., Abstr. PM223.

22. Diehl, V., Henle, G., Henle, W., and Kohn, G. (1968). Demonstration of a herpes group virus in cultures of peripheral leukocytes from patients with infectious mononucleosis. *J. Virol. 2*:663-669.

23. Rocchi, G., DeFelici, A., Ragona, G., and Heinz, A. (1977). Quantitative evaluation of Epstein-Barr virus infected mononuclear peripheral blood leukocytes in infectious mononucleosis. *N. Engl. J. Med. 296*:132-134.

24. Chang, R. S., Lewis, J. P., Reynolds, R. D., Sullivan, M. J., and Neuman, J. (1978). Oropharyngeal excretion of Epstein-Barr virus by patients with lympho-

proliferative disorders and by recipients of renal homografts. *Ann. Intern. Med.* *88*:34-40.

25. Bornkamm, G. W., Hudenwentz, J., Freese, U. K., Zimber, U. (1982). Deletion of the non-transforming Epstein-Barr virus strain P3HR-1 causes fusion of the large internal repeat to the DS$_L$ region. *J. Virol.* *43*:952-968.

26. Desgranges, C., Bornkamm, G. W., Zeng, Y. et al. (1982). Detection of Epstein-Barr viral DNA internal repeats in the nasopharyngeal mucosa of Chinese with IgA/EBV-specific antibodies. *Int. J. Cancer 29*:87-91.

27. Sumaya, C. V. (1985). Serological testing for Epstein-Barr virus—developments in interpretation. *J. Infect. Dis. 151*:984-987.

28. Lange, B., Henle, W., Meyers, J. D., Yang, L. C., August, C., Koch, P., Arbeter, A., and Henle, G. (1980). Epstein-Barr virus-related serology in marrow transplant recipients. *Int. J. Cancer 26*:151-157.

29. Joncas, J., Lapointe, N., Gervais, F., Leyrits, M., and Will, A. (1977). Unusual prevalence of antibodies to Epstein-Barr virus early antigen in ataxia telangiectasia. *Lancet 1*:1160.

30. Sullivan, J. L., Medveczky, P., Forman, S. J., Baker, S. M., Monroe, J. E., and Mulder, C. (1984). Epstein-Barr virus induced lymphoproliferation: Implications for antiviral chemotherapy. *N. Engl. J. Med. 311*:1163-1167.

31. Lipscomb, H., Tatsumi, E., Harada, S., Yetz, J., Davis, J., Bechtold, T. et al. (1983). Epstein-Barr virus and chronic lymphadenomegally in male homosexuals with acquired immunodeficiency syndrome. *AIDS Res. 1*:59-82.

32. Hirsch, M. S., Schooley, R. T., Ho, D. D., and Kaplan, J. C. (1984). Possible viral interaction in the acquired immunodeficiency syndrome. *Rev. Infect. Dis. 6*:726-731.

33. Moss, D. J., Rickinson, A. B., and Pope, J. H. (1979). Long-term T-cell-mediated immunity to Epstein-Barr virus in man. III. Activation of cytotoxic T cells in virus-infected leukocyte cultures. *Int. J. Cancer 23*:618-625.

34. Ablashi, D. V., Markham, P. D., Salahuddin, S. Z., Veronese, K. F., and Gallo, R. C. (1987). A possible role for epitopes other than CD4 in the receptor complex for HIV. *Proc. III Int. Conf. AIDS*. Washington, D.C., Abstr. TP20.

35. Colby, B. M., Shaw, J. E., Elion, G. B., and Pagano, J. S. (1980). Effect of acyclovir]9-(2-hydroxymethyl)guanine] in Epstein-Barr virus DNA replication. *J. Virol. 34*:560-568.

36. Datta, A. K., Colby, B. M., Shaw, J. E., and Pagano, J. S. (1980). Acyclovir inhibition of Epstein-Barr virus replication. *Proc. Natl. Acad. Sci. USA 77*: 5163-5166.

37. Pagano, J. S. and Datta, A. K. (1982). Perspectives on interactions of acyclovir with Epstein-Barr and other herpesviruses. *Am. J. Med. 73*(Suppl. 1A):18-26.

38. Hoagland, R. S. (1955). The transmission of infectious mononucleosis. *Am. J. Med. Sci. 229*:262.

39. Sixbey, J. W., Harmon, H., and Pagano, J. S. (1982). Epstein Barr virus transformation of human lymphocytes in the presence of acyclovir [9-(2-hydroxyethoxymethyl)guanine]. *Clin. Res. 30*:521A.

40. Nonoyama, M. and Pagano, J. S. (1972). Separation of Epstein-Barr virus DNA from large chromosomal DNA in non-virus-producing cells. *Nature 238*:169-171.
41. Sixbey, J. W., Vesterinen, E. H., Nedrud, J. G., Raab-Traub, N., Walton, J. A., and Pagano, J. S. (1983). Replication of Epstein-Barr virus in human epithelial cells infected in vitro. *Nature 306*:480-484.
42. Andersson, J., Britton, S., Ernberg, I., Andersson, U., Henle, W., Skoldenberg, B., and Tissel, A. (1986). Effect of acyclovir on infectious mononucleosis: A double-blind, placebo-controlled study. *J. Infect. Dis. 153*:283-290.
43. Richardson, E. P. (1961). Progressive multifocal leukoencephalopathy. *N. Engl. J. Med. 265*:815-823.
44. Krupp, L. B., Lipton, R. B., Swerdlow, M. L., Leeds, N. E., and Llena, J. (1985). Progressive multifocal leukoencephalopathy: Clinical and radiographic features. *Ann. Neurol. 17*:344-349.
45. Snider, W. D., Simpson, D. M., Nielsen, M. D., Gold, J. W. M., Metroka, C. E., and Posner, J. B. (1983). Neurological complications of acquired immune deficiency syndrome: Analysis of 50 patients. *Ann. Neurol. 14*:403-418.
46. Levy, R. M., Bredesen, D. E., and Rosenblum, M. L. (1985). Neurological manifestations of the acquired immunodeficiency syndrome: Experience at UCSF and review of the literature. *J. Neurosurg. 62*:475-495.
47. Blum, L. W., Chanbers, R. A., Schwartzman, R. J., and Streletz, L. J. (1985). Progressive multifocal leukoencephalopathy in acquired immune deficiency syndrome. *Arch. Neurol. 42*:137-139.
48. Padgett, B. L. and Walker, D. L. (1973). Prevalence of antibodies in human sera against JC virus, an isolate from a case of progressive multifocal leukoencephalopathy. *J. Infect. Dis. 127*:467.
49. Hogan, T. F., Borden, E. C., McBain, J. A. et al. (1980). Human polyomavirus infections with JC and BK virus in renal transplant patients. *Ann. Intern. Med. 92*:373.
50. Padgett, B. L., Walker, D. L., Su Rhein, G. M. et al. (1971). Cultivation of papova-like virus from human brain with progressive multifocal leukoencephalopathy. *Lancet 1*:1257.
51. Dorries, K., Johnson, R. T., and ter Meulen, V. (1979). Detection of polyoma virus DNA in PML-brain tissue by in situ hybridization. *J. Gen. Virol. 42*:49.
52. Silverman, L. and Rubenstein, L. F. (1965). Electron microscopic observations on a case of progressive multifocal leukoencephalopathy. *Acta Neuropathol. 5*:215.
53. Stoner, G. L., Ryschkewitsch, C. F., Walker, D. L., and Webster, H. deF. (1986). JC papovavirus large tumor (T)-antigen expression in brain tissue of acquired immune deficiency syndrome (AIDS) and non-AIDS patients with progressive multifocal leukoencephalopathy. *Proc. Natl. Acad. Sci. USA 83*:2271-2275.
54. Bernick, C. and Gregorios, J. B. (1984). Progressive multifocal leukoencephalopathy in a patient with acquired immune deficiency syndrome. *Arch. Neurol. 41*:780-782.

55. Berger, J. R. and Mucke, L. (1987). Neurological recovery and prolonged survival in progressive multifocal leukoencephalopathy with HIV infection. *Proc. III Int. Conf. AIDS.* Washington, D.C., Abstr. MP143.

56. Whelan, M. A., Kricheff, J. J., Handler, M. et al. (1983). Acquired immunodeficiency syndrome: Cerebral computed tomographic manifestations. *Radiology 149*:477-484.

57. Jarvik, J., Hesselink, J., Kennedy, C., Teschke, R., Wiley, C., and McCutchan, J. A. (1987). Patterns of magnetic resonance brain scanning of lesions in AIDS and ARC patients. *Proc. III Int. Conf. AIDS.* Washington, D.C., Abstr. TP158.

58. Houff, S. A., Katz, D., Kufta, C., Elder, G., Vacante, D., and Major, E. (1987). Progressive multifocal leukoencephalopathy in AIDS patients: Diagnostic considerations and pathologic findings. *Proc. III Int. Conf. AIDS.* Washington, D.C., Abstr. MP159.

59. Bauer, W. R., Turel, A. P., and Hognson, K. P. (1973). Progressive multifocal leukoencephalopathy and cytarabine: Remission with treatment. *JAMA 226*: 174-176.

60. Marriott, P. J., O'Brien, M. D., and MacKenzie, C. K. (1975). Progressive multifocal leukoencephalopathy: Remission with cytarabine. *J. Neurol. Neurosurg. Psychiatry 38*:205-209.

61. Hilleman, M. R. and Werner, J. H. (1954). Recovery of a new agent from patients with acute respiratory illness. *Proc. Exp. Biol. Med. 85*:183.

62. Huebner, J. R., Rowe, W. P., Ward, T. G., Parrott, R. H., and Bell, J. A. (1954). Adenoidal-pharyngeal-conjunctival agents: A newly recognized group of common viruses of the respiratory system. *N. Engl. J. Med. 251*:1077-1086.

63. Horwitz, M. S., Valderrama, G., Hatcher, V., Korn, R., deJong, P., and Spiglank, I. (1984). Characterization of adenovirus isolates from AIDS patients. *Ann. N.Y. Acad. Sci. 437*:161-174.

64. deJong, P. J., Valderrama, G., Spigland, I., and Horwitz, M. S. (1983). Adenovirus isolates from urine of patients with acquired immunodeficiency syndrome. *Lancet 2*:1293-1296.

65. Shields, V. F., Hackman, R. C., Fife, K. H., Corey, L., and Meyers, J. D. (1985). Adenovirus infections in patients undergoing bone-marrow transplantation. *N. Engl. J. Med. 312*:529-533.

66. Stalder, H., Heirholzer, J. C., and Oxman, M. N. (1977). New human adenovirus (candidate adenovirus 35) causing fatal disseminated infection in a renal transplant recipient. *J. Clin. Microbiol. 6*:257.

67. Tyms, A. S., Taylor, D. L., Davis, J. M., Taylor-Robinson, D., Pinching, A. J., and Jeffries, D. J. (1987). Cytomegalovirus and adenovirus infections: Response to DHPG. *Proc. III Int. Conf. AIDS.* Washington, D.C., Abstr. TH4.4.

68. Parkin, J., Tyms, S., Roberts, A., Burnell, R., Jeffries, D., and Pinching, A. (1987). "Cytomegalovirus" colitis: Can it be caused by adenovirus? *Proc. III Int. Conf. AIDS.* Washington, D.C., Abstr. TH8.3.

69. Straus, S. E., Dale, J. K., Tobi, M., Lawley, T., Preble, O., Blaese, M., Hallahan, C., Henle, W. (1988). Acyclovir treatment of the chronic fatigue syndrome. Lack of efficacy in a placebo-controlled trial. *N. Engl. J. Med. 319*:1692.

Part IV
Bacterial Infections

13
Bacterial Infections in Acquired Immunodeficiency Syndrome

Jane E. Koehler and Richard E. Chaisson* *University of California, San Francisco, California*

Infections caused by bacterial pathogens have been recognized as complications of the acquired immunodeficiency syndrome (AIDS) and human immunodeficiency virus (HIV) infection since early in the AIDS epidemic (Table 1). The incidence of certain infections, specifically pneumonias caused by encapsulated bacteria and enteritis and disseminated infections caused by *Salmonella*, is higher in HIV-infected populations. Clinical manifestations of bacterial infections in HIV-infected patients may differ from other populations, with an increased frequency of atypical presentations, including bacteremia, and high rates of relapse, despite appropriate therapy. In this chapter we will describe the pathogenesis, clinical features, and management of bacterial infections in patients with HIV infection and AIDS.

PATHOGENESIS

Bacterial pathogens can escape host defenses in AIDS patients because of selective defects in cellular and humoral immunity caused by HIV infection (Table 2). Qualitative and quantitative defects of CD4 + lymphocytes result in infections by organisms that require intact cell-mediated immunity for control, such as *Salmonella*, *Listeria*, and mycobacteria (1,2). Impaired phagocytic functioning of macrophages is also common in HIV-infected

Current affiliation: The Johns Hopkins University School of Medicine, Baltimore, Maryland

TABLE 1   Bacterial Pathogens Causing Disease in Patients with HIV Infection

	Site(s)	Comment
Gram-positive organisms		
Streptococcus pneumoniae	Lung, blood	Bacteremia common
Streptococcus species	Lung, skin	
Staphylococcus aureus	Skin, blood, lung	Increased incidence (?)
Listeria monocytogenes	Blood, meninges	Uncommon
Gram-negative organisms		
Salmonella species	GI tract, blood	Bacteremia > enteritis
Shigella	GI tract, blood	
Campylobacter	GI tract, blood	
Spirochetes		
Treponema pallidum	Integument, CNS	Accelerated course (?)

TABLE 2   Immunologic Defects Associated with Bacterial Infections in HIV-Infected Patients

Abnormality	Types of bacterial infections
Cellular immunity	
loss of CD4+ lymphocyte	*Salmonella, Listeria,* mycobacteria
impaired antigen presentation	
impaired phagocytosis	
decreased lymphokine production	
Humoral immunity	
impaired response to neoantigens	Encapsulated bacteria,
spontaneous B-cell proliferation	*Enterobacteriaciae* (?)
polyclonal immunoglobulin synthesis	

persons and can contribute to disease from organisms controlled by cellular immunity. Decreased production of γ-interferon, a macrophage-activating cytokine, probably contributes to this impairment, resulting in a high incidence of bacteremic pyogenic infections in this population. Localized disease in the gastrointestinal tract may result from derangements in cellular immune response in the intestinal mucosa of patients with HIV infection (3).

Alterations in humoral immunity can be documented in most AIDS patients and may be an early complication of HIV infection. Patients commonly demonstrate spontaneous B-cell proliferation, nonspecific immunoglobulin synthesis with a polyclonal gammopathy, and a lack of response to both T-cell-dependent and T-cell-independent neoantigens (4-6). Defects in B-cell-mediated immune responses are associated with infections caused by encapsulated bacteria, particularly *Streptococcus pneumoniae* and *Haemo-*

philus influenzae. The highest frequency of bacterial infections appears to be in infants and children with HIV infection (7,8), presumably because these patients lack specific antibodies to encapsulated bacteria, whereas most adults have circulating differentiated B cells capable of clonal expansion to produce adequate levels of antibodies to prevent development of disease.

Loss of granulocytes is generally not a consequence of AIDS or HIV infection, and infections common in neutropenic hosts do not usually occur in AIDS. However, several therapeutic agents used to treat HIV infection and opportunistic disease in AIDS patients are known to cause granulocytopenia and an increased frequency of infections caused by staphylococci and gram-negative bacilli. Zidovudine (AZT), ganciclovir (DHPG), and a number of antineoplastic agents used to treat Kaposi's sarcoma and lymphomas can cause granulocytopenia in AIDS patients (9). As the use of these agents increases, so will the infectious complications associated with neutropenia.

PULMONARY BACTERIAL INFECTIONS

Pneumonia caused by pyogenic bacteria was reported in AIDS patients early in the epidemic. In a series compiled by Murray et al. (10), bacterial pathogens were found in 2.5% of AIDS-related pneumonias. Simberkoff and associates (11) reported five AIDS patients with pneumococcal pneumonia, three of whom had bacteremia, and one of whom had been given type-specific pneumococcal vaccine 6 months before developing pneumococcal disease. Polsky and co-workers (12) reported 18 cases of pneumonia caused by the pneumococcus or *H. influenzae,* accounting for 10% of pneumonias in AIDS patients at Memorial-Sloan Kettering Cancer Center. These authors also reported a high relapse rate (4 of 13 patients) and a lack of specific antibody response following infection in several patients. Several other series have confirmed and extended these findings. Gerberding et al. (13) reported a high rate of bacteremia in AIDS patients with bacterial pneumonias at San Francisco General Hospital, and Witt and associates (14) found an increased rate of bacterial pneumonias in IV drug users and Haitians with AIDS, compared with homosexual men with AIDS. In a prospective study of HIV-seropositive IV drug users without AIDS, Selwyn and co-workers (15) reported a significantly greater frequency of bacterial pneumonia, primarily caused by *H. influenzae,* compared with seronegative controls.

Bacteremic infections without pneumonia have been reported in patients with AIDS, although a localized site of infection, such as a skin abscess or catheter infection, is usually found (16,16a).

Presentation and Diagnosis

Patients who are infected with HIV and have bacterial pneumonia typically present with the classic features of community-acquired pneumonia, including

of bacteremia, initial therapy should be given parenterally; oral therapy sudden onset of symptoms, fever, chills, productive cough, and pleuritic chest pain (13). In contrast, *Pneumocystis carinii* pneumonia (PCP) in this population tends to have a longer prodrome and is not usually associated with productive cough or pleurisy (17). Localizing physical findings may include dullness to percussion, decreased breath sounds, egophony, and crackles. Typical laboratory findings include leukocytosis commonly ranging from 6000 to 15,000/mm^3, with increased numbers of immature forms, respiratory alkalosis and hypoxemia, and radiographic evidence of pulmonary consolidation in a lobar, segmental, or subsegmental pattern. *Pneumocystis carinii* pneumonia is usually associated with a low white blood cell count (<4000/mm^3) and diffuse, interstitial infiltration on the chest radiograph (17). It has been suggested that *H. influenzae* pneumonia in AIDS patients is more likely to cause diffuse infiltrates than pneumococcal pneumonia, although few data are available to support this assertion (12). Microscopic examination of sputum generally shows many polymorphonuclear leukocytes (PMNs) and may reveal the causative bacteria. Cultures of sputum frequently grow the causative agent. In addition, blood cultures are positive in 50% to 80% of patients with bacterial pneumonia and HIV infection (12-16). Patients with *P. carinii* pneumonia may also have PMNs in sputum, and bacteria may be recovered from routine sputum culture. However, sputum from patients with pneumocystosis usually contains contaminants such as *Neisseria, S. aureus,* or streptococci. Isolation of pneumococci or *H. influenzae* suggests a bacterial bronchitis or pneumonia in addition to PCP. Other organisms included in the differential diagnosis of pneumonia in the HIV-infected or AIDS patient include the fungi *Cryptococcus, Histoplasma,* or *Coccidioides immitis*; viral infections, particularly CMV; or nonspecific pneumonitis in which no organism is identified. Evaluation of the patient with known HIV infection and respiratory symptoms is discussed elsewhere (see Chaps. 5 and 17).

Therapy

Patients suspected of having either *P. carinii* or a bacterial pathogen can be given trimethoprim-sulfamethoxazole (15 mg/kg of trimethoprim per day) empirically, a regimen that will adequately cover *P. carinii, H. influenzae,* other *Haemophilus* species, *S. pneumoniae,* and *S. aureus.* Patients suspected of having bacterial pneumonia, but not pneumocystosis, should be treated with a second- or third-generation cephalosporin (e.g., cefuroximine or ceftriaxone). For documented pneumococcal pneumonia, penicillin is the drug of choice (Table 3). Patients allergic to penicillin can be treated with a cephalosporin (although 5% to 15% of penicillin-allergic patients may cross-react to cephalosporins) or with erythromycin. Because of the high prevalence

TABLE 3 Treatment of Bacterial Infections in Patients with HIV Infection

Organism	Disease	Drug(s)
S. pneumoniae	Pneumonia, bacteremia	Penicillin G 6 million units/day IV Penicillin VK 2 g/day PO Cefuroxime 750 mg Q 8 hr IV Erythromycin 2 g/day PO or IV
H. influenzae	Pneumonia, bronchitis	Cefuroxime 750 mg Q 8 hr IV TMP (10 mg/kg per day)-SMX (50 mg/kg per day) PO or IV
L. monocytogenes	Bacteremia, meningitis	Ampicillin 4 g/day, plus gentamicin 1 mg/kg per day, or TMP (5-10 mg/kg per day)-SMX (25 mg/kg per day), all IV
T. pallidum	Primary, secondary, syphilis	Benzathine penicillin 2.4 million units IM
	Latent, early	Benzathine penicillin 2.4 million units IM
	late	Benzathine penicillin 2.4 million units/wk × 3 wk IM
	Tertiary	Procaine penicillin G 2.4 million units/day IM plus probenecid 2.0 g/day × 2 wk PO
Salmonella	Bacteremia, enteritis	Ampicillin 4 g/day PO or IV Chloramphenicol 2-3 g/day PO or IV TMP (5-10 mg/kg per day)-SMX (50 mg/kg per day) PO or IV Ciprofloxacin 500-750 mg b.i.d. PO
Shigella	Enteritis, bacteremia	TMP (5 mg/kg per day)-SMX (25 mg/kg per day) PO or IV Ampicillin 2-4 g/day PO or IV Ciprofloxacin 500-750 mg b.i.d. PO
Campylobacter jejuni	Enteritis, bacteremia	Erythromycin 2 g/day PO or IV Ciprofloxacin 500-750 mg b.i.d. PO
C. fennelliae *C. cinaedi*		Ampicillin, doxycycline, chloramphenicol, and rifampin show in vitro activity (61)

TMP, trimethoprim; SMX, sulfamethoxazole.

may be substituted when a clinical response is achieved. Documented *H. influenzae* pneumonia can be treated with ampicillin (for susceptible strains), amoxacillin and clavulanate potassium (Augmentin), trimethoprim-sulfamethoxazole, or a second- or third-generation cephalosporin. Trimethoprim-sulfamethoxazole may cause serious adverse reactions in up to 60% of AIDS patients, including rash, drug fever, hepatitis, neutropenia and nausea (18, 19). However, the shorter duration of therapy (1 to 2 weeks vs 3 weeks) and the lower doses employed for treatment of bacterial pneumonia, compared to pneumocytosis, may result in a lower frequency of serious adverse reactions.

AIDS patients with pneumonia caused by encapsulated bacteria usually fail to form specific antibody and have a high rate of relapse (11,12). HIV-infected children should receive prophylactic therapy with trimethoprim-sulfamethoxazole(5 mg and 25 mg/kg per day, respectively) and monthly injections of immune globulin (20). Additionally, the second-generation *H. influenzae* type b protein (diphtheria toxoid)-polysaccharide conjugate vaccine should be given to all children over 1 year of age. The efficacy of preventive therapy for adults with HIV infection and AIDS has not been established. Several studies have shown that subjects with advanced HIV infection and a low CD4 + lymphocyte count respond poorly to pneumococcal vaccine, and instances of vaccine failure have been reported (1,11,21). Administration of pneumococcal vaccine to asymptomatic HIV-infected patients with CD4 + lymphocyte counts above 450/mm^3 results in a satisfactory serologic response, although efficacy trials have not been conducted (22). Routine use of pneumococcal vaccine for all HIV-infected individuals cannot be recommended at this time. Most authorities agree that patients who have had two or more episodes of pneumococcal or *H. influenzae* pneumonia should receive antibacterial prophylactic therapy, either with penicillin, a first-generation oral cephalosporin, or trimethoprim-sulfamethoxazole. Initiating prophylactic treatment after a single episode of bacterial pneumonia is controversial, but may be indicated in some instances.

OTHER BACTERIAL PATHOGENS

Treponema pallidum

A series of recent case reports indicate that patients with HIV infection or AIDS may have atypical manifestations of syphilis (23-25). Five cases of rapid progression of secondary syphilis to tertiary neurosyphilis, even following appropriate theray, have been reported (23,24). A single case of secondary syphilis with negative serologic tests for syphilis in an HIV-infected patient has been reported (25). Other patients have had recurrences of syphilis, without reexposure, and abnormal serologic responses after appropriate therapy.

Because the populations at risk for HIV infection also include many persons with a high risk of syphilis, routine screening for syphilis (with a VDRL) is recommended for all HIV-seropositive individuals. Treatment of primary, secondary, and latent syphilis in HIV-infected patients should follow current guidelines promulgated by the Centers for Disease Control (CDC) (26). However, patients with any unexplained neurologic symptoms should also have a lumbar puncture; the CSF should be sent for protein determination, cell count and differential, and a VDRL test. Because 15% to 30% of patients with central nervous system infection caused by *T. pallidum* may have a negative CSF VDRL test result, symptomatic patients with an elevated CSF protein level, a lymphocytic pleocytosis, and serologic evidence of syphilis should be treated for neurosyphilis with 10 days of penicillin G (24 million units/day), regardless of the CSF VDRL result. Patients with a positive CSF VDRL test, but a normal protein level, and an acellular CSF, probably do not have active neurosyphilis, although some experts would recommend intravenous therapy in this circumstance. All HIV-infected patients treated for syphilis should have close clinical and serologic follow-up. Patients whose VDRL titers fail to fall should be re-treated, perhaps intravenously. Further studies of HIV and syphilis are urgently needed.

Listeria monocytogenes

Listeria monocytogenes is a gram-positive rod that is a frequent contaminant of dairy products and other foods. Patients with cellular immune deficiency, including infants and the elderly, have a propensity for listerial infections, which frequently present as meningitis. Case reports of listerial meningitis and bacteremia in patients with AIDS have appeared, but the incidence of AIDS-related listerial infections is surprising low (27,28). Patients with listerial meningitis present with acute or chronic meningitis, characterized by fever, headache, meningismus, and altered mentation. Conversely, a febrile illness, often preceded by gastrointestinal symptoms, may be the presenting complaint. Physical examination may reveal meningeal signs. A lumbar puncture shows an elevated opening pressure, elevated protein level, normal to low glucose level, and a mild to moderate pleocytosis (50 to 500 cells/mm^3), with either polymorphonuclear or mononuclear cells predominant. The Gram stain is usually negative, and blood and CSF cultures may take 3 to 7 days to grow listeria. Patients should be treated with penicillin or ampicillin, with or without an aminoglycoside; trimethoprim-sulfamethoxazole plus rifampin appears to be a satisfactory alternative for patients with severe penicillin allergy. Most patients are treated for 10 to 14 days and relapses appear to be uncommon. Prophylactic or maintenance therapy is not recommended.

TABLE 4 Infectious Causes of Diarrhea in AIDS Patients

Associated with enterocolitis
  Bacterial
    Campylobacter jejuni and other species
    Salmonella spp.
    Shigella flexneri
  Parasitic
    Cryptosporidium
    Entamoeba histolytica
    Giardia lamblia
    Isospora
  Viral
    cytomegalovirus
Associated with proctitis
  Bacterial
    Chlamydia trachomatis
    Neisseria gonorrhoeae
    Treponema pallidum
  Viral
    herpes simplex

BACTERIAL GASTROINTESTINAL INFECTIONS

The increased incidence of gastrointestinal infections in homosexual men was well documented before identification of HIV and the onset of the AIDS epidemic (29-32). The same infectious enteric pathogens frequently isolated from homosexual men and inhabitants of developing countries also cause major morbidity and mortality among patients with AIDS (Table 4). Persistent or recurrent infection with several of these agents may also result in an index AIDS diagnosis, according to the revised surveillance case definition for AIDS (e.g., recurrent nontyphoidal salmonella septicemia) (33). Additional gastrointestinal infectious agents may be associated specifically with patients who already have an AIDS diagnosis, as a result of severe immunocompromise (e.g., cytomegalovirus colitis or cryptosporidiosis). Gastrointestinal complaints, especially diarrhea, are common in patients with AIDS and require a systematic and thorough workup, with the goal of identifying any infection amenable to treatment or amelioration. The diverse group of organisms associated with lower gastrointestinal tract disease in AIDS patients is listed in Table 4.

Presentation

Bacterial agents implicated in disease of the gastrointestinal tract in HIV-infected patients include *Salmonella, Shigella, Campylobacter, Neisseria,*

T. pallidum, and *Chlamydia*. AIDS patients infected with these organisms may present with a wide range of findings, from mild diarrhea, with or without proctitis, to severe, systemic involvement with bacteremia; asymptomatic infection with all of these pathogens also may occur. Diarrhea in an AIDS patient may be associated with rectal pain or pruritus, abdominal cramping, myalgia, nausea, vomiting, tenesmus, bloating, fever, and abdominal tenderness. Tenesmus and rectal pain suggest proctitis caused by chlamydiae, gonococci, *T. pallidum*, or herpes simplex virus. Fever, fecal leukocytes, and gross or occult fecal blood suggest bacterial infection with *Campylobacter, Shigella,* or *Salmonella* spp., as well as amebic dysentary or cytomegalovirus colitis.

Diagnosis

The initial approach to the AIDS patient with gastrointestinal complaints should include a careful history and physical examination; evaluation of the stool for fecal leukocytes and blood, ova, and parasites (three separate specimens); and culture for bacterial pathogens (Table 5). If the patient is febrile, appears toxic, or has severe symptoms, blood cultures should be obtained. If the initial evaluation fails to identify a causal agent, additional procedures may be necessary, as outlined in Table 5. The patient may eventually require sigmoidoscopy, with biopsy for culture and tissue stains to identify infection with cytomegalovirus, *Chlamydia*, and *T. pallidum*, or a noninfectious process such as Kaposi's sarcoma or lymphoma. Patients who have multiple causes identified are common.

TABLE 5 Diagnostic Approach to Diarrhea in AIDS Patients

Physical examination
    fever, abdominal tenderness, rectal pain
Laboratory evaluation
    stool
        fecal leukocytes
        ova and parasites ($\times$ 3), including *Cryptosporidium*
        culture tests for *Salmonella, Shigella, Campylobacter* spp.
    serology
        VDRL
    blood cultures (if toxic or febrile)
Sigmoidoscopic evaluation
    biopsy to culture for *Chlamydia, Neisseria,* herpesvirus, cytomegalovirus
    biopsy to examine pathology for herpesvirus, cytomegalovirus

Salmonella

Salmonella species are ubiquitous aerobic gram-negative rods that are a common cause of enteric fever and enterocolitis. Nontyphoidal salmonellae are classified as belonging to two major species; the one most commonly isolated from humans is *S. enteritidis*. More than 1500 serotypes of the nontyphoidal salmonellae have been identified, and more than 30 serotypes are frequent causes of enterocolitis in humans. In the nonimmunosuppressed host salmonellosis is usually a self-limited enteritis associated with cramping, watery diarrhea, and fecal blood and leukocytes. The primary host defense against salmonellae is cellular immunity, especially activated T lymphocytes and macrophages, and severe or disseminated salmonellosis was previously known to complicate malignancy, immunosuppressive therapy, malaria, and bartonellosis (34,35). Therefore, the occurrence of salmonellosis in patients with HIV infection was expected.

Case reports of salmonellosis in AIDS first appeared in 1983 from Africa and in 1984 from the United States (36,37). By 1985 numerous cases had been reported (38-41). Common features of these cases were a high rate of bacteremic infections, severe clinical complications, including prolonged disease, and frequent recurrences in spite of appropriate antimicrobial therapy. A study by Celum and co-workers (42) showed that the incidence of salmonellosis was 20-fold higher in AIDS patients than in men 18 to 59 years old not known to have AIDS. By using population-based AIDS and Salmonella registry data, these investigators also showed that 46% of AIDS patients with salmonellosis were bacteremic, compared with 9% of controls. Common serotypes in AIDS patients include *S. typhimurium, S. enteritidis* and *S. dublin*. Infections caused by *Salmonella* serotypes occurred throughout the late stages of HIV infection, and one-third occurred before an AIDS-defining diagnosis. Unlike other opportunistic infections in AIDS, most salmonella infections are probably new, rather than reactivated, and common environmental sources of salmonellae are often identified, including snake powders, raw milk, inadequately cooked turkeys, pet turtles, and contaminated meats (43).

Salmonellosis in HIV-infected patients may present as an acute gastroenteritis or as a typhoidal syndrome with a predominance of constitutional symptoms. Common gastrointestinal symptoms include abdominal cramping and bloating, bloody stools, watery diarrhea, and anorexia; the usual constitutional symptoms are fevers, night sweats, headache, fatigue, and prostration. Many patients with bacteremic salmonellosis lack gastrointestinal symptoms. Fever, poor skin turgor, hyperactive bowel sounds, and abdominal tenderness are common findings. The white blood cell count is often normal or slightly elevated with a preponderance of immature forms; anemia and an elevated sedimentation rate are also common. Stool examination may show occult blood and fecal leukocytes, although the sensitivity of these tests has not been determined in patients with AIDS. Cultures of the stool or blood generally grow salmonella. Salmonellae have also been isolated from a variety of other sites in AIDS patients, such as urine, bone marrow, brain abscesses, and spleen. Coinfections with a variety of enteric and nonenteric pathogens may be found.

Whereas salmonellosis is frequently not treated in the immunocompetent host, all patients with HIV infection and salmonella enteritis or bacteremia should be treated for at least 10 to 14 days. Only a limited number of antimicrobials are known to be effective for salmonellosis: ampicillin, chloramphenicol, trimethoprim-sulfamethoxazole (TMP-SMX). Therapy should be guided by susceptibility testing. Recently, two fluoroquinolones, norfloxacin and ciprofloxacin, have been released and have proved highly effective against many enteric bacterial pathogens, including *Salmonella* spp. When the differential diagnosis includes both *Salmonella* and *Campylobacter*, empiric therapy with a quinolone (e.g., ciprofloxacin 500 to 750 mg orally b.i.d.) is recommended. Because high rates of relapse have been observed in AIDS patients with salmonellosis, prolonged therapy is usually required, and many physicians choose to give suppressive therapy with TMP-SMX or ampicillin. We have seen bacteremic breakthroughs in patients treated with suppressive doses of ampicillin and, therefore, we prefer to use ciprofloxacin (250 to 500 mg b.i.d.) as chronic suppressive therapy. An uncontrolled study of ciprofloxacin for treatment of salmonellosis in six patients with HIV infection has shown sustained clinical benefit and no relapses (S. Hahn and J. L. Gerberding, personal communication). Additional controlled clinical trials of the management of AIDS-related salmonellosis are necessary.

Campylobacter

Members of the genus *Campylobacter* are slender, curved gram-negative rods that have a characteristic darting motility when viewed under dark-field or phase microscopy (44). Although *Campylobacter* species were initially believed to affect primarily immunocompromised hosts, during the last 10 years *C. jejuni* has been recognized as a major gastrointestinal tract pathogen of the normal human host (45). Newly described *Campylobacter* species (*C. fennelliae, C. cinaedi*) have recently been recognized as pathogens in homosexual men and immunocompromised patients, including those with AIDS (46,47).

Campylobacter jejuni is a major cause of bacterial gastrointestinal disease worldwide, and may be the most common cause of bacterial diarrhea in the United States. In a recent laboratory-based surveillance study, *Campylo-*

bacter isolates outnumbered *Shigella* or *Salmonella* isolates in some states, despite underreporting (48).

Outbreaks of campylobacteriosis have been associated with contaminated poultry, fresh water, unpasteurized milk, and with zoonotic transmission (49). The infective dose of organisms may be quite small, perhaps as few as 500 organisms (50). The low infective dose would be expected to facilitate fecal-oral transmission as it does for shigella. The incubation period for *C. jejuni* is reported to be 1 to 7 days (48).

The most common manifestation of campylobacter infection in AIDS patients is probably diarrhea, as it is in immunocompetent individuals (51). Bacteremia and cholecystitis have also occurred (Table 6).

Dworkin et al. (52) reported a case of chronic diarrhea caused by multiply antibiotic-resistant *C. jejuni* in a woman with AIDS who presented with diarrhea, weight loss, oral candidiasis, and disseminated *Mycobacterium avium-intracellulare* infection. A stool culture grew *C. jejuni* without other pathogens. Over the subsequent 8 months, stool cultures were positive for *C. jejuni* on 11 occasions, despite multiple courses of oral and intravenous antibiotics.

TABLE 6   Severe Campylobacter Infections Reported in Patients with AIDS or ARC

Isolate	Signs, symptoms	Source	Relapse	Associated conditions	Treatment	Ref.
C. jejuni	Refractory diarrhea	Stool	Yes	AIDS, disseminated MAI, CMV	ERY, AG, TCN	52
C. fetus	Abdominal pain, fever	Blood, peritoneal fluid	Yes	AIDS, disseminated cryptococcosis	ERY/NAF, and tobra, then ERY	56, 57
C. cinaedi	Abdominal distention, fever, diarrhea	Blood	No	AIDS, lymphoma	Tobra, cefazolin, and ERY	54
C. cinaedi	[a]Fever	Blood	No	ARC	NAF, gent, CAM	55
C. fennelliae	[a]Fever, diarrhea	Blood	No	ARC	NAF, gent	55

[a]Same patient, with successive bacteremias due to two different *Campylobacter* spp.
Abbreviations: MAI, *Mycobacterium avium-intracellulare*; CMV, cytomegalovirus; AIDS, acquired immunodeficiency syndrome; ARC, AIDS-related complex.
Antibiotics: ERY, erythromycin; TCN, tetracycline; NAF, nafcillin; CAM, chloramphenicol; tobra, tobramycin; gent, gentamicin; AG, aminoglycoside.

The first isolate tested was resistant to multiple antibiotics, including erythromycin and tetracyline, drugs to which *C. jejuni* is nearly always susceptible (53).

Bacteremia with *C. cinaedi* was reported in a homosexual man with AIDS in 1987 (54). The index AIDS diagnosis in this patient was undifferentiated lymphoma, which developed 1 year before the bacteremic episode. When bacteremia was diagnosed, the patient was febrile and septic but not neutropenic. Several loose, bloody stools failed to grow any enteric pathogen; two aerobic blood cultures drawn on admission grew *C. cinaedi* on day 6. Erythromycin produced dramatic resolution of findings, and he was well 6 months later. Both *C. cinaedi* and *C. fennelliae* were reported as causing successive bacteremias in a bisexual male with AIDS-related complex, despite appropriate antimicrobial therapy (55). *Campylobacter fetus* spp. *fetus* bacteremia was associated with cholecystitis in another patient with AIDS (56,57). This patient was noted to have acalculus cholecystitis with perforation noted at laparotomy, and *C. fetus* and *Staphylococcus epidermidis* were cultured from his blood and peritoneal fluid. Cultures taken after 2 weeks of IV erythromycin, tobramycin, and nafcillin therapy were negative. Eight months later, the patient developed abdominal pain, and *C. fetus* spp. *fetus* was again recovered from blood cultures.

Recognition and diagnosis of campylobacter infections can be difficult because of their diverse clinical manifestations (Table 6) and the specialized culture techniques required to recover *Campylobacter* species (see Chap. 21).

Treatment   Whether or not *C. jejuni* diarrhea in normal persons should be treated is controversial, because the disease is self-limited, and many patients are asymptomatic or markedly improved by the time the organism is identified in stool (58). However, the mean duration of campylobacter shedding in the stool is significantly decreased by antibiotic treatment, from 2 weeks to 2 days (59), and very early antibiotic treatment (within 2 days of onset of symptoms) probably decreases the duration of symptoms (60). *Campylobacter jejuni* is usually resistant to trimethoprim-sulfamethoxazole and susceptible to erythromycin, ciprofloxacin, and chloramphenicol, although erythromycin-resistant strains have been reported. All campylobacterlike organisms tested by Flores et al. (61) were susceptible to ampicillin, tetracycline, nalidixic acid, rifampin, and ceftriaxone, and most were also susceptible to trimethoprim-sulfamethoxazole; approximately one-fourth of these strains were resistant to erythromycin.

In the immunocompromised patient with AIDS, symptomatic diarrhea caused by *C. jejuni* warrants antimicrobial therapy with erythromycin or ciprofloxacin for 7 to 10 days. Therapy should be altered depending on antimicrobial susceptibility patterns. Symptoms that persist after treatment should prompt a repeat stool culture and susceptibility testing. Susceptibility testing must be performed on all isolates of *C. jejuni, C. fetus,* and campylobacterlike organisms isolated from sterile sites (blood, etc.), and the patient should be treated with parenteral antibiotics.

Shigella

Four species of *Shigella* are responsible for disease in humans: *S. dysenteriae, S. flexneri, S. boydii,* and *S. sonnei,* also referred to as subgroups A, B, C, and D, respectively (62). Shigella was recognized as an important cause of dysentery before the turn of the century, and was reported as causing sexually transmitted enteritis in homosexual men in 1974 (63).

Incidence   The estimated incidence of *Shigella* infections in the United States is 200,000/yr. Enteric infection is most prevalent in children, with approximately 70% of the isolates in the United States noted to be *S. sonnei* (64). In one study of stools submitted from a young adult population, approximately 2% of the stool cultures were positive for *Shigella* species (48). The incidence of shigella enteritis in homosexual men, with or without AIDS, is apparently greater than in the heterosexual population, and the species most commonly isolated is *S. flexneri* (65). In a recent study of acute diarrhea by Siegal et al. (66) *Shigella* species were recovered from the stools of 67% of homosexual men who had a bacterial pathogen; the remaining 33% had *Campylobacter* species. In a study of intestinal infections in patients with AIDS (67), a bacterial pathogen was isolated in 40% of patients, and of these, 25% were *S. flexneri.* Shigella bacteremia occurs only rarely, most often in young children and less frequently in immunocompromised patients, including those with AIDS. The 27 adult cases of shigellemia reported in the English literature, and the six cases reported to date in patients with AIDS, have recently been reviewed (68-71).

Presentation   Shigella gastroenteritis presents with abdominal cramping, fever, and diarrhea that often contains gross blood and fecal leukocytes on microscopy (Table 7). Sigmoidoscopy often reveals ulcerated, friable, edematous mucosa. Rarely, *Shigella* spp. may be cultured from stool in the absence of symptoms, as noted in only one patient (of 243 asymptomatic patients) in a recent study of the prevalence of enteric pathogens in homosexual men with and without AIDS (72). In contrast, six asymptomatic homosexual patients had cultures positive for herpes simplex virus, six for *Campylobacter* spp., and seven for *Chlamydia* spp. Shigellae were more often associated with symptoms of diarrhea and proctitis, with a higher rate of isolation in the symptomatic group without AIDS when compared with the symptomatic group with AIDS. Persistent shigella infection with diarrhea in an HIV-infected patient has been reported (73).

TABLE 7 Severe Shigella Infections Reported in Patients with AIDS or Infection with HIV

Isolate	Signs symptoms	Colonoscopy	Source	Relapse	Associated conditions	Treatment	Ref.
S. flexneri	Severe diarrhea	Colitis	Blood	NA	Esophageal candidiasis, weight loss, AIDS	AMP for 10 days	71
S. flexneri	Severe diarrhea T = 39.5 °C	ND	Blood, stool	NA	SS, AIDS	Cefoxitin	69
S. flexneri	Fever, diarrhea	Proctocolitis	Blood	No	Disseminated histo-plasmosis. crypto-sporidiosis, scrofula, AIDS	AMP for 14 days	70
S. flexneri	Diarrhea T = 40.0 °C	Hyperemia, aphthous ulcers	Blood, then stool	Yes—Sx recurred after 1 wk, with positive stool cx	Subsequent PCP, CMV retinitis	AMP then T/S for 14 days	70
S. flexneri	Abdominal tenderness, T = 40.5 °C	ND	Blood	No	Miliary tuberculosis, AIDS	Gent and AMP, then T/S	70
S. flexneri	Diarrhea T = 40.0 °C	Colitis (postmortem exam)	Blood	Died from shigella sepsis	KS, angioimmuno-blastic lymphadeno-pathy, AIDS	PCN, CAM, at time of death	70
S. flexneri	Diarrhea T = 40.0 °C	ND	Blood and stool, then stool	Yes, 4 wk after Rx	Cryptosporidiosis. AIDS	AMP for 14 days, then T/S	70
S. flexneri	T = 38.3 °C	Colitis	Stool	No	HIV Ab present	T/S, then norfloxacin	73

Antibiotics: AMP, ampicillin; T/S, trimethoprim-sulfamethoxazole; TCN, tetracycline; gent, gentamicin; PCN, penicillin; CAM, chloramphenicol.

Abbreviations: ND, not done; T, temperature; SS, sickle cell disease; NA, not available; Sx, symptoms; cx, culture; PCP, Pneumocystis carinii pneumonia; CMV, cytomegalovirus; Rx, treatment; HIV, human immunodeficiency virus; Ab, antibody.

Presenting symptoms in AIDS patients with shigella bacteremia uniformly included diarrhea and high fever. One patient developed septic shock and ARDS and died, despite intravenous therapy with chloramphenicol (70). Table 7 summarizes the presenting signs and symptoms of severe shigella infections reported in patients with AIDS and HIV infection.

Diagnosis Gastrointestinal infection with *Shigella* spp. should be suspected and sought by culture of stools in all AIDS patients with diarrhea. Blood cultures should also be obtained in patients with high fever and other systemic symptoms. The organisms remain viable in stool for only a short period and, thus, stool specimens should be processed without delay (see Chap. 21). Recovery of *Shigella* and *Campylobacter* spp. from rectal swabs is excellent. Recovery of *Shigella* organisms is especially high from specimens taken from colonic ulcers seen with colonoscopy.

Treatment Studies have shown that antimicrobial therapy of immunologically normal patients with shigella infection shortens the duration of illness and excretion of organisms in the stool. AIDS patients with documented shigella infections should receive antibiotic therapy, including the rare, asymptomatic patient with positive stool cultures. Determination of antimicrobial susceptibilities is extremely important because of the increasing number of isolates resistant to conventionally used agents such as ampicillin and trimethoprim-sulfamethoxazole. The quinolone antibiotics, norfloxacin and ciprofloxacin, demonstrate excellent activity against most bacterial enteric pathogens and provide a logical choice for empiric therapy when infection with *Shigella*, *Campylobacter*, or *Salmonella* spp. is suggested. A quinolone should be considered for therapy of established infection with multiresistant or persistent *S. flexneri*. Suspected shigellemia should be treated with intravenous antibiotics, preferably trimethoprim-sulfamethoxazole (5 to 7.5 mg/ kg per day of trimethoprim), and treatment should be continued for 7 to 14 days. Cultures obtained after completion of antibiotic therapy can document eradication of the shigella infection.

REFERENCES

1. Bowen, D. L., Lane, H. C., Fauci, A. S. (1985). Immunopathogenesis of the acquired immunodeficiency syndrome. *Ann. Intern. Med. 103*:704-709.
2. Lane, H. C., Depper, J. M., Green, W. C. et al. (1985). Qualitative analysis of immune function in patients with the acquired immunodeficiency syndrome: Evidence for a selective defect in soluble antigen recognition. *N. Engl. J. Med. 313*: 79-84.
3. Rogers, V. D. and Kagnoff, M. F. (1987). Gastrointestinal manifestations of the acquired immune deficiency syndrome. *West. J. Med. 146*:57-67.
4. Ammann, A. S., Schiffman, G., Abrams, D. et al. (1984). B-cell immunodeficiency in acquired immune deficiency syndrome. *JAMA 251*:1447-1449.

5. Katz, I. R., Krown, S. E., Safai, B., Oettgen, H. F., and Hoffman, M. K. (1986). Antigen-specific and polyclonal B-cell responses in patients with acquired immunodeficiency disease syndrome. *Clin. Immunol. Immunopathol. 39*:359-367.

6. Lane, H. C., Masur, H., Edgar, L. C. et al. (1983). Abnormalities of B-cell activation and immunoregulation in patients with the acquired immunodeficiency disease syndrome. *N. Engl. J. Med. 309*:453-58.

7. Bernstein, L. J., Krieger, B. Z., Novick, B., Sicklide, M. J., and Rubinstein, A. (1985). Bacterial infection in the acquired immunodeficiency syndrome of children. *Pediatr. Infect. Dis. 4*:472-475.

8. Oleske, J., Minnefor, A., Cooper, R. Jr. et al. (1983). Immune deficiency syndrome in children. *JAMA 249*:2345-2349.

9. Richman, D. D., Fischl, M. A., Grieco, M. H. et al. (1987). The toxicity of azidothymidine (AZT) in the treatment of patients with AIDS and AIDS-related complex: A double-blind, placebo-controlled trial. *N. Engl. J. Med. 317*:192-197.

10. Murray, J. F., Felton, C. P., Garay, S. M. et al. (1984). Pulmonary complications of the acquired immunodeficiency syndrome: Report of a National Heart, Lung and Blood Institute Workshop. *N. Engl. J. Med. 310*:1682-1688.

11. Simberkoff, M. S., El Sadr, W., Schiffman, G., and Raha, J. J. Jr. (1984). *Streptococcus pneumoniae* infections and bacteremia in patients with acquired immunodeficiency syndrome, with report of pneumococcal vaccine failure. *Am. Rev. Respir. Dis. 130*:1174-1176.

12. Polsky, B., Gold, J. W. M., Whimbey, E. et al. (1986). Bacterial pneumonia in patients with the acquired immunodeficiency syndrome. *Ann. Intern. Med. 104*:38-41.

13. Gerberding, J. L., Krieger, J., and Sande, M. A. (1986). Recurrent bacteremic infection with *S. pneumoniae* in patients with AIDS virus (AV) infection. *Program Abstr. 26th Intersci. Conf. Antimicrob. Agents Chemother.* American Society for Microbiology, p. 177 (Abstr. 443).

14. Witt, D. J., Craven, D. E., and McCabe, W. R. (1987). Bacterial infections in adult patients with the acquired immune deficiency syndrome (AIDS) and AIDS-related complex. *Am. J. Med. 82*:900-906.

15. Selwyn, P. A., Feingold, A. R., Hartel, D., Schoenbaum, E. E., and Friedland, G. H. (1987). Bacterial pneumonia and HIV infection in parenteral drug users without AIDS. *Proc. III Int. Conf. AIDS.* Washington, D.C., Abstr. TH41.

16. Eng, R. H., Bishburg, E., Smith, S. M., Geller, H., and Kapila, R. (1986). Bacteremia and fungemia in patients with acquired immune deficiency syndrome. *Am. J. Clin. Pathol. 86*:105-107.

16a. Whimberg, E., Gold, J. W. M., Polsky, B. et al. (1986). Bacteremia and fungemia in patients with acquired immunodeficiency syndrome. *Ann. Intern. Med. 104*:511-514.

17. Kovacs, J. A., Hiemenz, J. W., Macher, A. M. et al. (1984). *Pneumocystis carinii* pneumonia: A comparison between patients with the acquired immunodeficiency syndrome and patients with other immunodeficiencies. *Ann. Intern. Med. 100*:663-671.

18. Gordin, F. M., Simon, G. L., Wofsy, C. B., and Mills, J. (1984). Adverse reactions to trimethoprim-sulfamethoxazole in patients with the acquired immunodeficiency syndrome. *Ann. Intern. Med. 100*:495-499.

19. Jaffe, H. S., Abrams, D. I., Ammann, A. J. et al. (1983). Complications of cotrimoxazole in treatment of AIDS-associated *Pneumocystis carinii* pneumonia in homosexual men. *Lancet* 2:1109-1111.

20. Calvelli, T. A. and Rubinstein, A. R. (1985). Intravenous gamma-globulin in infant acquired immunodeficiency syndrome. *Pediatr. Infect. Dis.* 5(suppl. 3): S207-210.

21. Pahwa, S. G., Quilop, M. T. J., Lange, M., Pahwa, R. M., and Griego, M. H. (1984). Defective B-lymphocyte function in homosexual men in relation to the acquired immunodeficiency syndrome. *Ann. Intern. Med.* 101:757-763.

22. Huang, K.-L., Ruben, F. L., Rinald, C. R. et al. (1987). Antibody responses after influenza and pneumococcal immunization in HIV-infected homosexual men. *JAMA* 257:2047-2050.

23. Berry, C. D., Hooton, T. M., Collier, A. C., and Lukehart, S. A. (1987). Neurologic relapse after benzathine penicillin therapy for secondary syphilis in a patient with HIV infection. *N. Engl. J. Med.* 316:1587-1589.

24. Johns, D. R., Tierney, M., and Felsenstein, D. (1987). Alteration in the natural history of neurosyphilis by concurrent infection with the human immunodeficiency virus. *N. Engl. J. Med.* 316:1569-1572.

25. Hicks, C. B., Benson, P. M., Lupton, G. P., and Tramont, E. L. (1987). Seronegative secondary syphilis in a patient infected with the human immunodeficiency virus (HIV) with Kaposi sarcoma: A diagnostic dilemma. *Ann. Intern. Med.* 107:492-495.

26. CDC (1985). 1985 STD treatment guidelines: Syphilis. *MMWR* 34(4S):945-995.

27. Jacobs, J. L. and Murray, H. W. (1986). Why is *Listeria monocytogenes* not a pathogen in the acquired immunodeficiency syndrome? *Arch. Intern. Med.* 146:1299-1300.

28. Mascola, L., Lieb, L., Chiu, J., Fannin, S. L., and Linnan, M. J. (1988). Listeriosis: An uncommon opportunistic infection in patients with acquired immunodeficiency syndrome. A report of five cases and a review of the literature. *Am. J. Med.* 84:162-164.

29. Kazal, H. L., Sohn, N., Carrasco, J. L., Robilotti, J., Jr., and Delaney, W. E. (1976). The gay bowel syndrome: Clinicopathologic correlation in 260 cases. *Ann. Clin. Lab. Sci.* 6:184-192.

30. Owen, W. F. (1980). Sexually transmitted diseases and traumatic problems in homosexual men. *Ann. Intern. Med.* 92:805-808.

31. Quinn, T. C., Corey, L., Chaffee, R. G., Schuffler, M. D., Brancato, F. P., and Holmes, K. K. (1981). The etiology of anorectal infection in homosexual men. *Am. J. Med.* 71:395-406.

32. Baker, R. W. and Peppercorn, M. A. (1982). Gastrointestinal ailments of homosexual men. *Medicine* 61:390-405.

33. CDC (1987). Revision of the CDC surveillance case definition for acquired immunodeficiency syndrome. *MMWR* 36(suppl. 1S):1S-16S.

34. Cherubin, C. E., Fodor, T., Denmark, L., Master, C., Fuerst, H. T., and Winter, J. (1969). The epidemiology of salmonellosis in New York City. *Am. J. Epidemiol.* 90:112-125.

35. Han, T., Sokal, J. E., and Neter, E. (1967). Salmonellosis in disseminated malignant diseases. A seven-year review (1959-1965). *N. Engl. J. Med.* 275:1045-1052.

36. Offenstadt, G., Pinta, P., Hericord, P., Jagueux, M., Jean, F., Amstutz, P., Valade, S., and Lesavre, P. (1983). Multiple opportunistic infection due to AIDS in a previously healthy black woman from Zaire. *N. Engl. J. Med. 308*:775.

37. Bottone, D. L., Lane, H. C., and Fauci, A. S. (1985). Immunopathogenesis of the acquired immunodeficiency syndrome. *Ann. Intern. Med. 103*:704-709.

38. Jacobs, J. L., Gold, J. W. M., Murray, H. W., Roberts, R. B., and Amstrong, D. (1985). Salmonella infections in patients with the acquired immunodeficiency syndrome. *Ann. Intern. Med. 102*:186-188.

39. Glaser, J. B., Morton-Kute, L., Berger, S. R., Weber, J., Siegal, F. P., Lopez, C., Robbins, W., and Landesman, S. H. (1985). Recurrent *Salmonella typhimurium* bacteremia associated with the acquired immunodeficiency syndrome. *Ann. Intern. Med. 102*:189-193.

40. Profeta, S., Forrester, C., Eng, R. H. K., Liu, R., Johnson, E., Palinkas, R., and Smith, S. M. (1985). Salmonella infections in patients with acquired immunodeficiency syndrome. *Arch. Intern. Med. 145*:670-672.

41. Fischl, M. A., Dickinson, G. M., Sinave, C., Pitchenik, A. E., and Cleary, T. J. (1985). Salmonella bacteremia as manifestation of acquired immunodeficiency syndrome. *Arch. Intern. Med. 146*:113-115.

42. Celum, C. L., Chaisson, R. E., Rutherford, G. W., Barnhart, J. L., and Echenberg, D. F. (1987). Incidence of salmonellosis in patients with AIDS. *J. Infect. Dis. 156*:998-1002.

43. Chaisson, R. E. (1988). Infections due to encapsulated bacteria, *Salmonella, Shigella,* and *Campylobacter. Infect. Dis. Clin. N. Am. 2*:475-84.

44. Morris, G. K. and Patton, C. M. (1985). *Campylobacter.* In *Manual of Clinical Microbiology*, 4th ed. (Lennette, E. H., Balows, A., Hausler, W., Jr., and Shadomy, H. J., eds.). Washington, D.C., American Society for Microbiology, pp. 302-308.

45. Skirrow, M. B. (1977). Campylobacter enteritis: A "new" disease. *Br. Med. J. 2*:9-11.

46. Quinn, T. C., Goodell, S. E., Fennell, C., Wang, S.-P., Schuffler, M. D., Holmes, K. K., and Stamm, W. E. (1984). Infections with *Campylobacter jejuni* and campylobacter-like organisms in homosexual men. *Ann. Intern. Med. 101*: 187-192.

47. Totten, P. A., Fennell, C. L., Tenover, F. C., Wezenberg, J. M., Perine, P. L., Stamm, W. E., and Holmes, K. K. (1985). *Campylobacter cinaedi* (sp.nov.) and *Campylobacter fennelliae* (sp.nov.): Two new *Campylobacter* species associated with enteric disease in homosexual men. *J. Infect. Dis. 151*:131-139.

48. Blaser, M. J., Wells, J. G., Feldman, R. A., Pollard, R. A., Allen, J. R., and Collaborative Diarrheal Disease Study Group. (1983). Campylobacter enteritis in the United States. *Ann. Intern. Med. 98*:360-365.

49. Blaser, M. J., Tayler, D. N., and Feldman, R. A. (1983). Epidemiology of *Campylobacter jejuni* infection. *Epidemiol. Rev. 5*:157-176.

50. Blaser, M. J. and Reller, L. B. (1987). Campylobacter enteritis. *N. Engl. J. Med. 305*:1444-1452.

51. Fennell, C. L., Totten, P. A., Quinn, T. C., Patton, D. L., Holmes, K. K., and Stamm, W. E. (1984). Characterization of campylobacter-like organisms isolated from homosexual men. *J. Infect. Dis. 149*:58-66.

52. Dworkin, B., Wormser, G. P., Abdoo, R. A., Cabello, F., Aguero, M. E., and Sivak, S. L. (1986). Persistence of multiply antibiotic-resistant *Campylobacter jejuni* in a patient with the acquired immune deficiency syndrome. *Am. J. Med.* *80*:965-970.

53. Vanhoof, R., Vanderlinden, M. P., Dierckx, R., Lauwers, S., Yourassowsky, E., and Butzler, J. P. (1978). Susceptibility of *Campylobacter fetus* subsp. *jejuni* to twenty-nine antimicrobial agents. *Antimicrob. Agents Chemother.* *14*:553-556.

54. Cimolai, N., Gill, M. J., Jones, A., Flores, B., Stamm, W. E., Laurie, W., Madden, B., and Shahrabadi, M. S. (1987). *Campylobacter cinaedi* bacteremia: Case report and laboratory findings. *J. Clin. Microbiol.* *25*:942-943.

55. Ng, V. L., Hadley, W. K., Fennell, C. L., Flores, B. M., and Stamm, W. E. (1987). Successive bacteremias with *Campylobacter cinaedi* and *Campylobacter fennelliae* in a bisexual male. *J. Clin. Microbiol.* *25*:2008-2009.

56. Costel, E. E., Wheeler, A. P., and Gregg, C. R. (1984). *Campylobacter fetus* ssp. *fetus* cholecystitis and relapsing bacteremia in a patient with acquired immunodeficiency syndrome. *South. Med. J.* *77*:927-928.

57. Wheeler, A. P. and Gregg, C. R. (1986). Campylobacter bacteremia, cholecystitis, and the acquired immunodeficiency syndrome. *Ann. Intern. Med.* *105*:804.

58. Anders, B. J., Lauer, B. A., Paisley, J. W., and Reller, L. B. (1982). Double-blind placebo controlled trial of erythromycin for treatment of campylobacter enteritis. *Lancet* *1*:131-132.

59. Pai, C. H., Gillis, F., Tuomanen, E., and Marks, M. I. (1983). Erythromycin in treatment of campylobacter enteritis in children. *Am. J. Dis. Child.* *137*:286-88.

60. Salazar-Lindo, E., Sack, R. B., Chea-Woo, E., Kay, B. A., Piscoya, Z. A., Leon-Barua, R., and Yi, A. (1986). Early treatment with erythromycin of *Campylobacter jejuni*-associated dysentery in children. *J. Pediatr.* *109*:355-360.

61. Flores, B. M., Fennell, C. L., Holmes, K. K., and Stamm, W. E. (1985). In vitro susceptibilities of campylobacter-like organisms to twenty antimicrobial agents. *Antimicrob. Agents Chemother.* *28*:188-191.

62. Kantor, H. S. (1986). Bacterial enteritis. In *Infectious Diseases and Medical Microbiology*, 2d ed. (Braude, A. I., Davis, C. E., and Fierer, J., eds). Philadelphia, W.B. Saunders, pp. 897-899.

63. Dritz, S. K. and Back, A. F. (1974). Shigella enteritis venereally transmitted. *N. Engl. J. Med.* *291*:1194.

64. Blaser, M. J., Pollard, R. A., and Feldman, R. A. (1983). Shigella infections in the United States, 1974-1980. *J. Infect. Dis.* *147*:771-775.

65. Dritz, S. K., Ainsworth, T. E., Garrard, W. F., Back, A., Palmer, R. D., Boucher, L. A., and River, E. (1977). Patterns of sexually transmitted enteric diseases in a city. *Lancet* *2*:3-4.

66. Siegel, D., Cohen, P. T., Neighbor, M., Larkin, H., Newman, M., Yajko, D., and Hadley, K. (1987). Predictive value of stool examination in acute diarrhea. *Arch. Pathol. Lab. Med.* *111*:715-718.

67. Smith, P. D., Lane, H. C., Gill, V. J., Manischewitz, J. F., Quinnan, G. V., Fauci, A. S., and Masur, H. (1988). Intestinal infections in patients with the acquired immunodeficiency syndrome (AIDS): Etiology and response to therapy. *Ann. Intern. Med.* *108*:328-333.

68. Morduchowicz, G., Huminer, D., Siegman-Igra, Y., Drucker, M., Block, C. S., and Pitlik, S. D. (1987). Shigella bacteremia in adults: A report of five cases and review of the literature. *Arch. Intern. Med. 147*:2034-2037.
69. Mandell, W. and New, H. C. (1986). Shigella bacteremia in patients with the acquired immune deficiency. *JAMA 255*:3116-3117.
70. Baskin, D. H., Lax, J. D., and Barenberg, D. (1987). Shigella bacteremia in patients with the acquired immune deficiency. *Am. J. Gastroenterol. 82*:338-341.
71. Glupczynski, Y., Hansen, W., Jonas, C., and Deltenre, M. (1985). *Shigella flexneri* bacteraemia in a patient with acquired immune deficiency syndrome. *Acta Clin. Belg. 40*:388-390.
72. Laughon, B. E., Druckman, D. A., Vernon, A., Quinn, T. C., Polk, B. F., Modlin, J. F., Yolken, R. H., and Bartlett, J. G. (1988). Prevalence of enteric pathogens in homosexual men with and without acquired immunodeficiency syndrome. *Gastroenterology 94*:984-993.
73. Gander, R. M. and LaRocco, M. T. (1987). Multiple drug-resistance in *Shigella flexneri* isolated from a patient with human immunodeficiency virus. *Diagn. Microbiol. Infect. Dis. 8*:193-196.

14
Mycobacterial Diseases

Gisela F. Schecter* *Department of Public Health, San Francisco, California*

Since the presence of a new cause of immunodeficiency in adults was first noted in 1981, it has been recognized that numerous infections generally handled by cell-mediated immunity were found with high prevalence in this population. Mycobacterial diseases are no exception. The first mycobacterial pathogen associated with the acquired immunodeficiency syndrome (AIDS) was *Mycobacterium avium* complex (MAC). Infection with this pathogen was found in some of the earliest reported AIDS cases and it was soon appreciated that widely disseminated MAC infection was fairly common in people with AIDS (1,2). In these patients the manifestations of MAC infection were radically different from the previously known chronic pulmonary disease found in patients with preexisting lung disease. Instead, *M. avium* was found in multiple sites within the body, typically the gastrointestinal tract, the blood, bone marrow, liver, and other sites. Other nontuberculous mycobacteria have been reported in patients with AIDS but with far less frequency than MAC. The association between *M. tuberculosis* and AIDS was first reported in 1984 (3). Although tuberculosis in AIDS patients commonly has pulmonary manifestations, disseminated disease caused by *M. tuberculosis* is seen much more frequently in these patients than in patients with normal immune function. Unlike *M. avium* complex, however, *M. tuberculosis* is highly communicable and, thus, has major public health implications. The presence of *M. tuberculosis* cultured from any nonpulmonary site in the presence of a positive human immunodeficiency virus (HIV) serologic test is now part of the surveillance definition of AIDS (4).

Current affiliation: University of California, San Francisco, California

MYCOBACTERIUM TUBERCULOSIS

Epidemiology

One hundred years ago, tuberculosis was the chief infectious cause of death in the United States. The twentieth century has seen a steady decline in tuberculosis morbidity that accelerated in the early 1950s after the introduction of effective chemotherapy. With the decline in new tuberculosis infections, the mean age of persons with tuberculosis has progressively increased. By 1980, tuberculosis in the United States had become a disease of high-risk groups such as the elderly, the homeless, alcoholics, refugees and recent immigrants, and racial and ethnic minority groups. Concurrent with and, in part, because of the advent of AIDS, the decline in tuberculosis morbidity has halted. In 1986, for the first time since data have been collected nationally (1953), there was an increase in the number of indigenous cases of tuberculosis reported to the Centers for Disease Control (CDC) (5,6). This was due to increased numbers of cases in cities such as New York City, Newark, and Miami (3,7). The increase in new cases has occurred primarily among young adults and reflects the age distribution of AIDS.

The prevalence of active tuberculosis among patients with AIDS has reflected patterns of previous infection with the tubercle bacillus. Tuberculosis has been most common in AIDS patients who are black, Hispanic, Haitian, intravenous drug abusers, or foreign-born (3,7-9) rather than white, homosexual, American-born men who have not been involved with intravenous drug use. The prevalence of active tuberculosis among patients with AIDS varies sharply, depending upon locale. The primary predictor of rates of tuberculosis in AIDS patients has been the underlying demographics of the AIDS patients themselves. For example, in San Francisco only 2% of AIDS patients have had, or currently have, tuberculosis (10). The overwhelming majority of patients with AIDS in San Francisco are white, American-born males without a history of intravenous drug abuse (11). In contrast, 34% of AIDS patients reported by Pitchenick et al. (3) in 1984 in Florida also had tuberculosis. In that state, more than half of the patients reported with AIDS were Haitian, and the high frequency of tuberculosis undoubtedly reflects the very high background prevalence of tuberculous infection in migrants from that country. Other reports have shown tuberculosis rates intermediate between these extremes in the United States (7,9,12).

Information about the epidemiology of tuberculosis in African AIDS patients is, as yet, sketchy, but the disease is likely to become a major problem for this continent where the prevalence of *M. tuberculosis* infection in the general population is above 50%. In one report from Zaire (13), it was noted that 40% of patients on a general tuberculosis ward were found to be HIV-positive.

The reported median ages of patients with AIDS and tuberculosis, ranging from the low to mid-30s, is younger than those of patients with tuberculosis but without AIDS (11,12). The male preponderance usually seen in tuberculosis is exaggerated in AIDS patients, with the percentage of male AIDS/tuberculosis patients ranging from 80% to 100%. In most published reports, American-born or Haitian-born blacks constitute the majority of patients with AIDS and tuberculosis (3,7). This is not true in San Francisco where two-thirds of patients with both diagnoses are noted to be non-Hispanic white. AIDS remains rare among Asians, both on the Asian continent and in the United States. For this reason, Asian patients with both tuberculosis and AIDS have been very uncommon.

Pathophysiology

Tuberculosis is spread almost exclusively by the respiratory route. A person with pulmonary lesions, through coughing, singing, or even talking, can aerosolize droplets containing *M. tuberculosis.* These droplets then condense and remain airborne for extended periods. When a susceptible individual inhales droplet nuclei (1 to 10 μm in size) they may lodge in the alveoli where they can proliferate unchecked. The intra-alveolar organisms are picked up by alveolar macrophages and transported to the regional nodes. From there, hematogenous dissemination occurs. Approximately 3 to 8 weeks after infection, specific cell-mediated immunity develops (manifested by a significant tuberculin skin test reaction) and multiplication of *M. tuberculosis* is halted or greatly reduced. Cell-mediated immunity is crucial to halting the progression of infection, and activated tissue macrophages are the primary effector cells. In most patients, a few quiescent organisms remain, forming a nidus of latent infection, which may reactivate later in life, most commonly at the lung apices. Because one end result of infection with HIV is profound depression of cellular immunity, cell-mediated immunity may be insufficient to halt the progression of infection during the primary hematologic dissemination phase, and the infected person may develop miliary or widely disseminated tuberculosis as part of the primary infection process. Because *M. tuberculosis* is an organism sufficiently virulent to cause disease in a normal host, reactivation of quiescent tuberculosis may occur before the detection of other processes that define AIDS such as *Pneumocystis carinii* pneumonia.

Clinical Findings

The clinical and radiographic presentation of tuberculosis as it occurs in patients with HIV infection is considerably different from the presentation typically associated with tuberculosis in immunocompetent persons. Most notably, extrapulmonary tuberculosis is much more common in patients with

AIDS (3,7,11). Sites of involvement include lymph nodes (including intra-thoracic nodes), central nervous system (parenchymal tuberculomas and meningitis), soft tissues, bone marrow, genitourinary tract, liver, and blood. Bacteremia with *M. tuberculosis* has not been described in immunocompetent persons, yet several instances have been observed in AIDS patients (14). The classic symptoms of tuberculosis, such as weight loss, fevers, night sweats, and fatigue, are seen in many patients with AIDS who do not have tuberculosis, and thus they do not specifically suggest tuberculosis. Because of the frequency of extrapulmonary tuberculosis in AIDS patients, respiratory signs and symptoms are relatively less frequent and, when present, are often due to other pulmonary processes.

Pulmonary

When pulmonary tuberculosis is present in patients with AIDS, the customary chest roentgenographic abnormalities found in patients without AIDS, such as apical focal infiltrates with or without cavities, are less frequently seen. In a recent series, the radiographs showed diffuse interstitial or miliary patterns present on x-ray in 44% of cases, with a focal infiltrate present in only 26% (15). Cavitation was not present in any of these cases, although it has been seen in other series (11). Intrathoracic adenopathy is a highly unusual finding in adult tuberculosis without AIDS, but was present in 15% of AIDS patients. A pleural effusion, although thought to be rare in patients with AIDS and tuberculosis, has also been found in up to 20% of patients (11). Symptoms have included cough with sputum production, shortness of breath, chest pain, and hemoptysis.

Lymphatic

Approximately one-third of patients with AIDS and tuberculosis have presented with lymphatic disease (3,11). Adenopathy is most commonly seen in cervical, axillary, and intrathoracic locations. The cervical lymphatic nodes tend to rapidly increase in size, frequently over a period of only 2 to 4 weeks. A relatively distinctive feature of tuberculosis in AIDS patients has been the high frequency of mediastinal, paratracheal, and hilar lymphadenopathy noted on chest x-ray films. Although the intrathoracic adenopathy has tended to be large and bulky, as in cervical or axillary disease, there have been no reported cases of bronchial constriction as a result of extrinsic pressure from tuberculous nodes. Intra-abdominal adenopathy as well as inguinal adenopathy secondary to tuberculosis have also been described.

Central Nervous System

Although central nervous system tuberculosis makes up less than 2% of cases of tuberculosis in the country as a whole, the frequency of central nervous system manifestations in AIDS patients with tuberculosis has been about

5% to 10% (3,11,16,17). Of particular note has been the finding that tuberculomas presenting as mass lesions have been noted with increased frequency in AIDS patients. On computed tomography (CT) scan, these lesions are ring enhancing and are difficult to distinguish on CT scan from the lesions of toxoplasmosis (16). Meningitis, although less common than tuberculomas in AIDS patients, has also been found (11,16).

Other Sites

Other sites of localized tuberculosis have been the musculoskeletal system, the skin, and the soft tissues. In addition, positive cultures for *M. tuberculosis* have been recovered from cultures of urine, blood, bone marrow, and liver, but often without concomitant symptoms or signs referable to those organ systems. Blood cultures in one series were found to be positive for *M. tuberculosis* in 11% of AIDS patients with tuberculosis (22). A positive culture for *M. tuberculosis* from an extrapulmonary site has been present in more than half of patients with tuberculosis and AIDS.

Diagnosis

The diagnosis of tuberculosis in AIDS patients can be difficult. The tuberculin skin test is reactive in only about 10% to 39% of patients in contrast with over 90% positive in tuberculosis patients without AIDS (8,11). In HIV-infected patients without other manifestations of AIDS, the skin test reactivity rate has been 79% in our series of tuberculosis cases in San Francisco (unpublished data). As mentioned earlier, chest radiographs rarely show classic upper-lobe infiltrates, but more often show diffuse interstitial changes with prominent hilar and paratracheal enlargement; cavitation is very unusual. Culture of appropriate specimens remains the most important diagnostic tool. Sputum cultures in particular have had a high yield for *M. tuberculosis*. However, examination of smears has not been as productive, and not all patients who have subsequently had positive sputum cultures for *M. tuberculosis* are also smear-positive. Many patients with AIDS and tuberculosis have difficulty in producing adequate sputum for examination. In such cases, sputum induction may be tried. Bronchoscopy is an invaluable tool in the diagnosis of pulmonary conditions in AIDS or suspected AIDS patients, and every patient in this setting who has bronchoscopy should have specimens examined for mycobacteria by smear and culture. For the diagnosis of extrapulmonary tuberculosis in AIDS patients, tissue samples generally have been necessary for diagnosis. The material obtained by biopsy or fine-needle aspiration should be submitted for histologic analysis and for culture material; either may show the organism.

Treatment

Although a number of regimens have proved to be effective in the treatment of tuberculosis, currently there are two regimens that are recommended by the CDC and American Thoracic Society for use in the United States (18). The first is a 6-month regimen of isoniazid (INH) at 300 mg/day and rifampin at 600 mg/day for 6 months, with the addition of pyrazinamide at 20 to 30 mg/kg per day for the initial 2 months of treatment. The second recommended regimen is a 9-month regimen of isoniazid and rifampin in the same dosages. The addition of ethambutol or streptomycin to either regimen at the outset of treatment pending results of sensitivity tests is optional. After the initial 2 months of daily treatment, twice-a-week therapy with isoniazid at 900 mg and rifampin at 600 mg may be substituted if the initial isolate is sensitive to both drugs. The predominant toxicity of these regimens is hepatic and occurs in 0.5% to 2% of patients. To date, there have been no tuberculosis treatment trials in AIDS patients. The American Thoracic Society and CDC recommend that at least three antituberculous drugs be used in the initial phase of treatment (19). In general, patients with AIDS and tuberculosis have a favorable response to antituberculosis treatment (3,11). For patients with initially positive sputum cultures, the sputum has converted to negative at approximately the same rate as in patients with tuberculosis and without AIDS (11). The patients have noted a general improvement in their sense of well-being shortly after beginning antituberculous medication, with weight gain, decrease in fever, decrease in cough (if that was part of the initial presentation), and decrease in the size of lymphatic swelling.

Adverse reactions to antituberculosis medications necessitating a change in therapy have occurred in about a quarter of patients begun on an initial regimen of either INH and rifampin, with or without ethambutol, or INH, rifampin, and pyrazinamide. This is a much higher rate of adverse reactions than in patients without AIDS. The most common adverse reaction has been a rash, with or without pruritus, that has been attributed to either INH or rifampin (11). Hepatitis has been noted, as has thrombocytopenia and gastrointestinal intolerance. Renal failure in a patient receiving rifampin has been described, but other potential causes of renal failure were present and a cause-effect relationship could not be established (11).

The duration of therapy remains controversial; the CDC and American Thoracic Society recommend that treatment be prolonged for a minimum of 9 months or 6 months after culture conversion (19,20). In our experience at San Francisco General Hospital, relapse has been documented in one patient treated with INH and rifampin who missed several months of therapy because of noncompliance. A second patient with an INH-resistant isolate developed central nervous system tuberculosis, despite sputum conversion and continuation of appropriate therapy. This patient was initially treated with INH, rifampin, and ethambutol, and was subsequently given rifampin, ethambutol, and pyrazinamide when high-level INH resistance was documented. Culture-positive tuberculous meningitis developed 3 months into treatment. The patient acknowledged becoming erratic in taking his drugs in the weeks before developing meningitis. A third patient who was unable to tolerate rifampin received an 18-month regimen of INH and ethambutol but 5 months after the end of treatment, during a terminal episode of *Pneumocystis carinii* pneumonia (PCP), he developed positive blood cultures for *M. tuberculosis*. Pulmonary relapse was not present in this case, as respiratory cultures done during his final hospitalization were negative for *M. tuberculosis*. In 68 other patients, there was no evidence of treatment failure or relapse.

Mortality in patients with tuberculosis and AIDS is high. Survival for AIDS patients with tuberculosis from the time of either the tuberculosis diagnosis or the AIDS diagnosis tends to follow the same general time course as survival after the diagnosis of PCP and is shorter than for patients for whom Kaposi's sarcoma is the sole initial manifestation of AIDS (11). The cause of death in these patients has generally been other AIDS-related diseases. The contribution of tuberculosis to mortality has been minor, perhaps because of the availability of highly efficacious chemotherapy.

Prevention

Because of the progressive immunosuppression that results from HIV infection, patients who have quiescent *M. tuberculosis* infection are at a very high risk of reactivation if they become superinfected with HIV. At earlier stages of infection, before the development of profound defects in cell-mediated immunity, the skin test remains a useful tool to diagnose preexisting tuberculosis infection (19-21). Patients who are tuberculin reactive (≥ 10 mm of induration) and have HIV infection should be given isoniazid daily for 6 to 12 months to prevent the development of active tuberculosis. At this time there are no data showing that this will prevent reactivation of tuberculosis, but no other effective preventive strategies have been studied. In areas where the prevalence of HIV infection is high and the difficulties of obtaining HIV test results are great, it may be useful to treat tuberculin-reactive patients with INH without an HIV test result if they are in the high-risk groups. Contact investigation is crucial in AIDS patients with tuberculosis. Many contacts, in addition to being at risk for contracting the disease from the patient, may also be in the same risk groups for HIV infection and the development of AIDS themselves. It is likely that some patients who have developed tuberculosis many months after the diagnosis of AIDS was made were infected subsequent to their AIDS diagnosis, at a time when they were not immunocompetent and unable to limit the initial spread of *M. tuberculosis*. These contacts should be given INH preventive therapy at the time the initial case of tuberculosis is discovered.

Although seldom used in the United States, BCG vaccination is specifically contraindicated in patients with AIDS, because of the danger of disseminated infection (22).

MYCOBACTERIUM-AVIUM COMPLEX

Epidemiology

Mycobacterium avium complex (MAC) (also sometimes referred to as *Mycobacterium avium-intracellulare*) occurs widely in nature, being endemic in many waterfowl species and commonly present in soil and water. For many years MAC has been a known cause of chronic, slowly progressive pulmonary disease, primarily in persons with a preexisting lung disease, such as emphysema (23). By the late 1970s, MAC had become a more frequent cause of lung disease than *M. tuberculosis* in certain portions of the southeastern United States. Skin test surveys using PPD-B, derived from MAC, show a high prevalence of infection in many parts of the United States (24). However, disseminated infection was very rare before the AIDS epidemic, with less than 100 cases reported in the literature (25).

In 1982, reports of disseminated MAC infections in AIDS patients were first published (1,2). It quickly became recognized as a common opportunistic pathogen in AIDS patients in every part of the country and in all groups at high risk for AIDS. Disseminated MAC was included in the first surveillance definition for reporting of AIDS established by the CDC. Estimates of the prevalence of disseminated MAC infection in AIDS are partly dependent on the extent of the search for the organism, with 15% to 20% being the usually accepted figures. Autopsy series, however, have reported infection in up to 50% of cases (26). This discrepancy probably reflects some underdiagnosis of MAC in life; because the lung often is not involved, other infections may be considered the cause of symptoms and signs, and appropriate cultures may not be performed.

Pathophysiology

It is generally accepted that person-to-person spread of infection is not the mode of acquisition of MAC infection (23). The organism is found in water and soil samples throughout the world. The portal of entry has not yet been established with certainty in persons with AIDS, but because the gastrointestinal tract is often heavily infected with MAC, ingestion of MAC with food or drink is perhaps the most likely source of infection. The ingested organisms replicate in the intestine, spreading by the lymphatics to regional, intra-abdominal lymph nodes, from which dissemination occurs. Blood cultures are frequently positive, as are bone marrow and stool cultures (27). The organism stimulates very little inflammatory response in the AIDS patient.

Clinical Findings

Symptoms that have been attributed to MAC are nonspecific. Fever and diarrhea, with substantial weight loss, are the most frequently noted symptoms. Malabsorption can occur with intestinal involvement. Abdominal pain is sometimes present and can be the result of the intestinal infection per se or because of sometimes massive intra-abdominal lymph node enlargement (28). The lymphatic involvement can cause obstructive symptoms as well. Hepatosplenomegaly may be seen.

Peripheral and intrathoracic lymph nodes can also be involved with MAC. Cervical nodes can be large and somewhat tender on palpation, but without fluctuance. The adenopathy generally appears over the course of several weeks.

Patients with extensive bone marrow infection may develop anemia, leukopenia, and thrombocytopenia. The association between the disseminated MAC infection and hematologic toxicity, particularly anemia, is notable, although the results of treatment have not been striking.

In many patients, recovery of MAC from the blood or finding a positive smear and culture from liver or bone marrow is fortuitous, with no specific signs or symptoms prompting the tests. In these clinically silent infections the presence of disseminated MAC contributes little, if at all, to morbidity, nor does it appear to hasten mortality.

Diagnosis

A diagnosis of MAC disease in an AIDS patient requires culture of the organism because smears alone cannot differentiate MAC from *M. tuberculosis* or other atypical mycobacteria. Positive cultures from the blood, bone marrow, liver, or from multiple sites document dissemination. Blood cultures have been frequent sources of this organism, but laboratories must be alerted to process specimens in such a way as not to miss the organism if present (see Chap. 21).

Stool smears and cultures are frequently positive in patients with biopsy-proved infection of the bowel (27). A Whipple's-like histologic picture may be present on biopsy. Histiocytes packed with acid-fast bacilli in the lamina propria of the small bowel, together with enlarged lymph nodes containing foamy macrophages engorged with acid-fast bacilli are characteristic. The histologic appearance of biopsy material from involved tissues simulates the appearance of lepra cells in lepromatous leprosy. Also, as in lepromatous leprosy, there is very little host inflammatory response and many organisms. Granulomas, if present, are poorly formed.

Treatment

Mycobacterium avium complex infection is a difficult infection to treat in the nonimmunocompromised host. Various 4-, 5-, and 6-drug regimens, usually including INH, rifampin, ethambutol, and streptomycin, with or without cycloserine and ethionamide, have been given to chronic pulmonary cases for 18 to 24 months, resulting in cure rates of 50% to 75% (23,29). Adjunctive surgery for localized cavitary lung disease has resulted in a some-what higher response rate. In AIDS patients, the response to treatment has been minimal. The organism is usually resistant to most of the commonly used antimycobacterial agents (27), and surgery is not an option because the infection is almost always disseminated. Rifabutin, a rifampin derivative, and clofazimine, a drug used in leprosy, have shown in vitro evidence of efficacy against MAC (20) and amikacin has been shown to be bactericidal. A drug regimen of rifabutin 300 mg q.d., clofazimine 100 mg q.d., INH 300 mg q.d., and ethambutol 25 mg/kg daily was evaluated by the CDC, but preliminary results suggest that, although some symptoms such as fever can be ameliorated, only a few patients experienced any microbiologic response. Because the contribution of MAC infection to mortality may not be significant, and treatment is largely ineffectual and potentially toxic, it would seem that treatment should be reserved for those patients with symptoms that are probably due to MAC, and that a simple regimen of INH (to cover for the possibility that *M. tuberculosis* is the causative acid-fast organism before definitive culture), rifampin (or rifabutin, available from CDC), and ethambutol, with or without clofazimine (available from CDC) be used initially (19,20). Treatment effective against *M. tuberculosis* should be continued until an acid-fast isolate is definitively shown to be MAC. A regimen of rifabutin, clofazimine, and parenteral amikacin might be predicted to have the greatest efficacy, but there is now no clinical evidence to warrant this approach. Ciprofloxacin has in vitro activity against MAC and may be efficacious in combination with antimycobacterial drugs. Imipenum also is active in vitro against MAC.

OTHER ATYPICAL MYCOBACTERIAL INFECTIONS

Disseminated *M. kanasii* has been seen in patients with AIDS and is an indicator disease for AIDS, without laboratory evidence for HIV infection.

Other mycobacterial species, such as *M. gordonae, M. chelonei, M. fortuitum,* and *M. xenopi,* have been reported to cause disease in AIDS patients, but these have been rare, isolated events. Treatment should be geared to the susceptibilities of the specific organism isolated.

REFERENCES

1. Fainstein, V., Bolivar, R., Mavligit, G., Rios, A., and Luna, M. (1982). Disseminated infection due to *Mycobacterium avium-intracellulare* in a homosexual man with Kaposi's sarcoma. *Ann. Intern. Med. 97*:539-546.
2. Azkowski, P., Fligiel, S., Berlin, G. W., and Johnson, L., Jr. (1982). Disseminated *Mycobacterium avium-intracellulare* infection in homosexual men dying of acquired immunodeficiency. *JAMA 248*:2980-2982.
3. Pitchenik, A. E., Cole, C., Russell, B. W. et al. (1984). Tuberculosis, atypical mycobacteriosis, and the acquired immunodeficiency syndrome among Haitian and non-Haitian patients in South Florida. *Ann. Intern. Med. 101*:641-645.
4. CDC (1987). Revision of the CDC surveillance case definition for acquired immunodeficiency syndrome. *MMWR 36*(suppl.):3S-15S.
5. CDC (1987). Tuberculosis provisional data—United States, 1986. *MMWR 36*: 254-255.
6. CDC (1986). Tuberculosis—United States, 1985 and the possible impact of human T-lymphotropic virus type III/lymphadenopathy-associated virus infection. *MMWR 35*:74-76.
7. Sunderam, G., McDonald, R. J., Maniatis, T. et al. (1986). Tuberculosis as a manifestation of the acquired immunodeficiency syndrome (AIDS). *JAMA 256*: 362-366.
8. Goedert, J. J., Weiss, S. H., Biggar, R. J. et al. (1985). Lesser AIDS and tuberculosis. *Lancet 2*:52.
9. Guarner, J., del Rio, C., and Slade, B. (1986). Tuberculosis as a manifestation of the acquired immunodeficiency syndrome. *JAMA 256*:3092.
10. Schecter, G., Rutherford, G., and Echenberg, D. (1986). Tuberculosis in AIDS patients in San Francisco, 1982-1985 [Abstr.]. *Am. Rev. Resp. Dis. 133*(suppl.): A184.
11. Chaisson, R. E., Schecter, G. F., Theuer, C. P. et al. (1987). Tuberculosis in patients with the acquired immunodeficiency syndrome: Clinical features, response to therapy, and survival. *Am. Rev. Respir. Dis. 136*:570-574.
12. CDC (1987). Tuberculosis and AIDS—Connecticut. *MMWR 36*:133-135.
13. Mann, J., Snider, D. E., Francis, H. et al. (1986). Association between HTLV-III/LAV infection and tuberculosis in Zaire. *JAMA 256*:346.
14. Saltzman, B. R., Motyl, M. R., Friedland, G. H. et al. (1986). *Mycobacterium tuberculosis* bacteremia in the acquired immunodeficiency syndrome. *JAMA 256*:490-491.
15. Pitchenik, A. E. and Rubinson, H. A. (1985). The radiographic appearance of tuberculosis in patients with AIDS and pre-AIDS. *Am. Rev. Resp. Dis. 131*: 393-396.

16. Bishburg, E., Sunderam, G., Reichman, L. B. et al. (1986). Central nervous system tuberculosis with the acquired immunodeficiency syndrome and its related complex. *Ann. Intern. Med. 105*:210-213.

17. Sunderam, G., Bishburg, E., Kapila, R., and Reichman, L. B. (1986). Central nervous system tuberculosis in patients with AIDS and ARC [Abstr.]. *Am. Rev. Resp. Dis. 133*(suppl.):A185.

18. American Thoracic Society, Centers for Disease Control. (1986). Treatment of tuberculosis and tuberculosis infection in adults and children. *Am. Rev. Respir. Dis. 134*:355-363.

19. American Thoracic Society, Centers for Disease Control (1987). Mycobacterioses and the acquired immunodeficiency syndrome. *Am. Rev. Resp. Dis. 136*: 492-496.

20. CDC (1986). Diagnosis and management of mycobacterial infection and disease in persons with human T-lymphotropic virus type III/lymphadenopathy-associated virus infection. *MMWR 35*:448-452.

21. Pitchenik, A. E., Burr, J., Suarez, M. et al. (1987). Human T-cell lymphotropic virus-III (HTLV-III) seropositivity and related disease among 71 consecutive patients in whom tuberculosis was diagnosed. *Am. Rev. Resp. Dis. 135*:875-879.

22. CDC (1985). Disseminated *Mycobacterium bovis* infection from BCG vaccination of a patient with acquired immunodeficiency syndrome. *MMWR 34*:227-228.

23. Wolinsky, E. (1979). Nontuberculous mycobacteria and associated diseases. *Am. Rev. Respir. Dis. 119*:107-159.

24. American Thoracic Society, Centers for Disease Control (1981). The tuberculin skin test. *Am. Rev. Respir. Dis. 124*:356-363.

25. Horsburgh, C. R., Jr., Mason, U. G., Farhi, D. C., and Iseman, M. D. (1985). Disseminated infection with *Mycobacterium avium-intracellulare*. A report of 13 cases and a review of the literature. *Medicine 64*:36-48.

26. Wallace, J. M. and Hannah, J. (1985). Pulmonary disease found at autopsy in patients with the acquired immunodeficiency syndrome (AIDS) [Abstr.]. *Am. Rev. Respir. Dis. 131*:A222.

27. Kiehn, T. E., Edwards, F. F., Brannon, P., Tsang, A. Y., Maio, M., Gold, J. W., Whimbey, E., Wong, B., McClatchy, J. K., and Armstrong, D. (1985). Infections caused by *Mycobacterium avium* complex in immunocompromised patients: Diagnosis by blood culture and fecal examination, antimicrobial susceptibility tests, and morphological and seroagglutination characteristics. *J. Clin. Microbiol. 21*:168-173.

28. Jeffrey, R. B., Jr., Nyberg, D. A., Bottles, K., Abrams, D. I., Federle, M. P., Wall, S. D., Wing, V. W., and Laing, F. C. (1986). Abdominal CT in acquired immunodeficiency syndrome. *AJR 146*:7-13.

29. Iseman, M. D., Corpe, R. F., O'Brien, R. J., Rosenzweig, D. Y., and Wolinsky, E. (1985). Disease due to *Mycobacterium avium-intracellulare*. *Chest 87* (suppl. 2):139S-149S.

Part V
Fungal Infections

15
Cryptococcosis in Patients with Acquired Immunodeficiency Syndrome

Michael S. Simberkoff, *New York Veterans Administration Medical Center, and New York University School of Medicine, New York, New York*

Abigail Zuger, *Albert Einstein College of Medicine, Bronx, New York*

CRYPTOCOCCUS NEOFORMANS

Cryptococcosis is one of the life-threatening infectious diseases seen in patients with acquired immunodeficiency syndrome (AIDS). The pathogen causing this disease is *Cryptococcus neoformans*, an encapsulated yeastlike fungus that is found throughout the world and is related to several other nonpathogenic species. All cryptococcal species have urease activity; however, *C. neoformans* can be distinguished from nonpathogenic species by its virulence for mice and growth at 37 °C.

There are two taxonomic varieties of *C. neoformans* (1). These are *C. neoformans* var. *neoformans* (serotypes A and D) and *C. neoformans* var. *gattii* (serotypes B and C). The former organism (*C. neoformans* var. *neoformans*) has been isolated from clinical and environmental sources, particularly from soil and the excreta of pigeons and other seed-eating birds, whereas the latter has been isolated principally from infected animals and humans. Cryptococci are not part of the normal flora of humans; their isolation almost always indicates clinical or subclinical infection.

Cryptococcus neoformans var. *neoformans* has been associated with most of the reported instances of human disease in the United States, except in southern California; there, *C. neoformans* var. *gattii* has accounted for approximately 40% of the clinical isolates (2). However, one report has indicated that *C. neoformans* var. *neoformans* may be the more prevalent pathogen among patients with AIDS in Los Angeles (3) as well as in northern California and other parts of the United States (4). There are data suggesting that *C. neoformans* var. *neoformans* is more virulent than are organisms of the *C. gattii* variety. The latter grow poorly at 37 °C compared with *C. neoformans* var. *neoformans*, and they are relatively avirulent for mice following intravenous injection (5).

The cryptococcal fungal cell is round or oval and is usually 4 to 6 μm in diameter. The organism reproduces asexually by budding both in vitro and in clinical infection. Sexual reproduction as *Filobasidiella* may permit survival of the organism among parasites in the soil. However, sexual forms of the organism are not pathogenic and do not cause disease in humans.

The dominant feature of cryptococcus is its polysaccharide capsule, which may vary in thickness from 1 to 30 μm. Capsular size of cryptococci can be influenced by a variety of environmental and nutritional conditions (6). No differences in mortality were observed when poorly encapsulated or thickly encapsulated cryptococci were injected intravenously into groups of mice. However, tissues obtained from all groups of experimental animals at periods after intravenous inoculation contained only encapsulated organisms. This suggests either that encapsulated variants of the organism will grow preferentially in vivo, whereas unencapsulated organisms are rapidly eliminated by the host, or that encapsulation of cryptococci can occur rapidly in vivo.

Carbon dioxide concentrations may also affect the production of cryptococcal polysaccharide. Granger et al. (7) have shown that maximal capsule production occurs at carbon dioxide concentrations of 40 torr, at or near the concentration found in blood and tissues under physiologic conditions. Mutant organisms that are incapable of increasing capsule size in response to carbon dioxide stimulus will not cause chronic infection in steroid-treated rabbits and are rapidly cleared from the meninges of experimental animals.

Some recent reports have suggested that small-colony variants (capsule-deficient strains) may be more commonly isolated from patients with AIDS than from other subjects (8-11). The most poorly encapsulated organisms were recovered from patients with the most profound immunodeficiency (11). Furthermore, mouse passage resulted in an increase in the capsular size of the deficient organisms. These findings imply that the profound defects in host defense mechanisms characteristic of AIDS patients may permit the persistence of poorly encapsulated cryptococci. However, other workers have reported recovery of weakly encapsulated or nonencapsulated cryptococcal strains from patients before the AIDS epidemic (12). They argue that recovery of unencapsulated cryptococci from cerebrospinal fluid is not unique to AIDS patients. Further studies relating the encapsulation of cryptococci to the integrity of host defense mechanisms may be necessary to resolve this controversy.

HOST DEFENSE MECHANISMS AGAINST CRYPTOCOCCUS

A variety of host defense mechanisms are active against *C. neoformans.* Cryptococci activate chemotactic factors in normal human sera (13). The opsonized organisms are ingested and killed within neutrophils and monocytes by both oxygen-dependent systems (14) and by cationic proteins (15). In addition, neutrophils and monocytes can kill large (thickly encapsulated) organisms by nonphagocytic mechanisms, in the presence of specific antibodies (16). Some patients with cryptococcal meningitis, however, appear to be incapable of mounting an antibody response to cryptococcal polysaccharides, and this specific immunologic unresponsiveness may last for several years (17).

Neutrophils are involved in the primary clearance of the small, relatively unencapsulated cryptococci, which are aerodynamically capable of reaching the alveoli of experimental mice after inhalation infection (18). Subsequently, after the organisms grow, encapsulate and disseminate, clearance by monocytes and macrophages predominates. Nonspecific activation of macrophages confers protection against in vivo and in vitro challenge by cryptococci (19).

There is considerable evidence to suggest that cell-mediated immunity (CMI) is crucial for adequate host defenses against cryptococcosis. First, 50% or more of the patients with cryptococcal meningitis have other diseases or are receiving treatments that are known to suppress CMI (20). Second, lymphopenia, defects in skin reactivity, and decreases in in vitro lymphocyte blastogenic responses to fungal antigens may be observed in patients without known coexisting disease who have recovered from cryptococcosis (21). Third, nude (congenitally athymic) mice succumb to cryptococcal infection more rapidly than animals with normal T cells (22). These animals can be protected by thymic transplantation (23). Finally, transfer of T cells from sensitized animals will protect unimmunized animals from lethal challenges of cryptococci (24).

In summary, it appears that although both humoral and cellular immunity are operative against cryptococcosis, the latter is more important. The absence of an effective cell-mediated immune response in patients with AIDS, as well as those with less advanced forms of human immunodeficiency virus (HIV) infection, predisposes them to cryptococcosis when they encounter this pathogen.

TABLE 1   Prevalence of Cryptococcosis Among AIDS Patients in the United States

Location (Ref.)	Number of AIDS patients evaluated	Cases of cryptococcosis (%)
San Francisco (25)	352	16 (4.6)
New Jersey (26)	145	10 (6.9)
National Institutes of Health (27)	150	10 (7.5)
New York City (28)	396	34 (8.6)

PREVALENCE AND ORGAN INVOLVEMENT IN CRYPTOCOCCOSIS IN AIDS

Although the prevalence of cryptococcosis in large series of patients with AIDS has varied, it is generally regarded as one of the more common life-threatening opportunistic infections seen. Cryptococcosis has been observed in 5% to 10% of patients with AIDS evaluated at medical centers across the United States (25-28; Table 1). No geographic variations in the prevalence of cryptococcosis have been observed in the United States, and the disease appears to occur equally among all risk groups.

Cryptococcosis is also among the most commonly recognized opportunistic infections in AIDS patients outside of the United States. The prevalence of cryptococcosis among Italian patients with AIDS has been estimated to be from 8.6% to 17.2% (29). Cryptococcal infection has also been reported to be very common among African AIDS patients (30).

The central nervous system (CNS) is the organ system most frequently clinically infected by *C. neoformans* in AIDS patients. Estimates of the prevalence of CNS manifestations of cryptococcosis in AIDS have ranged from 65% to 90% (26-28). However, other organs also have frequently been involved, including blood, bone marrow, lungs, lymph nodes, skin, liver, kidneys, prostate, adrenal glands, joints, myocardium, pericardium, and spleen.

Multiple organ systems may be involved simultaneously. For example, in one series of patients (31), 10 of 22 (45%) with proven CNS or disseminated cryptococcosis and AIDS had pulmonary infection. In another series (32), three of five (60%) AIDS patients with cryptococcosis examined at autopsy showed histologic evidence of cryptococcal hepatic infection; although involvement of the liver was extensive, no inflammatory reaction to the infection was observed. The same group (33) also reported adrenal involvement in three of four (75%) patients with cryptococcosis; again, little or no inflammatory reaction was observed. Finally, another group (27) has reported histologic evidence of cryptococcal brain or meningeal infection in 73%, lung in 60%, lymph node in 53%, adrenal in 20%, and kidney infection in 13% of the patients studied at autopsy.

Simultaneous infections with cryptococcus and other opportunistic pathogens also may occur in AIDS patients. Gal et al. (31), reported concurrent *Pneumocystis carinii* pneumonia in 5 of 11 patients with pulmonary cryptococcosis studied, whereas Bahls and Sumi (34) reported coincident cryptococcal meningitis and toxoplasma brain abscess in a single patient.

CLINICAL MANIFESTATIONS OF CRYPTOCOCCOSIS IN AIDS

Clinical manifestations of cryptococcosis depend on the organ systems involved. Fever is usually present but rarely exceeds 39 °C unless concurrent infections are present. Symptoms are often vague or nonspecific. Therefore, a high index of suspicion must be present to detect the infection.

Headache is the most common symptom associated with central nervous system (CNS) cryptococcosis (27,28). Other symptoms and signs of CNS infection have been comparatively infrequent. Nausea, vomiting, and focal neurologic abnormalities may be seen. Seizures, photophobia, and meningismus occur in a few patients (28). Cryptococcal infection of the CNS has been observed without symptoms, signs, or laboratory findings suggesting meningeal inflammation (35).

In patients without AIDS, cryptococcal meningitis is typically a chronic, slowly progressive infection. Patients with AIDS, however, vary enormously in their presentation. The duration of CNS symptoms in this population can range from days to months. Some patients present with a fulminant CNS infection that is clinically indistinguishable from bacterial meningitis. In others, the disease has been entirely asymptomatic, and the diagnosis has been established only as a result of a routine screening protocol (27,35).

The retina, an extension of the CNS, can also be involved by cryptococcosis in AIDS patients (36-38). In one series, retinal cryptococcosis was documented in 2 of 35 patients with AIDS coming to autopsy; these two cases occurred among five patients with systemic cryptococcosis (38). The infections were associated with cotton wool spots, retinal hemorrhage or necrosis and, in one case, Roth spots and retinal microaneurysms (37,38).

Extraneural cryptococcosis occurs alone or in combination with CNS infection in 40% to 50% of patients. Skin lesions may be present in 15% of patients with cryptococcosis. These may be persistent or nonhealing ulcers (39), herpetiform lesions (40), or papules resembling molluscum contagiosum (41). The skin lesions are the result of disseminated infection and should lead to other diagnostic tests and systemic therapy.

Pulmonary cryptococcosis in AIDS is often asymptomatic, but may be associated with minimal symptoms of cough, scant sputum production, or chest pain (42). In rare instances, it may be associated with severe hypoxia and an adult respiratory distress syndrome (43). Cryptococcosis can result in an interstitial, alveolar, or nodular pulmonary parenchymal infiltrate on chest radiography (44). Intrathoracic, adenopathy commonly accompanies this infection and cavitation may occur. Because these symptoms and signs are not unique for cryptococcal infection, appropriate diagnostic tests must be initiated promptly.

Cryptococcal myocarditis has been reported to be clinically silent in AIDS patients (45). In contrast, cryptococcal pericarditis has resulted in massive effusion and signs of tamponade (46).

Cryptococcal prostatitis has been documented in an AIDS patient and was associated with lower abdominal discomfort, dysuria, and difficulty in initiating a urine stream (47). Cryptococcal arthritis in an AIDS patient was associated with joint swelling, effusion, and limitation of motion (48).

DIAGNOSIS OF CRYPTOCOCCOSIS

Central Nervous System Disease

From 65% to 90% of cryptococcal infections in patients with AIDS involve the CNS, either alone or as part of a disseminated infection. In most, but not all, of these infections, a diagnosis is contingent upon culturing the organism from the cerebrospinal fluid (CSF). It is noteworthy that in two cases of cryptococcal brain abscess without meningitis, CSF cultures were repeatedly negative. Diagnosis of these infections ultimately required brain biopsy and culture of the organism from the biopsy specimen after an empiric course of treatment for toxoplasmosis failed (28). This observation further emphasizes the importance of brain biopsy in establishing the diagnosis and proper treatment for intracerebral mass lesions in patients with AIDS (49). Positive blood cultures for cryptococcus have been reported to accompany CNS disease in up to 56% of patients (50). However, the inevitable delay in culture and identification of the organism from any site, in conjunction with an often fulminant clinical presentation, makes more rapid diagnostic tests particularly important in CNS cryptococcal infection.

Unlike patients with cryptococcal meningitis without AIDS, patients with AIDS have relatively few nonspecific abnormalities in the CSF. Of 38 AIDS patients with cryptococcal meningitis reported in the literature, only 19 (50%) were found to have a low CSF glucose concentration, and only 15 (39%) an elevation in CSF protein (27,28). Opening pressure of the CSF was elevated in 9 of 13 (69%) primary infections (28). The CSF leukocyte counts have been variable, exceeding 5 WBC/cc in only 13 of 39 (34%) infections (27, 51). In fact, cryptococcal meningitis with entirely normal CSF occurred in 3 of 18 patients in one series (27).

Computed tomographic (CT) scans of the brain have also been relatively unhelpful in the diagnosis of this infection, despite the range of CT abnormalities often associated with it (52). In one series of 23 patients with CNS infection, all were reported to have normal scans (50). In another, CT scans were abnormal in 4 of the 13 patients in whom they were performed, including two patients with large, ring-enhancing abscesses subsequently proved to be cryptococcoma (28).

Other maneuvers have been more effective in the rapid diagnosis of CNS cryptococcosis. India ink preparations of the CSF have been positive in 72 of 85 (85%) AIDS patients with the infection (27,28,50,51). In contrast, India ink preparations are reported to be positive in only 50% of patients in the absence of AIDS (53). Although India ink preparations can result in diagnoses within minutes of lumbar puncture, care must be taken to avoid false-positive as well as false-negative results.

The most useful of all immediate diagnostic tests has been the commercially available latex agglutination test for soluble cryptococcal antigen. Cryptococcal antigen has been reported to be present in the CSF of 60 of 63 (95%) patients with AIDS and CNS infection (27,28,50), sometimes in extraordinarily high titers. Patients without CSF antigen despite culture-proved infection include one with an encapsulated CNS cryptococcoma without meningeal inflammation, and one with meningeal infection with a poorly encapsulated fungus. The determination of cryptococcal antigen titers in serum has had a similarly high yield in these patients: serum antigen was present in 28 of 29 (97%) AIDS patients with proven meningitis (27,28).

The incidence of false-positive cryptococcal antigen titers has not been specifically addressed in the AIDS population. Rare cases of patients with significantly elevated antigen titers, despite negative cultures, have been reported both in AIDS and in other populations (28,54,55). In these cases, however, because of uniform serologic and symptomatic response to therapy, cultures have been considered to be falsely negative, rather than serology falsely positive. In addition, false-positive antigen titers caused by rheumatoid factor or other confounders are generally quite low (<1:4), whereas patients with AIDS typically present with cryptococcal serum antigen titers of unusual magnitude. The etiology of their elevated antigen titers is not yet clear. One investigator has postulated that they may reflect an undefined inability to clear the polysaccharide, rather than an increased antigen load (26).

As summarized in Table 2, then, in patients with CNS cryptococcosis, determination of cryptococcal antigen titers in CSF or serum is most likely to

TABLE 2 Recommended Diagnostic Tests for Cryptococcosis

Suspected site of infection	Recommended	Other
Meninges	CSF cryptococcal antigen, serum cryptococcal antigen, CSF culture	CSF India ink preparation, blood culture
Brain	Fungal stain and culture of biopsy specimen	
Lungs	Fungal stain and culture of cell block from bronchoalveolar lavage fluid or of transbronchial biopsy specimen	
Skin	Fungal stain and culture of biopsy specimen	

lead to a rapid diagnosis of this infection. The CSF India ink preparations are likely to be positive in AIDS patients, but inexperienced individuals must interpret them with caution. Other abnormalities of CSF are less frequent, as are abnormalities of CT scan. In the rare cases of CNS cryptococcoma, all diagnostic modalities except histopathologic examination and culture of needle aspiration or brain biopsy material may be negative.

Extraneural Infection

In the minority of cryptococcal infections in AIDS without CNS involvement, histopathologic examination and culture have been the mainstays of diagnosis. Serologic tests appear to be relatively unhelpful in these cases: Kovacs et al. (27), reported negative blood cryptococcal antigen titers in four of nine patients with extraneural cryptococcal infections, including one with positive blood cultures for the organism.

Pulmonary infections are the most common extraneural manifestation of cryptococcosis in AIDS. In one series of 11 patients with pulmonary cryptococcosis, bronchoscopy was performed in eight for worsening nonspecific respiratory symptoms (31). A variety of pathologic abnormalities were seen in biopsy specimens. In most, fungal dissemination was predominantly interstitial and was accompanied by a minimal cellular infiltrate. Some specimens showed alveolar invasion as well, and in one, extensive vascular invasion was found. As five of the eight patients had concurrent *Pneumocystis carinii* pneumonia, it is not entirely clear how the cryptococcal infection contributed to these pathologic findings. Cryptococcal organisms were identified in seven of seven cell blocks prepared from bronchoalveolar lavage fluid, in six of eight transbronchial biopsy specimens, in five of eight bronchial brushing specimens, and in five of six bronchial lavage fluid smears. Thus, a relatively high diagnostic sensitivity can be claimed for all of these techniques, although it is noteworthy that histopathologic examination of a fluid cell block rather than a tissue specimen had the highest sensitivity in this small study.

In some extraneural cryptococcal infections in AIDS, including skin and joint infections, a diagnosis has been made by direct microscopy of the fluid aspirated from the infected area (40,48). In most others, a biopsy of the affected tissue and special stains of the biopsy are required. Hematoxylin and eosin stains are virtually useless for identification of this organism; periodic acid-Schiff or methenamine silver stains are more specific for the presence of fungal infection, whereas acid mucicarmine stains specifically for the capsule, and will distinguish between cryptococcus and other fungi (53). In addition, the use of a DAPI-fluorochrome stain has been successful in the rapid detection of cryptococcus in spleen tissue of a patient with AIDS (56). This stain identifies both the cell wall and the capsule of the organism, thus enabling the rapid identification of both normally encapsulated and poorly encapsulated cryptococci.

TREATMENT OF CRYPTOCOCCOSIS

As in other patient populations, intravenous amphotericin B is the only established therapy for cryptococcal infection in patients with AIDS. The addition of oral flucytosine, as is generally recommended in other patients, may not be attempted in AIDS patients because of preexisting leukopenia or renal dysfunction. When flucytosine therapy is begun, investigators have reported a 30% rate of complications, most commonly leukopenia, that require its discontinuation (27,28). This toxicity rate parallels that found in patients without AIDS (57). The toxicities of amphotericin B, itself, appear no different or more severe in AIDS patients, most commonly consisting of infusion-related fever, chills, and nausea, and renal dysfunction related to cumulative amphotericin dose.

The daily dosage of amphotericin B in patients with AIDS is the same as that used for cryptococcosis in other patients: 0.3 to 0.7 mg/kg per day in patients receiving flucytosine, 0.4 to 1.0 mg/kg per day in others. In addition, the administration of intraventricular amphotercin B through an indwelling intraventricular reservoir has been added to systemic amphotericin B treatment in rare instances (27,28). Such therapy has proved to be useful in patients with CNS cryptococcosis complicating malignant diseases (58). However, complications of intraventricular amphotericin B, including bacterial reservoir infection and chemical irritation of the meninges, have been reported in AIDS patients as well as in others (28,58).

Virtually no guidelines have been established for the optimum total dosage of amphotericin B or duration of therapy in patients with AIDS. Clearly, as in other patients, sterilization of the CNS and other affected sites is the primary goal of therapy. However, the amount of amphotericin B that should be administered after cultures of the CSF or other body fluids have become sterile is still undetermined. Furthermore, the significance of persistently positive India ink preparations of CSF and of persistently elevated CSF or serum cryptococcal antigen titers remains to be determined.

Cryptococcal antigen titers of serum and CSF have become convenient and routinely used indicators of therapeutic progress in non-AIDS patients (57). In patients with AIDS, some doubt has been cast on the usefulness of this practice. One study of antigen levels found that, whereas CSF titers in patients with AIDS fell at a rate similar to those seen in patients without AIDS, serum titers did not reliably fall in the former (26). In fact, we have observed that serum titers in patients with AIDS may rise by several dilutions during early weeks of therapy, despite otherwise improving clinical indicators. Serum antigen titers thus may be unreliable indicators of disease activity.

In the absence of guidelines for terminating therapy for cryptococcosis in AIDS, a variety of practices have evolved. In some centers, a goal of 2500-mg total administered dose of amphotericin B is set. In other centers, the length of treatment and total administered dose of amphotericin B depend entirely on the patient's clinical response to antifungal therapy. One such treatment strategy is shown in Figure 1. Patients with a prompt clinical response may proceed rapidly to weekly maintenance therapy, whereas patients with persistently positive cultures or elevated antigen titers may receive daily treatment for months: failure to sterilize the CSF after a total of 5000 mg of amphotericin B has been reported (27).

PROGNOSIS

Treatment for cryptococcosis in AIDS has been characterized by responses to first courses of therapy that parallel those among other groups of immunosuppressed individuals. Of 48 patients in two studies treated for first infections, 28 were considered to be disease-free at the end of therapy, a response rate of 58% (27,28). Total doses of amphotericin B ranging from 1000 to more than 2500 mg were administered to achieve this response.

Mortality from a first episode of cryptococcosis has been somewhat more difficult to establish in these patients, largely because of the presence of one or more concurrent life-threatening infections during their course of antifungal therapy. In a single series, mortality from active cryptococcosis was estimated at 17% despite treatment (28). In contrast, mortality rates for

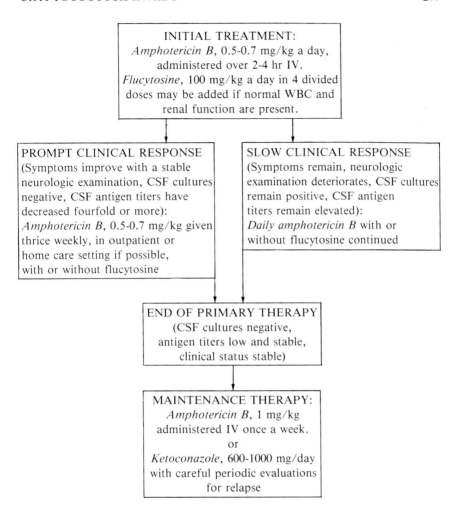

FIGURE 1   A therapeutic strategy for cryptococcosis in AIDS.

immunologically normal patients with cryptococcal meningitis have ranged from zero to 15%, and for patients who are immunocompromised by conditions other than AIDS, from 20% to 85% (57,59-61).

Efforts to identify poor prognostic factors in the AIDS population have been hampered by the small numbers of evaluable patients. In one study (27), no initial CSF variable, antigen titer, or treatment modality was found to correlate with eventual outcome of treatment. In another study (28), the height of both serum and CSF antigen titers appeared to correlate with an increased mortality, as did positive India ink preparation of the CSF at diagnosis. Initial CSF glucose levels, protein levels, opening pressure, and leukocyte count did not function as accurate predictors of treatment outcome, nor did the presence of extraneural disease or the addition of flucytosine to amphotericin B treatment. The administration of intraventricular amphotericin B appears to have little effect on mortality in this infection: of six patients treated with intraventricular amphotericin B, only one is reported to have survived the infection (27,28). This statistic may reflect the sicker patients selected for intraventricular therapy. Still, the increased morbidity associated with intraventricular amphotericin B therapy may outweigh its benefits in severely compromised patients.

Despite the fair response of AIDS patients to initial treatment for this infection, rates of relapse, as in other opportunistic infections in AIDS, have consistently exceeded those reported for other patient populations. Of 18 patients who appeared disease-free at the end of a first course of treatment, eight (44%) subsequently relapsed with active cryptococcal disease within 6 months of ending treatment (27,28). Efforts to identify factors that might predispose to relapse of infection have been stymied by the small number of patients studied. The CSF antigen titer height may have correlated with relapse in one study (28); most other clinical variables, including the presence of disseminated infection and the total amphotericin dose administered as primary therapy, did not correlate with risk of relapse.

Outcomes of second courses of therapy have been extremely poor in patients with relapsed infection. Only two of the nine patients retreated for a relapse of cryptococcal disease successfully completed a second treatment course.

MAINTENANCE TREATMENT

The high relapse rate in this disease, in conjunction with the high mortality of relapsed cases, has kindled a great deal of interest in long-term, low-dose antifungal therapy, or "maintenance treatment," for AIDS patients who have survived an initial cryptococcal infection. In 1984-1986, we studied the utility of weekly intravenous amphotericin B as maintenance treatment for approximately 20 AIDS patients. Because of poor patient compliance, only nine treatment courses could be adequately evaluated (62). Most patients received 100 mg of amphotericin B in a weekly 4-hr infusion; one patient received 40 mg twice weekly. Eight of nine patients followed for periods ranging up to 40 weeks were relapse-free, with declining or negative CSF and serum antigen titers, at the end of follow-up. One patient, distinguished from the others by particularly elevated antigen titers at the beginning of maintenance treatment (CSF titer 1:256, serum titer 1:1024), relapsed after 14 weekly treatments with amphotericin B and died with active infection.

Thus, although weekly intravenous amphotericin B appears useful in the management of these patients, it does not guarantee relapse-free survival. In addition, although the weekly infusion was well tolerated by most of our patients, two subjects suffered from prolonged hypotension during or shortly after an infusion. Problems with intravenous access and patient compliance further compromised the program.

Recent reports have claimed good success with high doses of oral keto-conazole in maintaining relapse-free survival in patients who have completed induction treatment with amphotericin B (63,64). Ketoconazole has no role in the primary treatment of cryptococcal infections; relapse of cryptococcosis has been documented in a patient receiving 400 mg/day of ketoconazole (51). However, in 15 patients who were given 1000 mg/day of ketoconazole after an initial 6- to 8-week induction course of amphotericin B, only one relapse was observed over periods of follow-up ranging from 6 to 11 months (64). Side effects of this regimen included nausea, abdominal pain, and hepatotoxicity that required termination of treatment in one instance.

FUTURE DIRECTIONS

Fluconazole and itraconazole, two new triazole compounds, have recently undergone evaluation in experimental cryptococcosis. In one study, a rabbit model of cryptococcal meningitis was employed (65). Itraconazole was more active than fluconazole against the cryptococcal strain studied. Fluconazole achieved excellent concentrations in the rabbit CSF, whereas CSF itraconazole concentrations were undetectable. Both drugs reduced yeast counts in treated animals, sterilizing the CSF in the majority. Fluconazole has also proved to be as effective as amphotericin B and more effective than ketoconazole in treating cryptococcal meningitis in experimental mice (66).

Clinical experience with these new drugs has been limited. Viviani et al. (67) reported intraconazole treatment of three patients with cryptococcosis and AIDS. Two were treated for relapse and the third for persistence of infection; all improved. Fluconazole has been used to treat 13 patients with cryptococcosis, some of whom had AIDS, who were failing conventional treatment regimens (68). Four out of nine of these patients converted their CSF cultures to negative with oral fluconazole administration. Fluconazole has, in addition, been used as a maintenance treatment for five patients after an initial course of amphotericin B; none of these patients had clinical relapses (69). These data suggest that the new triazole compounds may be useful adjuncts to conventional therapy for cryptococcosis in AIDS.

Further research in the area of cryptococcosis in AIDS should be directed toward two particular clinical goals. First, guidelines must be developed for determining the optimum drug or drug combination and duration of primary treatment for this infection in AIDS patients. Second, a safe, convenient, and effective long-term antifungal regimen is needed to prevent relapse of disease in these patients until some form of immune reconstitution is available for them.

REFERENCES

1. Kwon-Chung, K. J., Polacheck, I., and Bennett, J. E. (1982). Improved diagnostic medium for separation of *Cryptococcus neoformans* var. *neoformans* (serotypes A and D) and *Cryptococcus neoformans* var. *gattii* (serotypes B and C). *J. Clin. Microbiol.* *15*:535-537.
2. Kwon-Chung, K. J. and Bennett, J. E. (1984). Epidemiologic differences between the two varieties of *Cryptococcus neoformans*. *Am. J. Epidemiol.* *120*: 123-130.
3. Shimizu, R. Y., Howard, D. H., and Clancy, M. N. (1986). The variety of *Cryptococcus neoformans* in patients with AIDS. *J. Infect. Dis.* *154*:1042.
4. Rinaldi, M. G., Drutz, D. J., Howell, A., Sande, M. J., Wofsy, C. B., and Hadley, W. K. (1986). Serotypes of *Cryptococcus neoformans* in patients with AIDS. *J. Infect. Dis.* *153*:642.
5. Kwon-Chung, K. J., Bennett, J. E., and Rhodes, J. C. (1982). Taxonomic studies on *Filobasideilla* species and their anamorphs. *Antonie Leeuwenhoek J. Microbiol.* *48*:25-38.
6. Dykstra, M. A., Friedman, L., and Murphy, J. W. (1977). Capsule size of *Cryptococcus neoformans*: Control and relationship to virulence. *Infect. Immun.* *16*: 129-135.
7. Granger, D. L., Perfect, J. R., and Durack, D. T. (1985). Virulence of *Cryptococcus neoformans*: Regulation of capsule synthesis by carbon dioxide. *J. Clin. Invest.* *76*:508-516.
8. Bottone, E. J., Toma, M., Johannson, B. E., and Wormser, G. P. (1985). Capsule-deficient *Cryptococcus neoformans* in AIDS patients. *Lancet* *1*:400.
9. Bottone, E. J. and Wormser, G. P. (1985). Capsule-deficient cryptococci in AIDS. *Lancet* *2*:553.
10. Bottone, E. J., Toma, M., Johansson, B. E., and Wormser, G. P. (1986). Poorly encapsulated *Cryptococcus neoformans* from patients with AIDS. I. Preliminary observations. *AIDS Res.* *2*:211-218.
11. Bottone, E. J. and Wormser, G. P. (1986). Poorly encapsulated *Cryptococcus neoformans* from patients with AIDS. II. Correlation of capsule size observed directly in cerebrospinal fluid with that after animal passage. *AIDS Res.* *2*:219-225.
12. MacKenzie, D. W. R. and Hay, R. J. (1985). Capsule-deficient *Cryptococcus neoformans* in AIDS patients. *Lancet* *1*:642.

13. Diamond, R. D. and Erickson, N. F. (1982). Chemotaxis of human neutrophils and monocytes induced by *Cryptococcus neoformans. Infect. Immun. 38*:380-382.

14. Diamond, R. D., Root, R. K., and Bennett, J. E. (1972). Factors influencing killing of *Cryptococcus neoformans* by human leukocytes in vitro. *J. Infect. Dis. 125*:367-376.

15. Lehrer, R. I. and Ladra, K. M. (1977). Fungicidal components of mammalian granulocytes active against *Cryptococcus neoformans. J. Infect. Dis. 136*:96-99.

16. Diamond, R. D. and Allison, A. C. (1976). Nature of the effector cells responsible for antibody-dependent cell-mediated killing of *Cryptococcus neoformans. Infect Immun. 14*:716-720.

17. Henderson, D. H., Bennett, J. E., and Huber, M. A. (1982). Long-lasting, specific immunologic unresponsiveness associated with cryptococcal meningitis. *J. Clin. Invest. 69*:1185-1190.

18. Gadebush, H. H. (1972). Mechanisms of native and acquired resistance to infection with *Cryptococcus neoformans. CRC Crit. Rev. Microbiol. 1*:311-315.

19. Gentry, L. O. and Remington, J. S. (1972). Resistance against *Cryptococcus neoformans* conferred by intracellular bacteria and protozoa. *J. Infect. Dis. 123*: 22-32.

20. Lewis, J. L. and Rabinovich, S. (1972). The wide spectrum of cryptococcal infections. *Am. J. Med. 53*:315-322.

21. Graybill, J. R. and Alford, R. H. (1974). Cell-mediated immunity in cryptococcosis. *Cell. Immunol. 14*:12-21.

22. Cauley, L. K. and Murphy, J. W. (1979). Response of congenitally athymic mice (nude) and phenotypically normal mice to *Cryptococcus neoformans* infections. *Infect. Immun. 23*:644-651.

23. Graybill, J. R., Mitchell, L., and Drutz, D. J. (1979). Host defense in cryptococcosis: III. Protection of nude mice by thymus transplantation. *J. Infect. Dis. 140*:546-552.

24. Lim, T. S. and Murphy, J. W. (1980). Transfer of immunity to cryptococcosis by T-enriched splenic lymphocytes from *Cryptococcus neoformans* sensitized mice. *Infect. Immun. 30*:5-11.

25. Levy, R. M., Bredeson, D. E., and Rosenblum, M. L. (1985). Neurological manifestations of the acquired immunodeficiency syndrome (AIDS): Experience at UCSF and review of the literature. *J. Neurosurg. 62*:475-495.

26. Eng, R. H. K., Bishburg, E., Smith, S. M., and Kapila, R. (1986). Cryptococcal infections in patients with acquired immune deficiency syndrome. *Am. J. Med. 81*:19-23.

27. Kovacs, J. A., Kovacs, A. A., Polis, M. et al. (1985). Cryptococcosis in the acquired immunodeficiency syndrome. *Ann. Intern. Med. 103*:533-538.

28. Zuger, A., Louie, E., Holzman, R. S., Simberkoff, M. S., and Rahal, J. J. (1986). Cryptococcal disease in patients with acquired immunodeficiency syndrome. *Ann. Intern. Med. 104*:234-240.

29. Viviani, M. A. and Tortorano, A. M. (1986). Cryptococcosis in patients at risk or affected with AIDS: Proposal of a surveillance protocol. *Boll. Ist. Sieroter. Milan 65*:156-160.

30. Vandepitte, J., Verwilghen, R., and Zachee, P. (1983). AIDS and cryptococcosis (Zaire, 1977). *Lancet* *1*:925-926.
31. Gal, A. A., Koss, M. N., Hawkins, J., Evans, S., and Einstein, H. (1986). The pathology of pulmonary cryptococcal infection in the acquired immunodeficiency syndrome. *Arch. Pathol. Lab. Med.* *110*:502-507.
32. Glasgow, B. J., Anders, K., Layfield, L. J. et al. (1985). Clinical and pathologic findings of the liver in the acquired immune deficiency syndrome (AIDS). *Am. J. Clin. Pathol.* *83*:582-588.
33. Glasgow, B. J., Steinsapir, B. S., Anders, K., and Layfield, L. J. (1985). Adrenal pathology in the acquired immune deficiency syndrome. *Am. J. Clin. Pathol.* *84*:594-597.
34. Bahls, F. and Sumi, S. M. (1986). Cryptococcal meningitis and cerebral toxoplasmosis in a patient with acquired immune deficiency syndrome. *J. Neurol. Neurosurg. Psychiatry* *49*:328-340.
35. Roux, P., Touboul, J. L., Feuilhade de Chauvin, M. et al. (1986). Disseminated cryptococcosis diagnosed in AIDS patient by screening for soluble serum antigens. *Lancet* *1*:1154.
36. McCluskey, P. J. and Wakefield, D. (1985). Ocular involvement in the acquired immune deficiency syndrome (AIDS). *Aust. N.Z. J. Ophthalmol.* *13*:293-298.
37. Schuman, J. S. and Friedman, A. H. (1983). Retinal manifestation of the acquired immune deficiency syndrome (AIDS): Cytomegalovirus, *Candida albicans*, *Cryptococcus*, toxoplasmosis and *Pneumocystis carinii*. *Trans. Ophthalmol. Soc. U. K.* *103*:177-190.
38. Pepose, J. S., Holland, G. N., Nestor, M. S., Chochran, A. J., and Foos, R. Y. (1985). Acquired immune deficiency syndrome: Pathogenic mechanisms of ocular disease. *Ophthalmology* *92*:472-484.
39. Feldman, S. R. and Kuttner, B. J. (1986). Forehead ulcer in a homosexual man. *Arch. Dermatol.* *122*:822.
40. Borton, L. K. and Wintroub, B. U. (1984). Disseminated cryptococcosis presenting as herpetiform lesions in a homosexual man with acquired immunodeficiency syndrome. *J. Am. Acad. Dermatol.* *10*:;387-390.
41. Rico, M. J. and Penneys, N. S. (1985). Cutaneous cryptococcosis resembling molluscum contagiosum in a patient with AIDS. *Arch. Dermatol.* *121*:901-902.
42. Hollerman, J. J., Bernstein, M. A., and Beute, G. H. (1987). Thoracic manifestations of AIDS. *Am. Fam. Physician* *35*:109-118.
43. Perla, E. N., Mayan, S., Miller, S. N., Ramaswamy, G., and Eisenberg, H. (1985). Disseminated cryptococcosis presenting as the adult respiratory distress syndrome. *N.Y. State J. Med.* *85*:704-706.
44. Shuster, B., Akerman, M., Orenstein, M., and Wax, M. R. (1986). Pulmonary manifestations of AIDS: Review of 106 episodes. *Radiology* *161*:87-93.
45. Lewis, W., Lipsick, J., and Cammarosano, C. (1985). Cryptococcal myocarditis in acquired immune deficiency syndrome. *Am. J. Cardiol.* *55*:1240.
46. Shuster, M., Valentine, F., and Holzman, R. (1985). Cryptococcal pericarditis in an intravenous drug abuser. *J. Infect. Dis.* *152*:842.
47. Lief, M. and Sarfarazi, F. (1986). Prostatic cryptococcosis in acquired immune deficiency syndrome. *Urology* *28*:318-319.

48. Ricciardi, D. D., Sepkowitz, D. V., Berkowitz, L. B., Bienestock, H., and Maslow, M. (1986). Cryptococcal arthritis in a patient with acquired immune deficiency syndrome: Case report and review of the literature. *J. Rheumatol. 13*: 455-458.
49. Levy, R. M., Poss, V. G., and Rosenblum, M. L. (1983). Intracerebral mass lesions in the acquired immunodeficiency syndrome (AIDS). *N. Engl. J. Med. 309*:1454-1455.
50. Chernoff, D. N. and Sande, M. A. (1986). Cryptococcal infection in patients with the acquired immunodeficiency syndrome. *Proc. II Int. Conf. AIDS.* Paris, France, Abstr. 543.
51. Folansbee, S. E. and Busch, D. F. (1985). Cryptococcal meningitis complicating AIDS: Analysis of 22 cases. *Proc. I Int. Conf. AIDS.* Atlanta, Ga., Abstr. W17.
52. Daunt, N. and Jaysinghe, L. S. (1985). Cerebral torulosis: Clinical features and correlation with computed tomography. *Clin. Radiol. 36*:485-490.
53. Diamond, R. D. (1985). *Cryptococcus neoformans.* In *Principal and Practice of Infectious Disease*, 2nd ed. (Mandell, G. L., Douglas, R. G., and Bennett, J. E., eds.) New York, John Wiley & Sons, pp. 1460-1468.
54. Goodman, J. S., Kaufman, L., and Koenig, M. G. (1971). Diagnosis of cryptococcal meningitis: Value of immunologic detection of cryptococcal antigen. *N. Engl. J. Med. 285*:434-436.
55. Snow, R. M. and Dismukes, W. E. (1975). Cryptococcal meningitis: Diagnostic value of cryptococcal antigen in cerebrospinal fluid. *Arch. Intern. Med. 135*: 1155-1157.
56. Grossengebauer, K. and Pohle, H. D. (1986). *Cryptococcus neoformans*: Rapid detection in the spleen of an AIDS patient using DAPI-flurochrome. *Mykosen 29*:155-158.
57. Bennett, J. E., Dismukes, W. E., Duma, R. J. et al. (1979). A comparison of amphotericin B alone and combine with flucytosine in the treatment of cryptococcal meningitis. *N. Engl. J. Med. 301*:126-131.
58. Polsky, B., Depman, M. R., Gold, J. W. M., Galicich, J. H., and Armstrong, D. (1986). Intraventricular therapy of cryptococcal meningitis via a subcutaneous reservoir. *Am. J. Med. 81*:24-28.
59. Sarosi, G. A., Parker, J. D., Doto, I. L., and Tosh, F. E. (1969). Amphotericin B in cryptococcal meningitis: Long-term results of treatment. *Ann. Intern. Med. 71*:1079-1087.
60. Spickard, A., Butler, W. T., Andriole, V., and Utz, J. P. (1962). The improved prognosis of cryptococcal meningitis with amphotericin B therapy. *Ann. Intern. Med. 58*:66-83.
61. Kaplan, M. H., Rosen, P. P., and Armstrong, D. (1977). Cryptococcus in a cancer hospital: Clinical and pathological correlates in forty-six patients. *Cancer 39*:2265-2274.
62. Shuster, M., Zuger, A., Simberkoff, M. S., Rahal, J. J., and Holzman, R. S. (1986). Maintenance therapy of cryptococcal meningitis in patients with AIDS. *Proc. II Int. Conf. AIDS.* Paris, France, Abstr. 545.
63. Mess, T. P., Kadley, W. K., and Wofsy, C. B. (1986). Use of high dose oral ketoconazole in AIDS patients for prevention of relapse in cryptococcal infections. *Proc. II Int. Conf. AIDS.* Paris, France, Abstr. 544.

64. Mess, T. P., Hadley, W. K., and Wofsy, C. B. (1987). Use of high dose oral ketoconazole in AIDS patients for prevention of relapse in cryptococcal meningitis. *Proc. III Int. Conf. AIDS.* Washington, D.C., Abstr. TP219.
65. Perfect, J. R., Savani, D. V., and Durack, D. T. (1986). Comparison of itraconazole and fluconazole in treatment of cryptococcal meningitis and candida pyelonephritis in rabbits. *Antimicrob. Agents Chemother. 29*:579-583.
66. de Fernandez, E. P., Patino, M. M., Graybill, J. R., and Tarbit, M. H. (1986). Treatment of cryptococcal meningitis in mice with fluconazole. *J. Antimicrob. Chemother. 18*:261-270.
67. Viviani, M. A., Torotrano, A. M., Giani, P. C. et al. (1987). Itraconazole for cryptococcal infection in the acquired immunodeficiency syndrome. *Ann. Intern. Med. 106*:166.
68. Pfizer Central Research (1986). *Investigators' Reference Manual: Fluconazole.* November 1986 update. Groton, Connecticut.
69. Stern, J., Sharkey, K., Hartman, B., and Graybill, J. (1987). Fluconazole therapy in AIDS patients with cryptococcosis. *Program Abstr. 27th Intersci. Conf. Antimicrob. Agents Chemother.* New York City, Abstr. 948.

16
Endemic Mycoses

Michael G. Threlkeld and William E. Dismukes   *University of Alabama at Birmingham School of Medicine, Birmingham, Alabama*

The immunologic hallmark of the acquired immune deficiency syndrome (AIDS) is a marked reduction in the helper T-lymphocyte population associated with loss of nearly all cell-mediated defenses. It is, therefore, not surprising that individuals infected with the human immunodeficiency virus (HIV) should fall easy prey to organisms, such as the endemic fungi, that require intact lymphocyte/macrophage function for containment and eradication.

Organisms are designated endemic fungi because of their characteristic geographic ranges. Endemic fungi are important pathogens within their respective habitats, but they are an uncommon cause of disease among persons living outside the endemic areas. The major organisms in this group are *Histoplasma capsulatum, Blastomyces dermatitidis,* and *Coccidioides immitis. Sporothrix schenckii,* although not a true endemic fungus, is often included with them. Another nonendemic fungus, *Candida* species, and the syndrome of disseminated candidiasis will also be discussed. Although all of these organisms produce disease in normal individuals, they do not commonly cause progressive, disseminated disease in hosts with intact cellular immunity. Fulminant, multisystem disease is far more likely to develop in immunocompromised hosts, particularly patients with AIDS.

HISTOPLASMOSIS

Histoplasma capsulatum, the imperfect state of the sexually reproducing fungus *Emonsiella capsulatum* (1), is a dimorphic pathogenic fungus that readily converts from its environmental mycelial phase to a yeast phase at mammalian body temperature. The organism is primarily a soil saprophyte with a distinct preference for areas enriched by the nitrogenous waste products of birds or bats (2). It has often been isolated from the soil near starling roosts, chicken yards, and other similar environments. The species is widely distributed over much of the north and south central United States, and most persons living in the endemic area have been infected (3). Characteristic conidia are abundantly produced in nature and, when aerosolized, play a major role in the transmission of the organism to its incidental host, humans. Inhaled spores are deposited in the terminal airways where they germinate; organisms proliferate and are hematogenously distributed throughout the body. Specific cell-mediated immunity develops several weeks after infection and is usually successful in arresting fungal cell proliferation. Most normal individuals who are infected experience no symptoms and manifest only a positive skin test as evidence of the encounter (4). However, living organisms, with the potential for further proliferation, may persist in a dormant state for a prolonged period. Immunocompromised patients may develop symptomatic disease from reactivation of these latent foci or through progression of a newly acquired primary infection. The relative importance of these two mechanisms in the pathogenesis of disease in the immunocompromised patient has not been fully established, but there is evidence that either mechanism may be responsible (5).

More than 40 well-documented cases of histoplasmosis in AIDS patients have been reported from several medical centers, and this number probably represents only a fraction of the actual cases (6-16). Histoplasmosis appears to be the most frequently encountered of the endemic fungi in the HIV-positive population. Reported series of three or more cases are summarized in Table 1. In some highly endemic areas, *H. capsulatum* rivals *Pneumocystis carinii* as a cause of life-threatening opportunistic infection in AIDS patients. Three of the first four AIDS cases diagnosed in Birmingham, Alabama, presented with histoplasmosis, and 7 of 15 AIDS patients in Indianapolis, Indiana, between 1980 and 1985 developed symptomatic histoplasmosis during the course of their illness (6,7).

The HIV-seropositive individuals with disseminated histoplasmosis fulfill the current Centers for Disease Control (CDC) criteria for the diagnosis of AIDS (17). Thus, a subgroup of patients will present with histoplasmosis as their first manifestation of AIDS. A high index of suspicion for *Histoplasma* must be maintained in patients from endemic areas.

Clinical Presentation

In the patient with AIDS, histoplasmosis usually manifests itself as a subacute systemic illness with nonspecific signs and symptoms (6-10). In most patients, symptoms have been present for a period of weeks, although a precise date of onset may be difficult to establish. Fever, documented in nearly

TABLE 1 Reported Cases of Histoplasmosis in AIDS Patients[a]

Ref.	Age/sex	Risk factor[b]	Diagnosis[c]	Treatment[d]	Outcome[e]	Autopsy data[f]
8	26/M	Homosexual	CXR,L	AMB (476 mg); keto prophy	Improved; died 2 mo later with PCP and CMV	NA
	35/M	Homosexual	LB,LNB,BC	AMB (2500 mg)	Improved; died subsequently of other causes	NA
	49/M	Homosexual	CXR,BM,L	AMB (2500 mg); (1200 mg) on relapse	Improved; relapsed and died at 6 mo	H.c. in lungs, BM, CNS
	32/M	Homosexual	CXR,L,BM	AMB (2400 mg)	Improved	NA
	34/M	Homosexual	BM,SB	AMB (1000 mg); keto prophy	Improved	NA
	27/M	Homosexual, IVDA	CXR,BM,LNB	AMB (2500 mg); keto prophy	Improved; died at 1 yr with H.c., MAI, CMV	H.c. in lungs, adrenals
	28/M	Homosexual, IVDA	CXR,BC,BM,SP	Keto (400 mg/d)	Improved but lost to follow-up	NA
	35/M	Homosexual	CXR,BC	Keto (400 mg/d); AMB (1000 mg)	Improved once AMB started; died subsequently	NA
	30/M	Bisexual	BM	AMB (2000 mg)	Improved	NA
	29/M	Homosexual	CXR,BM,SB	AMB (2500 mg)	Improved	NA
	50/M	?	BM	AMB (2500 mg)	Improved	NA
	33/M	Homosexual	CXR,BM,L,SP	AMB (2000 mg); 1000 mg on relapse	Improved; relapsed and died at 5 mo	NA

Table 1 (continued)

TABLE 1 Continued

Ref.	Age/sex	Risk factor[b]	Diagnosis[c]	Treatment[d]	Outcome[e]	Autopsy data[f]
6,8	31/M	Homosexual	CXR,BM,SB,TB,S	AMB (2000 mg); 326 mg on relapse; keto prophy	Improved; relapsed at 5 and 13 mo; died subsequently	No H.c. found
6	36/M	Homosexual	CXR,BM,BS,TB,S	AMB (2000 mg); additional AMB at relapse; keto prophy	Improved; relapsed at 11 mos; improved with re-treatment	NA
	32/M	IVDA	LNB	Keto (800 mg/d) × 11 mos; AMB at relapse	Improved; relapsed when keto discontinued; improved on AMB	NA
7	26/F	IVDA	S,BC	AMB (11 mg)	Died with H.c.	H.c. in lungs, liver, ? brain
	26/M	Homosexual	S,LB,BM,BC	AMB (35 mg/kg); repeated upon relapse	Improved; relapsed at 3 mo and died with H.c. and MAI	H.c. widely disseminated
	30/M	Bisexual	S,BM	AMB (35 mg/kg); keto prophy	Symptoms persisted; died 1 mo later	NA
	30/M	IVDA, Homosexual	CXR,S,L,BC	None	Died suddenly	NA
	29/M	IVDA	CXR,BC,BM,S	AMB; AMB (2500 mg) on relapse; keto prophy	Improved; relapsed at 3 mo; improved upon retreatment	NA
	34/M	Hemophiliac	CXR,SP	Keto 400 mg/d	Improved	NA

10	26/F	Heterosexual exposure	CXR,BM,BC,BS,S	AMB (50 mg)	Died during therapy	H.c. in liver, spleen, kidneys, lungs
	31/M	Homosexual	LNB	AMB (30 mg/kg); keto prophy	Improved	NA
	19/F	Heterosexual exposure, IVDA	LB	AMB (30 mg/kg); keto prophy	Improved	NA
	33/M	IVDA	CXR,BM	AMB (35 mg/kg); keto prophy	Improved	NA
16	30/M	IVDA	CXR,BM	None	Died rapidly	NA
	37/M	IVDA	CXR,BM,BC,TB	AMB (300 mg)	Died	NA
	52/M	IVDA	CXR,BC,TB,UC	AMB (3 days)	Died	NA
	49/M	IVDA	CXR,BC,BM	None	Died	NA
	33/M	IVDA	CXR,BC,BM,TB,LB	AMB (2050 mg); keto prophy	Improved; died subsequently	NA
	28/M	IVDA	CXR,BC,TB	AMB (1700 mg); AMB (1900 mg); keto prophy	Improved but re-lapsed; improved upon retreatment, died subsequently	NA

[a]Summary of reported series of three or more cases.

Abbreviations:

[b]IVDA, intravenous drug abuse.

[c]BC, blood culture; BM, bone marrow (aspirate or biopsy); BS, peripheral blood smear; CXR, chest x-ray; L, lung (unspecified source); LB, liver biopsy; LNB, lymph node biopsy; S, positive serology; SB, skin biopsy; SP, sputum (culture or histology); TB, transbronchial biopsy.

[d]AMB, amphotericin B; keto, ketoconazole; prophy, prophylaxis.

[e]CMV, cytomegalovirus; H.c., *Histoplasma capsulatum*, MAI, *Mycobacterium avium-intracellulare*; PCP, *Pneumocystis carinii* pneumonia.

[f]CNS, central nervous system; NA, not available.

100% of reported cases, is the single most common clinical finding; daily temperatures often exceed 39 °C (8). Splenomegaly, another common finding, was observed in 9 of 12 patients reported by Johnson et al. (8) and four of seven cases described by Wheat et al. (7). Although lymphadenopathy is also found in a majority of patients with histoplasmosis, the adenopathy may be secondary to HIV infection, rather than to fungal disease. Additional frequently encountered symptoms and signs include weight loss, fatigue, night sweats, dyspnea, cough, abdominal pain, and hepatomegaly (6-10). Occasional patients present with a fulminant illness closely resembling bacterial sepsis (7). These individuals are hypotensive and rapidly develop renal, hepatic, and pulmonary insufficiency.

Neurologic symptoms may be prominent in cases where central nervous system invasion has occurred. In Houston, Texas, four AIDS patients presented with alterations in mental status or, in one instance, cranial nerve palsies (G. Sarosi, personal communication). In each case, *H. capsulatum* was isolated from cerebrospinal fluid or brain tissue. Focal lesions were detected by computed tomography of the head in two of the four patients.

Dermatologic manifestations of *H. capsulatum* are rare, even in most immunocompromised patients. In contrast, AIDS patients with disseminated histoplasmosis appear to manifest skin lesions with greater frequency. One of our three original patients developed a prominent maculopapular rash, which yielded *H. capsulatum* at biopsy, over the face, trunk, and upper extremities (6). Three of 12 cases reported from Houston, Texas, were also noted to have skin lesions that on biopsy were culture-positive (8). An AIDS patient in Pretoria, South Africa, developed multiple papulonecrotic skin lesions surrounded by red halos. Yeast cells were present histologically in biopsy specimens, and *H. capsulatum* was isolated at culture. Thus, a skin rash, when present, is an important diagnostic clue for disseminated histoplasmosis. Whitish, ulcerative lesions of the oral mucosa have also been reported (Fig. 1).

Disseminated histoplasmosis must be considered in the differential diagnosis of any unexplained febrile illness in an AIDS patient, especially individuals who have lived or traveled extensively in the endemic areas. Unfortunately, the symptoms of histoplasmosis in this group of patients can closely mimic the symptoms of infection with other opportunistic pathogens including mycobacteria, cytomegalovirus (CMV), *P. carinii*, or even HIV alone. A conclusive diagnosis based solely on clinical grounds, therefore, cannot be made. Although pulmonary infiltrates, splenomegaly, or skin rashes are suggestive findings of histoplasmosis, no presentation can be considered specific for this disease.

Similarly, routine laboratory studies seldom point toward a diagnosis of histoplasmosis, as the abnormalities most commonly encountered may be

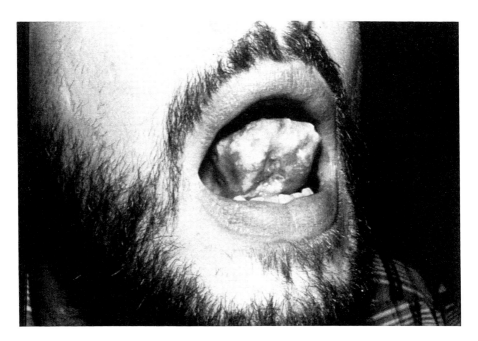

FIGURE 1   Oral lesions of histoplasmosis in a patient with AIDS.

caused by many opportunistic pathogens. Blood cytopenias are often reported with histoplasmosis and may reflect extensive bone marrow involvement or, in some patients, disseminated intravascular coagulation (7,8). Thrombocytopenia was present in five of seven Indianapolis cases (7), and 2 of 12 Houston patients developed petechiae secondary to depressed platelet counts (8).

Moderate liver function abnormalities (elevations of transaminases and alkaline phosphatase levels) have been described in AIDS patients with histoplasmosis (6-8). Although hepatic involvement with *H. capsulatum* is common, enzyme elevations are rarely striking and do not differentiate histoplasmosis from other conditions.

The radiographic presentation of histoplasmosis is quite variable. Although most patients have some abnormality seen on chest x-ray films, 12 of 39 cases for whom there is radiographic information reportedly had normal chest x-ray findings (6-10,14,16). Normal radiographic findings, therefore, do not exclude the diagnosis of histoplasmosis. The high frequency of normal chest radiographs argues for reactivation of latent systemic foci in the pathogenesis of this disease. Those patients who have abnormal chest x-ray films usually

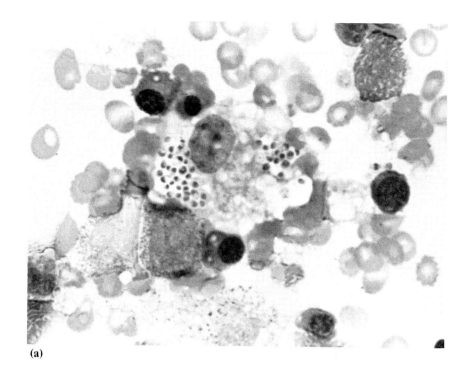

(a)

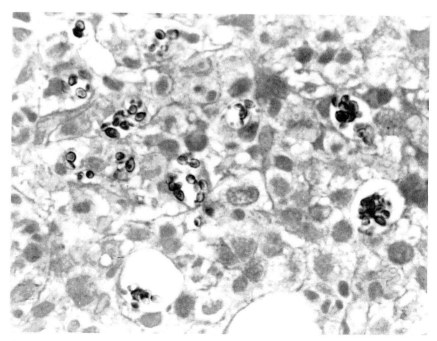

(b)

have bilateral or diffuse pulmonary involvement. The radiographic patterns are nonspecific and include interstitial, reticulonodular, alveolar, and nodular infiltrates (6-10). Similar radiographic findings can be produced by other opportunistic pathogens including CMV, mycobacteria, and *P. carinii*.

Laboratory Diagnosis

A number of special techniques are useful in establishing the diagnosis of histoplasmosis in patients with AIDS. Culture of bone marrow biopsy specimens appears to be the most sensitive method; positive results have been reported in over 70% of cases (8). However, identification of *H. capsulatum* by culture may take as long as 6 weeks. An immediate diagnosis can sometimes be made by histologic demonstration of yeast cells in bone marrow (Figs. 2a and 2b); Johnson et al. (8), Bonner et al. (6) and Mandell et al. (10) made definite histologic diagnoses from bone marrow in 1 of 10, 2 of 3, and 1 of 3 cases, respectively. By using methenamine silver staining of trephine bone marrow biopsy specimens, Davies et al. (18) were able to demonstrate fungi in 15 (68%) of 22 non-AIDS patients with disseminated histoplasmosis. Careful review of a number of tissue sections, stained specifically for fungi, probably improves sensitivity. Culture and histologic examination of specimens obtained by transbronchial biopsy are positive in 50% or more of patients with pulmonary involvement (8).

In addition, biopsy for culture and histopathology of focal sites of disease, such as skin, mucous membranes, lymph nodes, or liver, may be diagnostic (6-10). Specific tissue sampling should be performed whenever clinical or laboratory abnormalities suggest probable histoplasma disease (e.g., liver biopsy in the setting of markedly abnormal liver function tests). The yield from fungal cultures of peripheral blood is also significant, perhaps reflecting the large organism burden in this group of patients. Positive blood cultures have been reported in 16 of 42 published cases (6-11,16). The lysis centrifugation blood culture technique appears to be the most sensitive method. Typical yeast cells may even be seen occasionally on stained peripheral blood or buffy coat smears (Fig. 3) (11).

Because definitive identification of *H. capsulatum* may take several weeks and failure to observe yeast cells in histologic specimens does not exclude the diagnosis, a sensitive and specific serologic test for histoplasmosis would be particularly useful. The most commonly used serologic methods are complement fixation (CF) titers for yeast and mycelial antibodies and the immunodiffusion (ID) test for H and M precipitins. The CF test is generally more

---

FIGURE 2   (a) Clusters of *H. capsulatum* in bone marrow aspirate (Wright's stain, original magnification 1000×). (b) *H. capsulatum* in bone marrow biopsy specimen (Methenamine silver stain, original magnification 1000×).

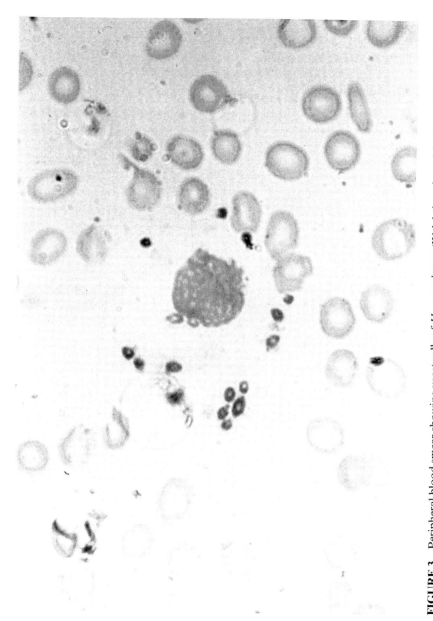

FIGURE 3   Peripheral blood smear showing yeast cells of *H. capsulatum* (Wright's stain, original magnification 1000 ×).

sensitive, whereas ID is more specific for disseminated disease (19). Newer enzyme-linked assays and radioimmunoassays for histoplasma antibody are also becoming available. The detection of specific *H. capsulatum* antigens in urine or serum holds great promise as a future diagnostic technique. Wheat and co-workers (20) have successfully demonstrated histoplasma antigen in the urine by radioimmunoassay during 20 of 22 episodes of documented disseminated histoplasmosis in a mixed patient population. Blood antigen measurement was somewhat less sensitive, detecting 11 of the 22 episodes.

To date, results of serologic testing for histoplasmosis in patients with AIDS have been inconsistent. Wheat (7) noted positive CF or ID tests in six of seven AIDS patients with disseminated histoplasmosis. The single patient with negative serologies had a strongly positive radioimmunoassay for anti-histoplasma IgG. In contrast, Mandell et al. (10) reported negative CF results in all three of their patients. Johnson and associates (8) stated that serologic testing was not useful in their group of 12 cases, but they did not report the specific results for individual patients. At our institution, we find serologic testing to be specific, although relatively insensitive, for diagnosis of histoplasmosis in AIDS patients. A positive result in a severely ill patient is highly suggestive of histoplasmosis. A negative result, however, does not exclude the diagnosis. Larger numbers of patients and standardized methods of testing will be required to fully evaluate the usefulness of serodiagnosis in the HIV-positive population.

Treatment

Amphotericin B is the drug of choice for histoplasmosis in the immunocompromised patient. Kauffman and coauthors (21) summarized the clinical outcomes of 58 histoplasmosis patients with a variety of underlying illnesses, including Hodgkin's disease and chronic lymphocytic leukemia. The mortality for the 15 patients treated with a total dose of amphotericin B greater than 1000 mg was only 6.7%. In contrast, mortality was 100% among 35 patients who received no therapy or less than 1000 mg of amphotericin B. Although ketoconazole alone is an effective drug for histoplasmosis in the normal host, results of primary therapy in immunocompromised individuals have been unimpressive. In the National Institute of Allergy and Infectious Disease (NIAID) Mycoses Study Group evaluation of ketoconazole therapy for histoplasmosis (22), 11 of the 14 treatment failures occurred in immunocompromised hosts. This group included one patient with AIDS who appeared to improve during therapy but promptly relapsed once the drug was discontinued.

The treatment of AIDS patients with disseminated histoplasmosis is unsatisfactory. Relapse rates have been unacceptably high, despite aggressive management. Of the 31 patients summarized in Table 1, at least 17 have died. Although the cause of death could not always be determined, five of six patients for whom autopsy data are available had evidence of active histoplasmosis. Twenty-three of the 31 patients temporarily improved with treatment, but at least nine of these apparent responders developed recurrent histoplasmosis within the first year after treatment. The true relapse rate is probably higher than the statistics indicate because some patients were lost to follow-up.

The most effective treatment regimen for histoplasmosis in AIDS patients has not been determined. We currently favor an induction course of amphotericin B with a minimum total dose of approximately 1 g given over several weeks. If the fungal disease is controlled, this induction therapy is followed by lifelong suppressive therapy with ketoconazole, 400 mg/day, or intermittent (i.e., weekly) amphotericin B in an effort to prevent relapse. Patients must be followed closely because recurrent disease has been reported despite long-term ketoconazole (14). If a patient does relapse, he should be re-treated with a course of parenteral amphotericin B; five of the patients shown in Table 1 had relapses that were successfully treated. Ketoconazole alone should be reserved for treatment of AIDS patients who cannot, or will not, take amphotericin B. Large clinical trials comparing the efficacy of different primary treatment and suppressive regimens are needed.

Newer triazole compounds, such as itraconazole and fluconazole, are currently undergoing investigation for the treatment of systemic fungal diseases. Itraconazole has a broader antifungal spectrum than ketoconazole, whereas fluconazole is unique because of its excellent penetration into the cerebrospinal fluid. Animal studies have shown that both drugs are active in vivo against *H. capsulatum* (23,24). These agents may prove to be superior to ketoconazole in the treatment or prophylaxis of disseminated histoplasmosis.

COCCIDIOIDOMYCOSIS

Coccidioides immitis is a dimorphic soil-inhabiting fungus primarily endemic to the hot, arid regions of North and South America. In the United States, the organism is largely restricted to the Southwest, particularly Arizona, New Mexico, Nevada, and southern California, including the San Joaquin valley. In its natural environment, *C. immitis* exists in a mycelial phase that produces easily fragmented and highly infectious arthrospores; these spores are aerosolized when colonized soil is disturbed by construction, digging, or even walking. After inhalation and subsequent germination of arthrospores, the pathogenic form, an endosporulating spherule, develops in the pulmonary alveolae. Thereafter, a granulomatous inflammatory tissue response by immunocompetent hosts usually contains the infectious process. Persons compromised by lymphoproliferative disorders, such as lymphoma and Hodgkin's disease, immunosuppressive therapy, or organ transplantation, are at particular risk of progression of primary infection with dissemination (25). Earlier studies suggested an increased incidence of disseminated disease among blacks and persons of Filipino ancestry, but several recent analyses have failed to confirm this association (26,27).

In normal hosts, primary infection with *C. immitis* is often asymptomatic or indistinguishable clinically from a viral respiratory tract infection (so-called valley fever) (25). Occasionally, patients present with a subacute pneumonia, but most recover from their influenzalike illness without specific therapy. In contrast, immunocompromised hosts are much more prone to develop severe pulmonary as well as progressive, widely disseminated disease (25).

Although coccidioidomycosis has not been reported with as great a frequency in AIDS patients as has histoplasmosis, in highly endemic areas, coccidioidomycosis is a significant cause of morbidity and mortality. For example, in Pima County, Arizona, between 1979 and 1986, coccidioidomycosis was diagnosed in 7 of 27 AIDS patients (29). There is evidence for both reactivation of latent disease as well as progressive primary infection in AIDS patients. One patient developed disseminated disease within 3 months of moving to Arizona from a nonendemic part of the United States (29). Another patient in Michigan developed disseminated coccidioidomycosis 2 years after recovery from a minimally symptomatic infection acquired during a visit to the Southwest (30). Clearly, physicians caring for AIDS patients in nonendemic areas should obtain a careful history of travel and prior places of residence to avoid overlooking the possibility of *C. immitis* as an opportunistic pathogen.

Clinical Presentation

Typically, coccidioidomycosis is a subacute systemic illness in patients with AIDS (29-33). Autopsy data from seven fatal cases have demonstrated spherules in a variety of organs including kidneys, liver, spleen, brain, lymph nodes, in addition to lung (29,31,33). Despite the extent of disease, symptoms are usually nonspecific, and frequently resemble those caused by other opportunistic pathogens or HIV infection alone. Patients typically have high fever (often over 39 °C), cough, dyspnea, fatigue, weight loss, and lymphadenopathy (29-33). The lung is the organ most consistently involved, and the majority of 11 reported cases (summarized in Table 2) had some type of respiratory symptom or sign (29-33). Focal lesions of skin, soft tissue, joint, and bone, which are often seen in disseminated coccidioidomycosis, have been uncommon in patients with AIDS (29).

TABLE 2 Reported Cases of Coccidioidomycosis in AIDS Patients

Ref.	Age/sex	Risk factor[a]	Diagnosis[b]	Treatment[c]	Outcome[d]	Autopsy data[e]
26	56/M	Homosexual	CXR,S,BC	Keto initially; AMB (930 mg); keto prophy	Died with PCP and MAI	NA
	31/M	IVDA	CXR,SC,BM,UC, BC,S	AMB (2500 mg); keto prophy	Improved; relapsed and died when keto prophy discontinued	C.i. in spleen, liver, lungs, kidneys
	25/M	Homosexual	CXR,LB,S	AMB (1000 mg); keto prophy	Improved; relapsed and died when keto prophy discontinued	C.i. in lungs and lymph nodes
	24/M	Homosexual	CXR,TB,BC,UC,S	AMB (1600 mg)	Improved; died subsequently	NA
	58/M	Bisexual	CXR,TB,S	AMB (900 mg) CMV, PCP, after	Died with C.i., liver, spleen, lymph initial stabilization	C.i. in lungs, nodes, thyroid, kidneys, CNS

26/M	Homosexual	CXR,TB	AMB (30 mg)	Died with C.i., KS	C.i. in lungs, liver, spleen
35/M	Homosexual	CXR,TB	AMB (1100 mg)	Died with C.i., lymphoma, CMV, aspergillus	C.i. in lungs, liver, spleen, kidney, heart
27	23/M	IVDA	LNB,SC,S	AMB (2230 mg)	Improved; died subsequently	NA
28	30/M	Homosexual	CXR,SC,LNB,UC,S	AMB (1400 mg)	Improved; relapsed and died after therapy discontinued	C.i. in lungs, LN
29	39/M	IVDA	CXR,TB,SC	AMB	Died	NA
30	30/M	Homosexual	CXR,LB,BC	AMB	Died with C.i.	C.i. in lungs, liver, spleen, LN

Abbreviations:

[a]IVDA, intravenous drug abuse.

[b]BC, blood culture; BM, bone marrow (aspirate or biopsy); CXR, chest x-ray; LB, liver biopsy; LNB, lymph node biopsy; S, positive serology; SC, sputum culture; TB, transbronchial biopsy; UC, urine culture.

[c]AMB, amphotericin B; keto, ketoconazole; prophy, prophylaxis.

[d]C.i., *Coccidioides immitis*; CMV, cytomegalovirus; KS, Kaposi's sarcoma; MAI, *Mycobacterium avium-intracellulare*; PCP, *Pneumocystis carinii*.

[e]CNS, central nervous system; LN, lymph node; NA, not available.

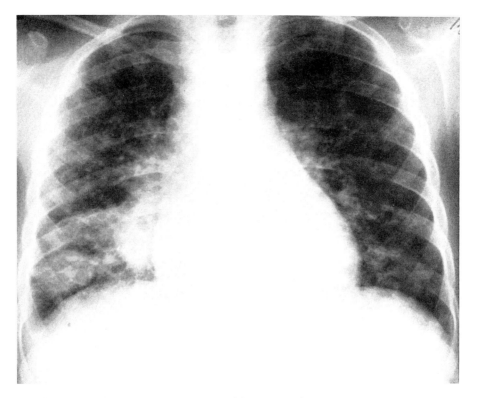

FIGURE 4 Chest x-ray of an HIV positive hemophiliac with disseminated cocci-dioidomycosis (Courtesy John N. Galgiani).

Routine laboratory studies in AIDS patients with coccidioidomycosis are generally not helpful. Abnormalities in levels of transaminases and alkaline phosphatase, reflecting hepatic dysfunction, are occasionally noted (29-33). Peripheral blood cytopenias have been described in some patients (29-33).

The chest radiograph may be the most helpful test to suggest the diagnosis of disseminated coccidioidomycosis in an AIDS patients with the appropriate exposure history (Fig. 4). Virtually all reported cases have had some detectable abnormality on chest x-ray (29-33). Diffuse reticulonodular infiltrates are seen most commonly; this pattern was described in six of the seven patients reported by Bronniman et al. (29). However, occasional patients may have only hilar or mediastinal adenopathy or isolated pulmonary nodules (29-31). In one reported case, the chest radiograph showed "no active disease," but nodules were present on computerized tomograms of the chest

(30). The value of a normal chest x-ray film in excluding the diagnosis of coccidioidomycosis cannot be estimated from the relatively small number of reported cases.

Laboratory Diagnosis

The most efficient method of proving the diagnosis of coccidioidomycosis in AIDS patients has not been established. However, evaluation of respiratory tract specimens appears to be quite sensitive. Culture of sputum or transbronchial biopsy specimen was diagnostic in 9 of 11 reported cases (29-33). In 5 of these 11 patients, a rapid diagnosis was made from histologic demonstration of *C. immitis* spherules in sputum or lung tissue (Fig. 5). In addition, the organism has been cultured or identified histologically in lymph node, liver, bone marrow, blood, and urine.

Complement fixation titers are quite useful in the diagnosis of disseminated coccidioidomycosis in most patient populations, including those with AIDS (34). However, several reports indicate that AIDS patients have lower CF titers than other patients (26-31). In addition, rare AIDS patients with proven coccidioidomycosis and negative CF titers have been described (32). Serologies should be routinely checked whenever a diagnosis of coccidioidomycosis is considered in an HIV-positive individual. Even a weakly positive test should arouse suspicion, but a negative result does not exclude the diagnosis.

Treatment

Amphotericin B has long been the standard therapy for life-threatening cases of coccidioidomycosis. Winn, in 1959 (35), described successful treatment with amphotericin B of 10 patients with severe or disseminated coccidioidal disease. Sarosi and co-workers (36) reported the clinical course of 20 individuals with chronic pulmonary coccidioidomycosis. Eleven patients were managed with amphotericin B alone; all 7 of the patients who received 30 mg/kg or more of the drug were cured. In contrast, the prognosis of immunocompromised patients with overwhelming coccidioidal disease is poor despite aggressive therapy. Ampel et al. (26) recently described 15 patients with *C. immitis* isolated from peripheral blood cultures. Thirteen of the patients were significantly immunosuppressed, with underlying conditions, including organ transplantation, malignancy, and AIDS. Only five of these individuals were alive 1 month after the fungemic episode. Moreover, a review of 21 previously reported cases of *C. immitis* fungemia revealed only three survivors.

The treatment of coccidioidomycosis in AIDS patients is difficult at best. As with most other infections in these patients, therapy is rarely curative;

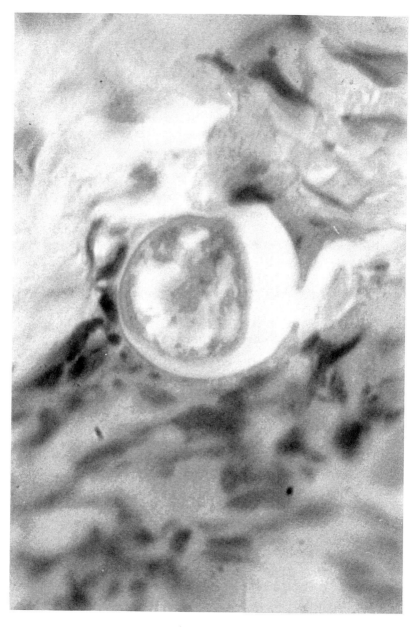

FIGURE 5 Spherule of *C. immitis* in tissue section.

relapse is a major problem whenever treatment is discontinued. Seven of 11 reported cases (see Table 2) had evidence of active coccidioidal disease at the time of autopsy, despite prior aggressive antifungal therapy with amphotericin B. However, most cases did improve, at least temporarily, after receiving parenteral amphotericin B.

Although ketoconazole is active against *C. immitis* in vitro and has been used with mixed results to treat coccidioidomycosis in normal hosts, two reported AIDS patients actually developed disseminated coccidioidomycosis while receiving ketoconazole for chronic candidal infections (29). There is one report in which ketoconazole was administered as primary therapy for coccidioidomycosis in an AIDS patient (29). Symptoms and radiographic abnormalities persisted until therapy with amphotericin B was initiated. Ketoconazole may have a role, however, in the long-term maintenance therapy of patients who have responded to initial treatment with amphotericin B. Two cases receiving such suppressive therapy relapsed promptly when ketoconazole was discontinued (29). Intermittent amphotericin B may also prove useful as a suppressive agent. Until controlled trials establish the most effective treatment regimen, AIDS patients with coccidioidomycosis should receive an initial course of 1 to 2 g of amphotericin B followed by either maintenance ketoconazole 400 mg/day or maintenance amphotericin B weekly. The future role of itraconazole or fluconazole in the management of this disease has not been determined.

SPOROTRICHOSIS

Sporothrix schenckii is found worldwide in soil, most often in association with plants or their organic debris (37). The pathogenic form of this dimorphic fungus is a cigar-shaped yeast (Fig. 6). The organism is a sporadic cause in humans of granulomatous lymphocutaneous disease, which usually results when a colonized thorn or splinter punctures the skin. Extracutaneous disease occurs uncommonly by contiguous spread to soft tissue, bone, or joints. Primary pulmonary infection has been reported, presumably from the direct inhalation of spores (38). Pulmonary sporotrichosis commonly mimics chronic pulmonary tuberculosis. A few cases of widely disseminated disease, with or without pulmonary involvement, have been described in immunocompromised individuals (39).

There have been two reported cases of sporotrichosis in HIV-infected patients in the United States (40,41). One patient, a 34-year-old heroin abuser, presented with purple, ulcerating, subcutaneous nodules on the extremities and trunk, associated with synovitis of the joints of both hands. Cultures of skin lesions (Fig. 7) and joint fluid grew *S. schenckii* (40). There was no specific history of exposure to the organism, but the percutaneous route of infection

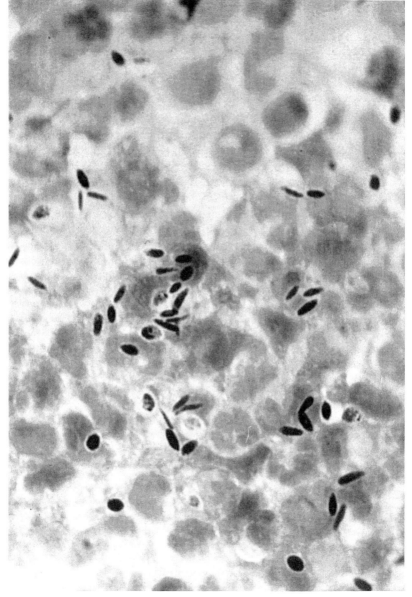

FIGURE 6 Cigar-shaped yeast cells of *S. schenckii* in tissue section.

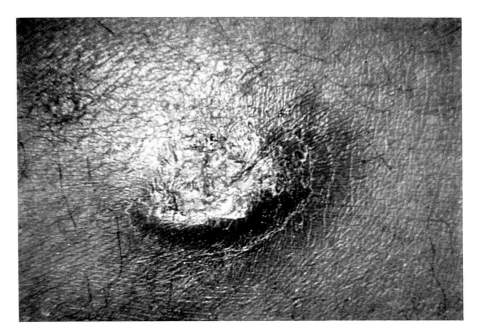

FIGURE 7   Ulcerative skin lesion of sporotrichosis in an AIDS patient.

was judged likely, given the absence of pulmonary symptoms. The patient's lesions improved significantly during an 8-week course of amphotericin B (total dose of 1900 mg). Less than a week after therapy was discontinued, however, the patient developed severe disturbances in mentation and died. Autopsy demonstrated extensive involvement of lung, spleen, skin, and liver with *S. schenckii*.

Disseminated disease was also reported in a 71-year-old woman who acquired HIV during factor VIII concentrate therapy for an acquired factor VIII inhibitor (41). This patient presented with multiple ulcerating skin lesions which grew *S. schenckii*. Results from chest x-ray examination were normal at the time of presentation. Despite marked improvement in her skin lesions during treatment with amphotericin B (total dose of 950 mg), the patient died from multiple opportunistic infections. An autopsy was not performed, but sporotrichosis was not felt to be the immediate cause of her death.

These two cases demonstrate that AIDS patients are at risk for disseminated sporotrichosis. Although skin and soft tissues were extensively affected in the two reported patients, there have been too few cases to fully define the clinical spectrum of this disease in patients with AIDS.

Laboratory Diagnosis

Sporotrichosis was diagnosed in the two reported patients by biopsy and culture of skin lesions; organisms may also be demonstrated in tissue by immunofluorescent staining (42). If future AIDS patients with sporotrichosis present with pulmonary or other visceral organ involvement, invasive diagnostic procedures, such as bronchoscopy, may be necessary. Serologic testing for *S. schenckii* antibodies has been evaluated, but it has not received widespread clinical use. Roberts and Larsh (43) achieved 100% sensitivity using CF and agglutination tests in three patients with disseminated disease, and Karlin and Nielson (44) reported positive agglutination titers in all eight of their patients with disseminated sporotrichosis. The sensitivity of serologic tests for sporotrichosis among AIDS patients, however, remains unknown. Additional patients must be evaluated before specific recommendations can be made about the usefulness of different diagnostic methods for sporotrichosis in the HIV-infected population.

Treatment

Amphotericin B is the mainstay of therapy for patients with disseminated sporotrichosis. Parker et al. (45) noted that five of seven patients with pulmonary and 8 of 14 patients with disseminated extrapulmonary disease responded well to treatment with amphotericin B alone. In addition, these authors suggested that patients who received more than 2 g of amphotericin B were more likely to recover. Results of primary ketoconazole therapy for sporotrichosis have been disappointing. The NIAID Mycoses Study Group in 1983 showed that only one of seven patients with skin, bone, articular, or soft tissue sporotrichosis was cured with ketoconazole as a single agent (46). Until further data are available, amphotericin B in a total dose of 2000 mg should be used as initial therapy for AIDS patients with sporotrichosis. Ketoconazole may have some role as a maintenance suppressive agent.

BLASTOMYCOSIS

Blastomyces dermatitidis is a thermally dimorphic fungus that exists in nature and in culture as a mycelium and as a yeast in humans at 37 °C. During a recent outbreak among environmental campers in Wisconsin, the organism was isolated from soil in and around a beaver lodge (47). This finding together with data from other point-source outbreaks indicate that the ecologic niche of *B. dermatitidis* is soil enriched with organic material such as animal or bird droppings (48). Because blastomycosis occurs primarily in persons living in the north and south central United States, the causative organism is considered an endemic fungus (49).

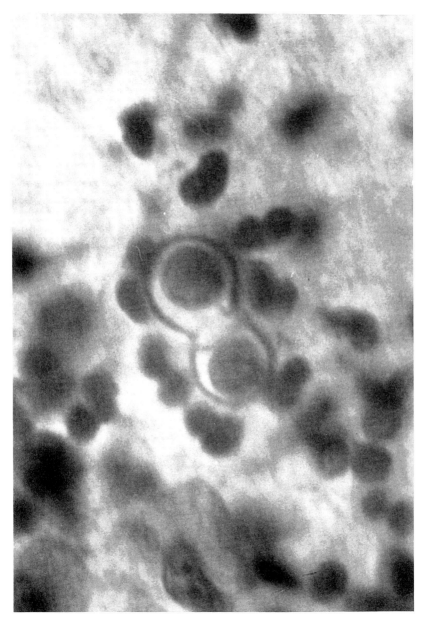

FIGURE 8 *B. dermatitidis* demonstrating refractile cell wall and broad-based budding.

The early stages of blastomycosis closely resemble those of histoplasmosis. Conidia are presumably inhaled and germinate in the terminal airways. The pathogenic yeast form has a characteristic morphology—a highly refractile cell wall and distinctive broad-based budding (Fig. 8) (50). An initial inflammatory response that includes large numbers of neutrophils as well as macrophages is usually successful in containing the infection. Primary infection in most individuals is asymptomatic or a mild influenzalike illness. Progressive disease in the normal host primarily involves the lung, skin, skeletal system, and prostate gland (30).

Blastomycosis differs from histoplasmosis and coccidioidomycosis in its strikingly low prevalence in immunocompromised patients. During a recent evaluation by the Mycoses Study Group, NIAID, none of 80 blastomycosis patients were receiving corticosteroids or immunosuppressive drugs (22). Over a 7-year period, Recht and co-workers (51) treated 78 individuals with symptomatic blastomycosis; only six patients were immunosuppressed (three with hematologic malignancies and three receiving corticosteroids). Clinical findings at presentation in these patients did not differ significantly from the nonimmunocompromised group. However, others have suggested that compromised hosts with blastomycosis are somewhat predisposed to develop widely disseminated disease. Stelling et al. (52) analyzed six cases of blastomycosis presenting with diffuse miliary infiltrates; three of these patients were considered immunosuppressed with underlying diseases including multiple myeloma, jejunoileal bypass, and lymphoma. To date, there have been no cases of blastomycosis reported in patients with AIDS, and the frequency of exposure in persons with HIV infection is unknown. Latent infection leading to reactivation may be less common in blastomycosis than in histoplasmosis and coccidioidomycosis. Alternatively, primary infection may require heavy exposure to an environmental site.

Blastomyces dermatitidis will probably infect and cause disease in an AIDS patients at some time in the future; hence, we might speculate about the nature of the resulting illness. The patient would likely present subacutely with fever and focal or diffuse pulmonary infiltrates. Early dissemination to skin and visceral organs would be expected. Although some immunocompromised patients with blastomycosis are cured with therapy, AIDS patients would probably relapse once treatment was discontinued. The therapeutic regimen of choice would be an induction course of amphotericin B followed by chronic maintenance suppressive ketoconazole, much as in the therapy of histoplasmosis in this population. (See note added in proof at the end of this chapter.)

DISSEMINATED CANDIDIASIS

Candida is a genus of yeasts that colonize mammalian gastrointestinal and genitourinary tracts. These normally commensal organisms have emerged as important opportunistic pathogens and may cause disease ranging from limited mucocutaneous involvement to widespread dissemination and invasive disease. A variety of host defense mechanisms interact to contain and eradicate candida infections (53); therefore, no single immunologic defect predisposes patients to all forms of candidal disease. For example, individuals with a defect in T-lymphocyte function and chronic mucocutaneous candidiasis rarely present with disseminated candidiasis. In contrast, patients who are myelosuppressed from hematologic malignancies and chemotherapy are at high risk for candidemia. Among 797 acute leukemia patients, 11% developed systemic candidiasis (54). In addition to granulocyte and lymphocyte function, intact skin and mucosal barriers appear to be important in the host defense against these organisms, as candida is a major cause of nosocomial fungemia in all types of critically ill patients with percutaneous intravascular catheters (55).

Candida is well recognized as a cause of mucous membrane disease in patients with AIDS. Esophageal candidiasis in HIV-positive patients fulfills the CDC case definition of AIDS, and oral candidiasis is often the first indication of waning immune function in these patients (17). However, as in patients with chronic mucocutaneous candidiasis, disseminated candidiasis has rarely occurred in patients with HIV infection. When candidemia or disseminated candidiasis occurs in AIDS patients, it is typically in the hospital setting among individuals with many of the usual risk factors for disseminated disease including neutropenia, intravascular catheters, and prior antimicrobial therapy. Whimbey and associates (13) described 49 episodes of bacteremia or fungemia occurring among 33 of 336 AIDS patients in New York City. Only four of these episodes were caused by C. albicans. In each case, the patient was terminally ill, and an infected vascular catheter was considered the source of the fungemia.

The subset of HIV-positive individuals who abuse intravenous drugs are also at risk for systemic disease caused by Candida species because of injection of contaminated material. These patients have an increased frequency of candidal osteomyelitis, endocarditis, endophthalmitis, and tissue abscesses (56,57). Such infections do not necessarily relate to the patient's HIV status, they merely reflect the association of both HIV infection and fungal disease with intravenous drug abuse.

Systemic candidiasis presents nonspecifically in individuals with or without AIDS. Patients are typically quite ill from an underlying condition and often have central venous and arterial lines in an intensive care unit setting. Such patients often manifest fever unresponsive to antibacterial therapy and may have initially negative blood cultures. Onset may be fulminant, resembling gram-negative bacteremia, or subacute with "failure to thrive." In occasional patients, focal organ involvement may dominate the clinical picture (e.g., brain or liver abscesses).

Diagnosis of disseminated candidiasis requires a high index of suspicion. Blood cultures are useful when positive, but when negative, they do not exclude the diagnosis. Careful retinal examination may reveal white exudates typical for candidal endophthalmitis. Neutropenic patients with disseminated candidiasis commonly develop maculopapular skin lesions that may yield organisms upon biopsy. In the appropriate clinical setting, computerized tomography of abdomen or head may detect lesions amenable to biopsy and culture.

The therapy of choice for disseminated candidiasis in immunocompromised individuals is amphotericin B. Most AIDS patients with candidemia have died rapidly from other infections, hence, the results of therapy cannot be fully evaluated. Removal of colonized intravascular lines and devices is an important adjunct to antifungal drug therapy. Invasive disease and focal lesions, particularly endocarditis, may require longer therapy and surgical management. Chronic suppressive therapy with ketoconazole may be prudent for AIDS patients who complete parenteral treatment.

PREVENTION

Because endemic fungi, particularly *H. capsulatum, C. immitis,* and *B. dermatitidis,* have discrete environmental habitats, prevention by avoidance of these areas by HIV-positive individuals has been suggested. It is known that persons who never venture into endemic areas are at very low risk of acquiring one of the endemic mycoses. Similarly, it seems prudent for HIV-positive persons who live in or visit endemic areas to avoid potential sites of intense exposure such as bird roosts (histoplasmosis), construction sites and farms in arid regions of the Southwest (coccidioidomycosis), and moist wooded areas (blastomycosis).

CONCLUSIONS

Endemic mycoses are an increasingly serious threat to patients with AIDS. A high index of suspicion is crucial to the diagnosis of any of these diseases because their clinical presentations are usually nonspecific. A careful travel history and review of prior places of residence should be a part of the initial evaluation of every AIDS patient. AIDS patients are prone to develop multiple concomitant opportunistic infections. Thus, establishing the presence of one pathogen does not exclude the presence of another. Patients not responding to therapy for a nonfungal infection should be evaluated for the possibility of a concomitant, opportunistic fungal disease.

Transbronchial and bone marrow biopsies appear to be the most useful techniques for diagnosis of disseminated fungal disease in AIDS patients.

Skin and other superficial mucosal lesions, when present, should be biopsied for culture and histologic examination. Blood cultures are occasionally diagnostic and should be obtained routinely. Additional invasive procedures may be necessary for diagnosis in some patients.

There is, as yet, no curative therapy for any serious fungal disease in AIDS patients. Although many patients will respond to treatment with amphotericin B, relapse predictably occurs once the drug is discontinued. Lifelong suppressive or maintenance therapy with either ketoconazole or intermittent amphotericin B appears necessary once primary therapy has been completed. Newer antifungal azoles, such as itraconazole and fluconazole, are currently being investigated.

NOTE ADDED IN PROOF

Since the preparation of this chapter, blastomycosis has been documented in several patients with AIDS, including one at our institution. These patients presented with manifestations similar to those proposed in the text.

REFERENCES

1. Kwon-Chung, K. J. (1972). Sexual stage of *Histoplasma capsulatum*. *Science* *175*:326.
2. Ajello, L. (1964). Relationship of *Histoplasma capsulatum* to avian habitats. *Public Health Rep. 79*:266.
3. Edwards, L. B., Acquaviva, F. A., Livesay, V. T. et al. (1969). An atlas of sensitivity to tuberculin, PPD-B, and histoplasmin in the United States. *Am. Rev. Resp. Dis. 99*:1-18.
4. Goodwin, R. A., Loyd, J. E., and Des Prez, R. M. (1981). Histoplasmosis in the normal host. *Medicine 60*:231-265.
5. Davies, S. F., Khan, M., and Sarosi, G. A. (1978). Disseminated histoplasmosis in immunologically suppressed patients. Occurrence in a nonendemic area. *Am. J. Med. 64*:94-100.
6. Bonner, J. R., Alexander, J., Dismukes, W. E. et al. (1984). Disseminated histoplasmosis in patients with the acquired immune deficiency syndrome. *Arch. Intern. Med. 144*:2178-2181.
7. Wheat, L. J., Slama, T. G., and Zeckel, M. L. (1985). Histoplasmosis in the acquired immune deficiency syndrome. *Am. J. Med. 78*:203-210.
8. Johnson, P. C., Sarosi, G. A., Septimus, E. J. et al. (1986). Progressive disseminated histoplasmosis in patients with the acquired immune deficiency syndrome: A report of 12 cases and a literature review. *Semin. Resp. Infect. 1*:1-8.
9. Taylor, M. N., Baddour, L. M., and Alexander, J. R. (1984). Disseminated histoplasmosis associated with the acquired immune deficiency syndrome. *Am. J. Med. 77*:579-580.

10. Mandell, W., Goldberg, D. M., and Neu, H. C. (1986). Histoplasmosis in patients with the acquired immune deficiency syndrome. *Am. J. Med. 81*:974-978.

11. Henochowicz, S., Sahovic, E., Pistole, M. et al. (1985). Histoplasmosis diagnosed on peripheral blood smear from a patient with AIDS. *JAMA 253*:3148.

12. Small, C. B., Klein, R. S., Friedland, G. H. et al. (1983). Community-acquired opportunistic infections and defective cellular immunity in heterosexual drug abusers and homosexual men. *Am. J. Med. 74*:433-441.

13. Whimbey, E., Gold, J. W. M., Polsky, B. et al. (1986). Bacteremia and fungemia in patients with the acquired immunodeficiency syndrome. *Ann. Intern. Med. 104*:511-514.

14. Gustafson, P. R. and Henson, A. (1985). Ketoconazole therapy for AIDS patients with disseminated histoplasmosis [Letter]. *Arch. Intern. Med. 145*:2272.

15. Hazelhurst, J. A. and Vismer, H. F. (1985). Histoplasmosis presenting with unusual skin lesions in acquired immunodeficiency syndrome (AIDS). *Br. J. Dermatol. 113*:345-348.

16. Huang, C. T., McGarry, T., Cooper, S. et al. (1987). Disseminated histoplasmosis in the acquired immunodeficiency syndrome: Report of five cases from a nonendemic area. *Arch. Intern. Med. 147*:1181-1184.

17. CDC (1985). Revision of the case definition of acquired immunodeficiency syndrome for national reporting—United States. *MMWR 34*:373-375.

18. Davies, S. F., McKenna, R. W., and Sarosi, G. A. (1979). Trephine biopsy of the bone marrow in disseminated histoplasmosis. *Am. J. Med. 67*:617-622.

19. Davies, S. F. (1986). Serodiagnosis of histoplasmosis. *Semin. Res. Infect. 1*: 9-15.

20. Wheat, L. J., Kohler, R. B., and Tewari, R. P. (1986). Diagnosis of disseminated histoplasmosis by detection of *Histoplasma capsulatum* antigen in serum and urine specimens. *N. Engl. J. Med. 314*:83-88.

21. Kauffman, C. A., Israel, K. S., Smith, J. W. et al. (1978). Histoplasmosis in immunosuppressed patients. *Am. J. Med. 64*:923-932.

22. National Institute of Allergy and Infectious Diseases Mycosis Study Group (1985). Treatment of blastomycosis and histoplasmosis with ketoconazole. Results of a prospective randomized clinical trial. *Ann. Intern. Med. 103*:861-872.

23. Kobayashi, G. S., Travis, S., and Medoff, G. (1986). Comparison of the in vitro and in vivo activity of the bistriazole derivative UK 49,858 with that of amphotericin B against *Histoplasma capsulatum*. *Antimicrob. Agents Chemother. 19*: 660-662.

24. Van Cutsem, J., Van Gerven, F., and Janssen, P. A. J. (1987). Activity of orally, topically, and parenterally administered itraconazole in the treatment of superficial and deep mycoses: Animal models. *Rev. Infect. Dis. 9*:S15-S32.

25. Deresinski, S. C. and Stevens, D. A. (1984). Coccidioidomycosis in compromised hosts. Experience at Stanford University Hospital. *Medicine 54*:377-395.

26. Ampel, N. M., Ryan, K. J., Carry, P. J. et al. (1986). Fungemia due to *Coccidioides immitis*. An analysis of 16 episodes in 15 patients and a review of the literature. *Medicine 65*:312-321.

27. Sievers, M. L. (1980). Racial susceptibility to coccidioidomycosis [Letter]. *N. Engl. J. Med. 302*:58-59.

28. Smith, C. E., Beard, R. R., Whiting, E. G., and Rosenberger, H. G. (1946). Varieties of coccidioidal infection in relation to the epidemiology and control of disease. *Am. J. Public Health 36*:1934.
29. Bronniman, D. A., Adam, R. D., Galgiani, J. N. et al. (1987). Coccidioidomycosis in patients with the acquired immunodeficiency syndrome. *Ann. Intern. Med. 106*:372-379.
30. Salberg, D. J. and Venkatachalam, H. (1986). Disseminated coccidioidomycosis presenting in AIDS. *VA Practitioner 3*:89-93.
31. Kovacs, A., Forthal, D. N., Kovacs, J. A. et al. (1984). Disseminated coccidioidomycosis in a patient with acquired immune deficiency syndrome. *West. J. Med. 140*:447-449.
32. Roberts, C. J. (1984). Coccidioidomycosis in acquired immune deficiency syndrome. Depressed humoral as well as cellular immunity. *Am. J. Med. 76*:734-736.
33. Abrams, D. I., Robia, M., Blumenfeld, W. et al. (1984). Disseminated coccidioidomycosis in AIDS. *N. Engl. J. Med. 310*:986-987.
34. Smith, C. E. and Saito, M. T. (1957). Serologic reactions in coccidioidomycosis. *J. Chronic Dis. 5*:571.
35. Winn, W. A. (1959). The use of amphotericin B in the treatment of coccidioidal disease. *Am. J. Med.* 617-634.
36. Sarosi, G. A., Parker, J. D., Doto, I. L. et al. (1970). Chronic pulmonary coccidioidomycosis. A National Communicable Disease Center Cooperative Mycoses Study. *N. Engl. J. Med. 283*:325-329.
37. Travassos, L. R. and Lloyd, K. O. (1980). *Sporothrix schenckii* and related species of ceratocystis. *Microbiol. Rev. 44*:683.
38. Pluss, J. L. and Opal, S. M. (1986). Pulmonary sporotrichosis: Review of treatment and outcome. *Medicine 65*:143-153.
39. Lynch, P. J., Voorhees, J. J., and Harrell, E. R. (1970). Systemic sporotrichosis. *Ann. Intern. Med. 73*:23-30.
40. Lipstein-Kresch, E., Isenberg, H. D., Singer, C. et al. (1985). Disseminated *Sporothrix schenckii* infection with arthritis in a patient with acquired immunodeficiency syndrome. *J. Rheumatol. 12*:805-808.
41. Bibler, M. R., Luber, H. J., Glueck, H. I., and Estes, S. A. (1986). Disseminated sporotrhicosis in a patient with HIV infection after treatment for acquired factor VIII inhibitor. *JAMA 256*:3125-3126.
42. Kaplan, W. and Kraft, D. E. (1969). Demonstration of pathogenic fungi in formalin fixed tissues by immunofluorescence. *Am. J. Clin. Pathol. 52*:420-432.
43. Roberts, G. D. and Larsh, H. W. (1971). Serologic diagnosis of extracutaneous sporotrichosis. *Am. J. Clin. Pathol. 56*:597-600.
44. Karlin, J. V. and Nielsen, H. S. (1970). Serologic aspects of sporotrichosis. *J. Infect. Dis. 121*:316-327.
45. parker, J. D., Sarosi, G. H., and Tosh, F. E. (1970). Treatment of extraceutaneous sporotrichosis. *Arch. Intern. Med. 125*:858-863.
46. Dismuikes, W. E., Stamm, A. M., Graybill, J. R. et al. (1983). Treatment of systemic mycoses with ketoconazole: Emphasis on toxicity and clinical response in 52 patients. *Ann. Intern. Med. 98*:13-20.

47. Klein, B. S., Vergeront, J. M., Weeks, R. J. et al. (1986). Isolation of *Blastomyces dermatitidis* in soil associated with a large outbreak of blastomycosis in Wisconsin. *N. Engl. J. Med. 314*:529-534.
48. Dismukes, W. E. (1986). Blastomycosis: Leave it to beaver. *N. Engl. J. Med. 314*:575-576.
49. Fulcolow, M. L., Balows, A., Menges, R. W. et al. (1986). Blastomycosis: An important medical problem in central United States. *JAMA 198*:529-532.
50. Chandler, F. W., Kaplan, W., and Ajello, L. (1986). *Histopathology of Mycotic Diseases.* Chicago, Year Book Medical Publishers, pp. 39-41.
51. Recht, L. D., Davies, S. F., Eckman, M. R., and Sarosi, G. A. (1982). Blastomycosis in immunosuppressed patients. *Am. Rev. Respir. Dis. 125*:359-362.
52. Stelling, C. B., Woodring, J. H., Rehm, S. R. et al. (1984). Miliary pulmonary blastomycosis. *Radiology 150*:7-13.
53. Kirkpatrick, C. H. (1984). Host factors against fungal infections. *Am. J. Med. 77*:1-12.
54. Maksymiuk, A. W., Thongprasert, S., Hopfer, R. et al. (1984). Systemic candidiasis in cancer patients. *Am. J. Med. 77*:20-27.
55. McGowan, J. E. (1985). Changing etiology of nosocomial, bacteremia and fungemia and other hospital-acquired infections. *Rev. Infect. Dis. 7*:5357-5370.
56. Rubinstein, E., Noviega, E. R., Simberkoff, M. S. et al. (1975). Fungal endocarditis: Analysis of 24 cases and review of the literature. *Medicine 54*:331-334.
57. Colligan, P. J. and Sorrell, T. C. (1983). Disseminated candidiasis: Evidence of a distinctive syndrome in heroin abusers. *Br. Med. J. 287*:861-862.

Part VI
Protozoal Infections

17
Pneumocystis carinii Pneumonia

Constance B. Wofsy *University of California and San Francisco General Hospital , San Francisco, California*

Pneumocystis carinii has been a relatively infrequent cause of pneumonia in non-AIDS immunocompromised patients, and treatment with either of the two available therapies, trimethoprim-sulfamethoxazole (TMP-SMX) or pentamidine isethionate cured most patients with acceptable levels of toxicity. In the setting of the acquired immunodeficiency syndrome (AIDS), *P. carinii* pneumonia (PCP) has become a routinely encountered infection. *Pneumocystis carinii* pneumonia constitutes the index acquired immunodeficiency syndrome (AIDS) diagnosis in approximately 60% of patients and occurs at some time during the course of the illness in 80% to 85% of all AIDS patients. This infection is almost exclusively restricted to the lungs in contrast with the other AIDS-defining opportunistic infections that tend to be widely disseminated. The frequency of PCP in AIDS has generated considerable research into in vitro cultivation techniques, new therapeutic regimens, adult prophylaxis, and mechanisms of transmission. A number of excellent reviews have been published (1-5).

EPIDEMIOLOGY

Pneumocystis carinii is found widely in the animal kingdom. The organisms found in the lungs of rat and man are morphologically identical by electron microscopy; however, serologic studies using monoclonal antibodies have shown that they are antigenically distinct (6,7). This raises very real questions about the primary source of infections in humans. Most children demonstrate antibodies to *P. carinii* by the age of 4 years (8,9), presumably from environmental exposure, although evidence of naturally occurring pneumocystis pulmonary disease in wild rodents and other animals is lacking. Despite serologic evidence of widespread exposure to *P. carinii*, disease in normal hosts is exceedingly rare. Pneumonia is widely thought to result from activation of latent infection following development of immunocompromise. Aerosol transmission in rats was demonstrated by the development of PCP in germ-free, immunosuppressed rats that were exposed to air from a laboratory that housed actively infected rats (10). Human-to-human transmission of *P. carinii* has never been documented; however, several reports have suggested this may occur. Several clusters of pneumocystis infection exceeding the expected frequency in a specific immunocompromised population have been reported from several pediatric leukemia wards (11,12). Immunocompromised human immunodeficiency virus (HIV)-infected individuals frequently mingle with coughing, *P. carinii*-infected patients socially, in clinic waiting rooms and during hospital visits. Fortunately, there are no reports of suspected aerosol transmission in AIDS. However, because of the remote possibility of aerosol transmission, patients with PCP should not share a hospital room with immunocompromised patients without PCP.

Extrapulmonary pneumocystis infection is exceedingly rare. However, several well-documented cases of AIDS patients with *P. carinii* in the ear, sinus, mastoid, and skin suggest that dissemination beyond the lung may be seen with increased frequency in this population (13,14).

DIAGNOSIS

Symptoms

Pneumocystis carinii pneumonia has many features of other atypical pneumonias. Patients almost always have a dry, paroxysmal nonproductive cough with associated dyspnea; a striking decrease in usual exercise tolerance, and fever are present in over 80% of all patients. Chest pain, although infrequent, may occasionally be the only major clinical symptom. A productive cough is unusual but does not exclude the diagnosis. AIDS patients with PCP often have gradually increasing symptoms, which begin weeks to months before diagnosis (median 25 days) in contrast with the more abrupt presentation of PCP characteristic of other immunocompromised populations (15). However, even in AIDS patients, the onset of PCP may also be very abrupt and the course fulminant. Suspicion of PCP is easily aroused in a high-risk population (e.g., homosexual men or IV drug users); however, as AIDS becomes more widespread, suspicion must be heightened in traditionally non-high-risk group patients (e.g., heterosexual men and women) in whom symptoms may mimic other pulmonary interstitial processes such as mycoplasma pneumonia.

Initial Evaluation of Pulmonary Symptoms in a Patient Suspected of *Pneumocystis carinii* Pneumonia

The clinician should first determine the presence of pulmonary disease using chest radiographs, pulmonary function testing, gallium scans, and serum lactate dehydrogenase (LDH) levels, or some combination thereof. Figure 1 is an algorithm of this evaluation. If the clinical and laboratory picture are consistent with PCP, histologic examination for the organism should follow.

The initial diagnostic study should be a chest x-ray. It is abnormal in more than 90% of documented PCPs, typically revealing bilateral interstitial infiltrates (Fig. 2). Occasionally, the infiltrates may be unilateral, lobar, nodular, or may mimic other diseases. Miliary or apical infiltrates suggesting tuberculosis (5,16), cavitary lesions, pneumatoceles, and nodules have all been described (17). Pleural effusions are extremely rare and, if present, should suggest other disorders such as Kaposi's sarcoma or fungal infection. Hilar adenopathy is not seen in PCP. Spontaneous pneumothorax has been noted in patients with PCP and no preexistent pulmonary disorder (5). If the chest x-ray is normal, pulmonary function studies and a gallium citrate lung scan may provide evidence of infection (see section on identification of etiology).

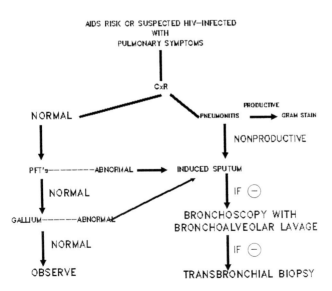

FIGURE 1   Evaluation of pulmonary symptoms when *P. carinii* is considered.

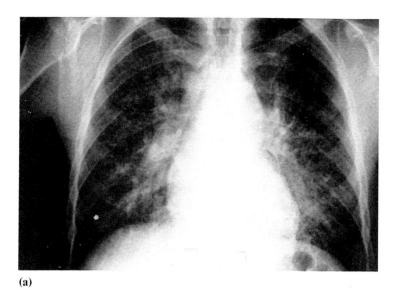

(a)

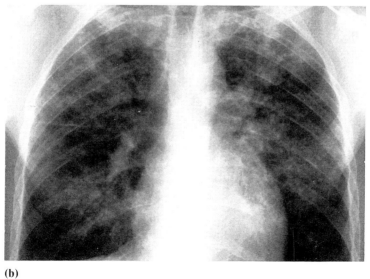

(b)

FIGURE 2 (a) Typical bilateral interstitial infiltrate; (b) upperlobe and apical infiltrates mimicking tuberculosis; (c_1) interstitial changes with pneumatocele; (c_2) spontaneous pneumothorax 5 days into therapy; (d) upper-lobe mass presentation of *P. carinii*.

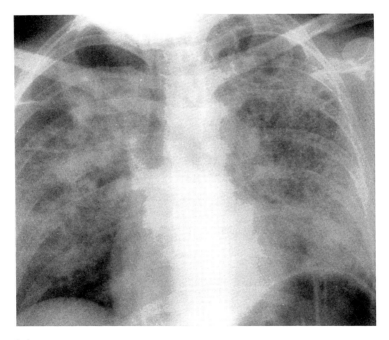

(c₁)

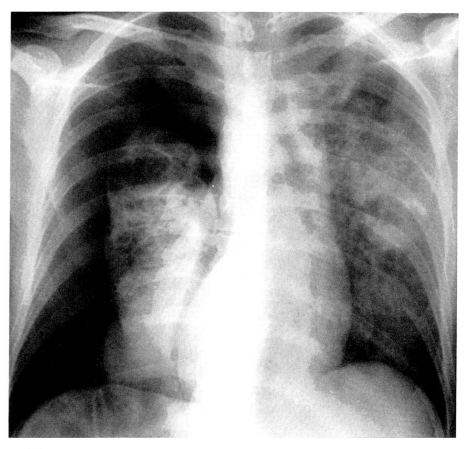

(c₂)
FIGURE 2 (Continued)

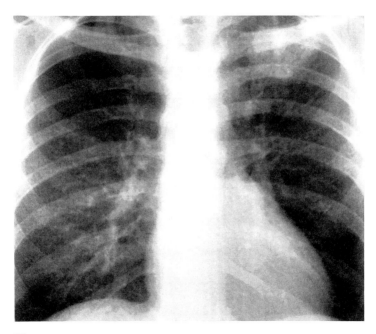

(d)

Identifying the Presence of Pulmonary Disease: Evaluation of the Patient with Suspicious Symptoms but with Normal Chest X-Ray Findings

When the chest x-ray is normal or the radiographic findings are ambiguous, several adjunctive diagnostic steps may be utilized to define the need for definitive diagnosis (see Fig. 1). Pulmonary function tests (PFTs) typically reveal a triad of decreased diffusing capacity of carbon monoxide ($D_L CO$), normal pulmonary flow rates, and reduced vital capacity. Such studies can usually be obtained within 24 hr. Next, if PFTs are normal or ambiguous, a gallium scan is obtained at our institution. Because it requires 48 to 72 hr from gallium injection to imaging, this study delays the diagnosis and the isotope requirement adds considerable cost to the workup. It thus should be reserved for patients in whom *P. carinii* pneumonia is suspected but the chest x-ray and PFTs do not suggest PCP. Gallium citrate scanning has a sensitivity of more than 90%, but a specificity of only 40% in the diagnosis of PCP (5). Other pulmonary inflammatory disorders such as *Mycobacterium avium-intracellulare* (MAI) infection will result in gallium uptake but usually with less intensity and often focal. If the chest x-ray, $D_L CO$ and gallium scan are negative, however, the diagnosis of PCP can be virtually excluded. If these studies reveal either an abnormal diffusing capacity or pulmonary uptake of gallium, histologic examination of induced sputum or bronchoscopy is in order. The exercise-facilitated A-a gradient is another adjunctive study used routinely in some medical centers; however, this requires the additional services of the pulmonary function and blood gas laboratories. The erythrocyte sedimentation rate (ESR) and serum LDH values are usually elevated in *P. carinii* pneumonia (18). Thus, if both of these are normal, the likelihood of diagnosis of PCP is remote.

Some patients fall into a gray zone in which the clinical symptoms suggest bronchitis but are also consistent with PCP (e.g., a productive cough, an ambiguous x-ray, and dyspnea). Our practice is to observe such patients closely, to counsel them regarding symptoms that should bring them to immediate medical attention, and to give a short course of a broad-spectrum antibiotic appropriate for pneumococcal or *Haemophilus influenzae* disease [e.g., amoxacillin + clavulinic acid (Augmentin 500 t.i.d.)] with revaluation at 7 to 14 days.

Identifying the Etiology of Pulmonary Disease: Induced Sputum and Bronchoscopy

If results of the chest x-ray suggests *P. carinii* pneumonia and the patient is known or suspected to be infected with HIV, proceeding directly to a specific diagnostic procedure is the most efficacious and cost-effective approach.

Multiple studies have confirmed that bronchoalveolar lavage (BAL) is virtually equal to transbronchial biopsy in diagnosing PCP (5), as well as the other opportunistic infections that may coexist with or mimic PCP. The BAL avoids the potential of bleeding in patients who have thrombocytopenia or other bleeding diatheses and avoids the risk of biopsy-induced pneumothorax.

More recently, the induced sputum method, which is noninvasive and easy to conduct, has proved to be highly sensitive (19). The only complication is cough and exacerbation of bronchospasm. After gargling and toothbrushing with physiologic saline, the patient inhales 3% to 5% nebulized saline. This procedure induces deep coughing, productive of bronchoalveolar fluid diluted with saline that must be concentrated before staining for *P. carinii* with a modified Giemsa stain or toluidine blue. Because the trophozoites (the predominant form of *P. carinii* in pneumonia) may look like artifact or cellular debris, laboratory personnel must be specially trained to make the diagnosis from induced sputum. The more easily identified cyst form with eight internally staining sporozoites is more readily detected in bronchoalveolar lavage fluid. Because sputum induction is only 80% sensitive, even in the most experienced laboratories, the decision to do an induced sputum must be coupled with a commitment to proceed to bronchoscopy if the sputum induction is negative. Bronchoscopy will reveal *P. carinii* in half of these cases. Twenty percent of patients with a chest x-ray film suggestive of PCP have induced sputum and bronchoscopy results that are both negative for *P. carinii*. In these patients, no specific treatable causes have emerged. Some of these patients may have lipoid interstitial pneumonia (LIP) or the nonspecific interstitial pneumonitis that has recently been described in AIDS patients (20).

Sputum or BAL specimens should also be cultured for viruses, bacteria, fungi, and legionallae (19); transbronchial biopsy tissue should be examined histologically with special stains for *P. carinii*, fungi, and acid-fast organisms. Open-lung biopsy is not necessary in all but the most unusual circumstances because an otherwise undetected, treatable diagnosis is virtually never encountered (5,21,22). Although open-lung biopsy provides a better means of diagnosis of Kaposi's sarcoma, pulmonary Kaposi's sarcoma can usually be deduced from external evidence, the chest x-ray pattern or occasionally direct visualization during bronchoscopy. If the BAL specimen does not reveal *P. carinii* organisms, repeat bronchoscopy with transbronchial biopsy (TBBx) may identify an additional small percentage of patients with *P. carinii* or another process such as LIP. A negative TBBx virtually rules out the possibility of *P. carinii* pneumonia. A repeat bronchoscopy with transbronchial biopsy within the first month of an initially negative TBBx is rarely diagnostic of another infectious process (23).

Empiric Diagnosis

Current tests for *P. carinii* antigen or antibody are not sufficiently sensitive or specific for noninvasive diagnosis and, at this time, play no role in evaluation of patients with suspected PCP. The toxicity of existing therapies, possible alternate or simultaneous infections, and ambiguity of diagnosis makes empiric therapy unwise unless the patient is very sick, and a definitive diagnostic procedure must be delayed, or the patient refuses diagnostic procedures. Until recently, tissue confirmation of *P. carinii* was required to establish an AIDS diagnosis definitively for reporting to the public health authorities and to gain access to azidothymidine (AZT). In the revised definition of AIDS, published in August 1987 (24), the presumptive diagnosis of PCP is accepted but strongly discouraged. A definitive diagnosis should always be established if PCP constitutes the index diagnosis of AIDS.

TREATMENT

AIDS Patients Contrasted with Other Immunocompromised Patients

Trimethoprim-sulfamethoxazole or pentamidine isethionate have been the established therapies for PCP in all immunocompromised patients, including those with AIDS. Equivalent effectiveness has been demonstrated in animal model studies and prospective and retrospective studies in adults and children with non-AIDS-related immunosuppression. Trimethoprim-sulfamethoxazole has been the preferred therapy because of its established efficacy, infrequent serious or permanent toxicity, oral absorption, and ready availability. Pentamidine must be given parenterally, induces major side effects in approximately 50% of treated patients, and may induce permanent diabetes mellitus or fatal hypoglycemia. One major adverse effect of pentamidine, painful, sterile abscesses at the intramuscular injection sites, has been eliminated now by routine intravenous administration. Pentamidine was thus reserved for trimethoprim-sulfamethoxazole failures or for patients with sulfonamide allergy. However, in contrast with other immunocompromised populations, several retrospective therapeutic studies have shown that more than 50% of AIDS patients with PCP develop major adverse reactions to trimethoprim-sulfamethoxazole, sufficient to require a switch to pentamidine (2,25-27).

Parenteral Therapy: Trimethoprim-Sulfamethoxazole and Pentamidine Isethionate

Clinical Studies

A prospective study conducted at San Francisco General Hospital compared the efficacy and toxicity of trimethoprim-sulfamethoxazole (TMP-SMX)

TABLE 1 Treatment Trials for First-Episode *P. carinii* in AIDS, San Francisco General Hospital

Trial therapy	Route	N	Efficacy (%)	Major toxicity requiring change (%)	Ref.
TMP-SMX[a]	IV	20	75	50	26
Pentamidine[a]	IV	20	95	55	
DAP-TMP	p.o.	15	100	13	34
DAP alone	p.o.	18	59	0	35
TMP-SMX[b]	p.o.	30	93	57[c]	27
DAP-TMP[b]	p.o.	30	90	30[c]	
Pentamidine	aerosol	15	86	0	44

[a]Randomized comparative trial.
[b]Randomized double-blind comparative trial.
[c]$p < 0.05$ between groups.
Abbreviations: DAP-TMP, dapsone plus trimethoprim; TMP-SMX, trimethoprim-sulfamethoxazole; IV, intravenous; p.o., oral.

with pentamidine (Table 1; 26). AIDS patients with first-episode PCP were randomly assigned to receive either trimethoprim-sulfamethoxazole (20/100 mg/kg per day) or pentamidine isethionate (4 mg/kg per day) intravenously for 3 weeks. Toxicity severe enough to require discontinuation of the drugs was found in 50% of the trimethoprim-sulfamethoxazole group and 55% of the pentamidine group. The two drugs were equally effective in the 40 patients evaluated, although a nonstatistically significant trend toward improved survival was seen with pentamidine. Major adverse reactions occurred after a mean of 11 days of therapy, with a range of 6 to 16 days. This finding of major toxicity occurring predominantly in the second week of therapy has been corroborated in other trials (26,27). Overall mortality was 15%, comparable with mortality observed in a number of series of AIDS and non-AIDS populations (5,15). The clinical, radiographic, and pulmonary function responses were comparable for the two treatment groups, but strikingly, two-thirds of patients in either group had persistence of *P. carinii* in their follow-up bronchoscopy specimens, a finding noted in other AIDS series and in striking contrast to the rapid eradication of *P. carinii* cysts in other populations after the onset of therapy. The persistence of *P. carinii* does not appear to alter survival.

Toxic Effects

The adverse reactions found in this prospective study (26) and other retrospective studies are outlined in Table 2. The toxicity criteria used to define

TABLE 2 Guidelines for PCP Drug Therapy

	Trimethoprim-sulfamethoxazole (TMP-SMX)	Pentamidine	Dapsone (Dap)-trimethoprim (TMP)
Dosage studied	TMP 20 mg/kg/d SMX 100 mg/kg/d	4 mg/kg/d	Dap 100 mg/d TMP 20 mg/kg/d[c]
Schedule	Four divided daily doses	Once daily	Dap one daily TMP four daily doses
Route	Oral or IV	IV	Oral
Common toxicity[a]	Nausea, vomiting, hyponatremia, neutropenia, LFTs abnormal, elevated creatinine, generalized rash, and fever	Same as TMP-SMX (no rash and fever)	Same as TMP-SMX (neutropenia rare)
Monitor[b]	CBC, platelets, LFTs, creatinine	Same as TMP-SMX and blood glucose	Same as TMP-SMX and G6PD pretherapy Hct, methemoglobin
Unique toxicity		Hypoglycemia, hypotension	Hemolytic anemia, methemoglobinemia

[a]Frequency 50% with TMP-SMX or pentamidine, 30% with Dap-TMP.
[b]Indications to discontinue or switch treatment include: PMN < 750; platelets < 40 K; LFTs > 5× normal level; creatinine > 3.0.
[c]TMP at 10 or 15 mg/kg/d may be adequate but has not been studied.
Source: AIDS File: June 1987, Vol 2, No. 2, reproduced with permission.

when therapy should be discontinued are given in parentheses. Toxicities common to both trimethoprim-sulfamethoxazole and pentamidine were neutropenia, (PMNs < 750/mm^3), thrombocytopenia (platelets < 40,000/mm^3), azotemia (creatinine > 3 mg/dl), hepatitis (LFTs over five times normal), and nausea and vomiting (unable to hold food down despite maximal antiemetic therapy for 24 hr). A generalized erythematous rash was the most common toxicity encountered with trimethoprim-sulfamethoxazole, but it was very rarely seen with pentamidine. Severe skin rashes often accompanied by fevers up to 104 °F (25,26) have been found in 8% to 50% of patients treated with trimethoprim-sulfamethoxazole. Subsequent investigations have shown that in many patients, the rash and fever will resolve within 48 to 72 hr if they are maintained on trimethoprim-sulfamethoxazole with or without antihistamines or a change in dosage (27,28). Thus, the drug should be discontinued only if the rash involves mucous membranes, is intolerable to the patient, is associated with severe hematologic or other organ system disease, or it fails to improve within 72 hr.

Neutropenia is frequently encountered with both trimethoprim-sulfamethoxazole and parenteral pentamidine. Fortunately, this complication fails to recur when the patient is switched to the alternate therapy, suggesting different mechanisms of toxicity. Antineutrophil antibodies have been demonstrated in AIDS patients in conjunction with adequate myeloid precursors in bone marrow studies (29). There is no concrete evidence that administration of folinic acid will decrease the incidence of neutropenia. The neutropenia appears to be relatively unique to AIDS, as it was not reported in non-AIDS patients with PCP treated with trimethoprim-sulfamethoxazole (30) or in 74 non-AIDS patients who received 12 or more days of pentamidine therapy (31). Chemical hepatitis is somewhat more frequent with trimethoprim-sulfamethoxazole than with pentamidine, and the etiology is not known. An elevated serum creatinine value while the patient is receiving pentamidine therapy is common; however, it seldom exceeds 3 mg/dl. There are no established guidelines for administration of pentamidine in renal failure, although the pharmacokinetic parameters of the drug are not altered by azotemia (32).

Hypoglycemia is well described with pentamidine, and a few patients may progress to insulin-dependent diabetes (29). Hypoglycemia usually occurs well into the course of therapy; it is not associated with the time of injection; it may be sudden in onset with rapid progression to coma or death; and it may occur after all therapy has been completed. Symptomatic patients should be treated with 10% dextrose in water and pentamidine should be discontinued.

Other side effects not usually requiring discontinuation of either trimethoprim-sulfamethoxazole or pentamidine therapy but commonly encountered are hyponatremia, which may be due to the large volume of free water administered with trimethoprim-sulfamethoxazole or to serum inappropriate ADH secretion associated with pulmonary disease itself; nausea and vomiting, which may occur with either oral or intravenous trimethoprim-sulfamethoxazole but can usually be controlled by antiemetics; and hypotension, which may develop late in the course of pentamidine therapy and is unresponsive to fluid intervention. The etiology is unclear and patients must be very well instructed about taking orthostatic precautions. Torsade de pointes is a rare, but potentially fatal arrhythmia seen with parenteral pentamidine therapy. Routine laboratory monitoring studies should include complete blood count with platelet counts; electrolyte concentrations, liver function tests, creatinine, and fasting blood sugar levels; and blood pressure monitoring, with observation for fever or skin rash. The patient should be monitored two to five times per week, and this monitoring should be particularly aggressive during the second week of therapy when the major toxic effects are most frequently encountered (1,26).

Oral Therapies: Trimethoprim Plus Dapsone and Trimethoprim-Sulfamethoxazole

Clinical Trials

To limit toxicity and to decrease time in the hospital, additional therapies, especially those that can be given by mouth, are needed (see Table 1). Trimethoprim plus dapsone, a sulfone currently licensed for the treatment of leprosy, was effective therapy in a well-established rat model of PCP (33). In an open study of 15 patients with mild to moderate first-episode PCP (expected to survive for at least 1 week even if untreated) oral therapy with dapsone 100 mg/day plus trimethoprim 20 mg/kg per day (divided into four doses) was clinically effective in all patients, and only 2 of the 15 patients developed rash requiring discontinuation of the study medication (34).

Because of the attractiveness of a once-a-day therapy, dapsone alone (100 mg by mouth once a day) was then used to treat an additional 18 patients with mild to moderate first-episode PCP (35). No severe adverse reactions requiring cessation of dapsone therapy were encountered. However, 7 of the 18 patients failed to improve, and response was slower than customary in several others. Additionally, several successfully treated patients relapsed within 3 months after discontinuation of therapy, in striking contrast with no relapses within 3 months with other therapeutic modalities (36). Dapsone alone at a dosage of 100 mg/day was thus considered suboptimal treatment.

To define the most effective and least toxic oral therapy, a randomized prospective double-blind trial of dapsone, 100 mg once a day plus trimethoprim (20 mg/kg per day divided into four doses), versus trimethoprim-sulfamethoxazole (20 and 100 mg/kg per day, respectively, divided into four doses) given orally for 21 days to first-episode PCP patients with $pO_2 > 60$ mmHg was conducted (27). Thirty patients were in each group. The two therapies were equally effective with clinical failure in three trimethoprim-sulfamethoxazole and two dapsone plus trimethoprim-treated patients. Dapsone plus trimethoprim induced significantly less neutropenia and hepatitis than did trimethoprim-sulfamethoxazole alone. The major toxic effects occurred in the second week of therapy, as had been shown in previous studies of parenteral pentamidine and trimethoprim-sulfamethoxazole (26). The toxic effects unique to dapsone plus trimethoprim were hemolytic anemia and methemoglobinemia. Severe methemoglobinemia of greater than 20% occurred in 1 of the 30 patients treated with dapsone plus trimethoprim. Because dapsone can induce severe hemolysis in persons with glucose-6-phosphate dehydrogenase (G6PD) deficiency, a G6PD screen must be done before initiation of therapy. One G6PD-deficient patient, who was not part of this study, was inadvertently started on a dapsone regimen before being screened for G6PD and had massive hemolysis, after several days of therapy, that required repeated blood transfusion and prolonged hospitalization (C.B. Wofsy, unpublished data). A lower dose of trimethoprim-sulfamethoxazole may be equally effective. In a double-blind study comparing trimethoprim-sulfamethoxazole (15-20 mg/kg per day of the trimethoprim component) with pentamidine (4 mg/kg), survival was 86% in the trimethoprim-sulfamethoxazole group, even when dosage adjustments were made to keep trimethoprim levels at 5 to 7 mg/ml (28).

Laboratory Monitoring

Routine studies are the same as those for trimethoprim-sulfamethoxazole or pentamidine, as discussed earlier (see Table 2). In addition, a G6PD screen must be obtained before initiating dapsone plus trimethoprim treatment, and hematocrit and methemoglobin levels must be monitored during therapy, in addition to white blood cell counts, platelet counts, electrolyte levels, liver function tests, serum creatinine, and fasting blood sugar levels.

Other Therapies: Trimetrexate, Difluoromethylornithine, Primaquine plus Clindamycin

Alternate therapies under investigation include potent dihydrofolate reductase (DHFR) inhibitors, such as trimetrexate and piritrexim, that are much more active in vitro against *P. carinii* than trimethoprim and permit single-drug therapy or provide improved efficacy over trimethoprim when combined with a sulfonamide or a sulfone. Trimetrexate, now available only for intravenous administration, was used effectively alone or in combination with a sulfonamide drug in a small group of patients with PCP studied at the NIH (37). However, these therapies have not been compared with standard therapies; they require massive amounts of concomitant and costly leucovorin; and the drug remains investigational at this time. In addition, early reports showed that trimetrexate-treated patients had a relapse rate of 35% at a mean of 38 days after completion of therapy (range 21 to 66 days) (F. Sattler and H. Masur, personal communication). Further clinical trials evaluating trimetrexate and another oral DHFR inhibitor, piritrexim, are in progress. Difluoromethylornithine (DFMO; eflornithine), a polyamine synthesis inhibitor used for trypanosomiasis, has been used in AIDS patients with PCP with evidence of clinical benefit (38,39). However, many of the patients studied had been clinical failures with other therapies, and DFMO's true efficacy is hard to evaluate. Major toxic effects are frequent, and relapse after cessation of therapy is the rule. Thus, it remains investigational.

Primaquine combined with clindamycin exhibits efficacy in treatment and prophylaxis of *P. carinii* in the rat model and will soon be evaluated in clinical trials (40).

Aerosol Pentamidine

Preliminary evidence of effectiveness of aerosol pentamidine for treatment of *P. carinii* pneumonia prophylaxis comes from rat model studies and several clinical trials (41-44). In an open study at San Francisco General Hospital, 15 patients with first-episode PCP were given daily aerosol pentamidine as short-term therapy (600 mg in a Marquest Respirgard II nebulizer given for a half hour daily; estimated inhaled dose 300 mg for 21 days) (42). Thirteen of the 15 patients responded clinically within about the same time as patients in similar open trials of other effective therapies. The major adverse reactions were cough and mild bronchospasm. Aerosol pentamidine thus offers considerable advantage over parenteral pentamidine because patients are spared the 50% frequency of serious side effects seen with parenterally administered pentamidine, which preferentially accumulates in liver, spleen, and adrenals. The optimal dose, frequency of administration, and optimal aerosol delivery device for aerosol pentamidine have not been established. Commercially available nebulizers that meet the optimal particle size of 1 to 4 μm are being evaluated for safe and successful therapy. A multicenter, prospective double-blind treatment trial comparing aerosol pentamidine with trimethoprim-sulfamethoxazole for patients with first-episode of PCP is underway.

APPROACH TO THERAPY

Mild to Moderate Disease

For the patient with mild symptoms, a $pO_2 > 60$ mmHg, a moderately abnormal A-a O_2 gradient (< 30 mg/mmHg), and ability to tolerate oral medications, the options include dapsone, 100 mg once daily plus trimethoprim 10 to 15 mg/kg per day divided into four doses (three 100-mg tablets given q.i.d. for a 70-kg person); or oral trimethoprim-sulfamethoxazole, 15 to 20 mg/kg per day of trimethoprim given in four divided doses (three single-strength or two double-strength tablets four times a day for a 70-kg person); or if available, aerosol pentamidine, 600 mg/day, the only dose studied to date using a nebulizer system capable of delivering a particle size of 1 to 4 μm (42). Trimethoprim-sulfamethoxazole is the only oral therapy currently licensed for treatment of PCP. A new drug application has been submitted for dapsone plus trimethoprim.

Careful laboratory and clinical monitoring are required, particularly during the second week of therapy when most of major adverse reactions occur. Patients with first-episode PCP need time to adjust to the diagnosis and may do best if hospitalized during the first 5 to 7 days to be sure there are no other associated pulmonary infections, to evaluate other AIDS-related problems, and to adjust to their new diagnostic situation. Patients who have a well-established outpatient support system, or who have a second episode of PCP and are otherwise clinically able, can be treated as outpatients from the onset of their disease, with careful monitoring. Because of the severe hypoglycemia, hypotension, and occasional cardiac arrhythmias with pentamidine, outpatient intravenous pentamidine should be avoided. Azidothymidine can be continued during PCP treatment but should be withheld if neutropenia develops (neutrophils < 1000 mm^3).

Moderate to Severe Disease

Patients who are clinically sick, have a pO$_2$ value of less than 60 mmHg, an LDH level > 350 IU (18), a respiratory rate $> 35/$min, or who are unable to maintain themselves at home, should be considered for admission to the hospital. Most clinicians initiate therapy with trimethoprim-sulfamethoxazole or, for those who are allergic to that drug, pentamidine isethionate, 3-4 mg/kg per day given intravenously slowly over 2 hr. Parenteral therapy should be continued until symptoms are under control. The remainder of the therapy can then be given orally using either trimethoprim-sulfamethoxazole or dapsone plus trimethoprim. If a serious adverse reaction develops or the patient's clinical condition markedly deteriorates over 4 to 5 days or fails to improve after 7 to 10 days, a switch should be made to the alternate regimen. We do not give trimethoprim-sulfamethoxazole and pentamidine simultaneously because of the high frequency of toxicity and because of failure to demonstrate added efficacy in the animal model. For those patients whose therapy fails, despite a switch, several reports have suggested that a short course of high-dose steroids (45,46) has been useful as an adjunctive therapy. However, this treatment is unproved. A controlled double-blind trial of steroids versus placebo is underway for patients with PCP and a pO$_2$ value of < 50 mm Hg. The expected survival until hospital discharge after a first episode of PCP is 75% to 95%; mean survival after a first episode of PCP has increased from 10 months to 14 months over the last 2 years.

Use of the Intensive Care Unit

All patients should be given the opportunity to review life-support decisions early in the course of infection. It can be presented as a "routine" part of the discussion about PCP therapy. Those who are in the first 4 to 5 days of therapy may benefit from intensive care to allow time to respond to therapy. Those who have not responded in 7 to 10 days are not likely to respond, even with respiratory support and intensive care (47), and this should be taken into account when reviewing life-support decisions with these patients. Patients are often relieved to designate a durable power of attorney to make decisions if they become to ill. Because azidothymidine does not alter the treatment outcome for PCP, recommendations for intensive care are not altered by the availability of this drug.

Duration of Therapy, Cross Toxicity

The optimal duration of therapy for PCP cannot be determined from current studies. Most clinical trials have used 3 weeks as the duration of therapy (26,27,34), yet two-thirds of successfully treated patients still have *P. carinii* organisms seen on posttreatment bronchoscopy (26). Therefore, most clinicians treat for 3 weeks and always for a minimum of 2 weeks. Some centers have used 2 weeks of therapy and describe an outcome similar to that of centers using 3 weeks, but no comparative studies have been done. There is little evidence that treatment beyond 3 weeks improves response or alters the outcome.

Treatment of a second or third peisode of PCP requires consideration of allergic reactions encountered during the previous course of therapy. Fortunately, toxic effects encountered with one course of pentamidine therapy may not recur; hence, treatment with pentamidine for a second bout of PCP is warranted, even if there were serious adverse reactions during initial therapy. A recent study compared cross toxicity between various sulfonamides and sulfones and found that patients treated with either trimethoprim-sulfamethoxazole or dapsone plus trimethoprim for a first episode had a zero to 33% likelihood of having a major adverse reaction to the alternate therapy given at least 3 months after for a subsequent episode of PCP (48). However, the adverse reactions to the second course of therapy invariably occurred more than 7 days after institution of therapy, suggesting a de novo toxicity, rather than exacerbation of the previous hypersensitivity. Thus, patients treated with one drug for one episode may be carefully rechallenged with another drug during a second episode if monitored closely. Severe hypotension and pulmonary infiltrates have been described in several trimethoprim-sulfamethoxazole allergic patients upon immediate rechallenge (49).

PREVENTION

Relapse of PCP is very common in patients with AIDS. When 74 patients with first-episode PCP were evaluated, relapse rates were 18% at 6 months,

TABLE 3 Pneumocystis Prophylaxis Options

Treatment	Route	Dosage	Limitation	Ref.
Dapsone	Oral	100 mg/d	Anemia, MetHb	56
TMP-SMX	Oral	1 DS b.i.d.	Frequent rash	51,52
Pentamidine	IV	4 mg/kg q 4 wk	Office time for administration	53
Pentamidine	Aerosol	30-300 mg q 2-4 wk	Dose, interval investigational	44
Fansidar	Oral	Once weekly	Rash, Stevens-Johnson	54

Abbreviations: TMP-SMX, trimethoprim-sulfamethoxazole; MetHb, methemoglobin; DS, double strength.

46% at 9 months, and 65% at 18 months when no suppressive therapy was given (36). Prophylaxis (Table 3) may be primary (before an episode of infection has occurred) or secondary (after completion of therapy for an acute episode of infection). There is considerable variability in the use of primary prophylaxis for PCP; however, there is agreement that secondary prophylaxis should be instituted in most patients.

Trimethoprim-Sulfamethoxazole

In non-AIDS immunocompromised populations, particularly in leukemic children, prophylactic treatment with trimethoprim-sulfamethoxazole, initially one double-strength tablet daily and, more recently, one double-strength tablet three times a week (50), has prevented virtually all cases of PCP with virtually no side effects. The success of trimethoprim-sulfamethoxazole as prophylaxis in AIDS populations is confirmed by a study by Fischl et al. (51), in which 60 patients with Kaposi's sarcoma were given either trimethoprim-sulfamethoxazole or no therapy and followed for 18 months. Sixteen of 30 untreated patients developed PCP compared with none of the treated group. Adverse reactions while on prophylaxis required discontinuation of therapy in five (17%) of the patients taking trimethoprim-sulfamethoxazole. Four of these developed severe erythroderma. However, more frequent and severe intolerance to low-dose trimethoprim-sulfamethoxazole was encountered in a double-blind, randomized study of trimethoprim-sulfamethoxazole versus placebo in patients with Kaposi's sarcoma (52). Eighty-six percent of the treated group developed severe reactions, including rash or fever at a median of 11.5 days after starting treatment.

Thus, the high frequency of adverse reaction to trimethoprim-sulfamethoxazole is not dose-related and, thereby, limits the usefulness of this therapy for primary prophylaxis. It is appropriate for secondary PCP prophylaxis for the 40% of patients who are able to complete a full course of initial therapy with trimethoprim-sulfamethoxazole.

Pentamidine, Fansidar, Dapsone, and Aerosol Pentamidine

Pentamidine (4 mg/kg IV or IM) given once a month is an alternative that is well tolerated and appears to be reasonably effective. Only 2 of 10 patients maintained for 6 months had a recurrence of PCP compared with seven patients with no prophylactic therapy (53). In 60 patients given weekly Fansidar (pyrimethamine-sulfadoxine) after an initial episode of PCP and followed for 11 months, only five developed PCP, three of whom had no detectable level of sulfonamide. Six of 50 developed a significant rash, but none were life-threatening (54). However, severe life-threatening hypersensitivity reactions to Fansidar (e.g., Steven-Johnson syndrome) have been described in other AIDS patients and, hence, limit the usefulness of this therapy as a routine prophylactic regimen (55). A large AIDS Treatment and Evaluation Unit study comparing trimethoprim-sulfamethoxazole, Fansidar, and aerosol pentamidine is now underway.

Dapsone, 25 mg four times a day or 100 mg once a day, was administered to 156 patients with AIDS-related complex or a history of PCP, only one of whom developed a new episode of PCP (56). Fourteen of 19 patients who chose not to receive prophylaxis developed the disease. However, a major complication of therapy was anemia; 25% of the patients required one or more transfusions. The toxicity and the striking inconvenience of taking a four-times-a-day medication limit the usefulness of dapsone at this dosage schedule for standard chemoprophylaxis.

Aerosolized pentamidine has excellent potential as a prophylactic regimen. It offers the advantages of infrequent administration, low toxicity with high efficacy, and excellent patient acceptance. It was initially used in secondary prophylaxis studies in New York where it was administered in a low dosage of 30 mg every 2 weeks; however, the nebulizer system used resulted in suboptimal pulmonary distribution. An ongoing community-based study in San Francisco compared the prophylactic efficacy of 30 mg and 150 mg doses given every 2 weeks with 300 mg every 4 weeks. In February 1989, based on these studies, the FDA approved a treatment Investigational New Drug (IND) to allow use of a pentamidine at 300 mg every 4 weeks, using the Respirguard II nebulizer for prevention of PCP in patients who have already experienced an episode of PCP or who have a T4 cell count less than 200.

REFERENCES

1. Kaplan, L. D., Wofsy, C. B., and Volberding, P. A. (1987). Treatment of patients with acquired immunodeficiency syndrome and associated manifestations. *JAMA* *257*:1367-1374.

2. Wofsy, C. B. (1987). Use of trimethoprim-sulfamethoxazole in the treatment of *Pneumocystis carinii* pneumonitis in patients with acquired immunodeficiency syndrome. *Rev. Infect. Dis. 9*:S184-S194.
3. Mills, J. (1986). *Pneumocystis carinii* and *Toxoplasma gondii* infections in patients with AIDS. *Rev. Infect. Dis. 8*:1001-1011.
4. Leoung, G. S. and Hopewell, P. (1987). Pneumocystis carinii *Pneumonia in San Francisco General Hospital AIDS Knowledge Base* (computerized data base). (Cohen, C., Sande, M., and Volberding, P., eds.). New York, BRS Saunders.
5. Hopewell, P. C. and Luce, J. M. (1986). Pulmonary manifestations of the acquired immunodeficiency syndrome. *Clin. Immunol. Allergy 6*:489-518.
6. Kovacs, J. A., Swan, J. C., Parillo, J. E., and Masur, H. (1986). Monoclonal antibodies against rat and human *Pneumocystis carinii*. *Clin. Res. 34*:523A.
7. Gigliotti, F., Stokes, D. C., Cheatham, A. B., Davis, D. S., and Hughes, W. T. (1986). Development of murine monoclonal antibodies to *Pneumocystis carinii*. *J. Infect. Dis. 154*:315-322.
8. Pifer, L. L., Hughes, W. T., Stango, S., and Woods, D. (1978). *Pneumocystis carinii* infection: Evidence for high prevalence in normal and immunosuppressed children. *Pediatrics 61*:35-41.
9. Meuwissen, J. H. E. T., Tauber, L., Leeuwenberg, A. D. E. M., Beckers, P. J. A., and Sieben, M. (1977). Parasitologic and serologic observations of infection with pneumocystis in humans. *J. Infect. Dis. 136*:43-49.
10. Hughes, W. T., Bartley, D. L., and Smith, B. M. (1983). A natural source of infection due to *Pneumocystis carinii*. *J. Infect. Dis. 147*:595.
11. Singer, C., Armstrong, D., Rosen, P. P., and Schottenfeld, D. (1974). *Pneumocystis carinii* pneumonia: A cluster of eleven cases. *Ann. Intern. Med. 82*:772-777.
12. Brazinsky, J. H. and Phillips, J. E. (1969). Pneumocystis pneumonia transmission between patients with lymphoma [Letter]. *JAMA 209*:1527.
13. Schinella, R. A., Breda, S. D., and Hammerschlag, P. E. (1987). Otic infection due to *Pneumocystis carinii* in an apparently healthy man with antibody to the human immunodeficiency virus. *Ann. Intern. Med. 106*:399-400.
14. Coulman, C. U., Greene, I., and Archibald, R. W. R. (1987). Cutaneous pneumocystis. *Ann. Intern. Med. 106*:396-398.
15. Haverkos, H. W. (1984). Assessment of therapy for *Pneumocystis carinii* pneumonia: PCP Therapy Project Group. *Am. J. Med. 76*:501-508.
16. Barrio, J. L., Suarez, M., Rodriguez, J. L., Saldana, M. J., and Pitchenik, A. E. (1986). *Pneumocystis carinii* pneumonia presenting as cavitating and noncavitating solitary pulmonary nodules in patients with the acquired immunodeficiency syndrome. *Am. Rev. Respir. Dis. 134*:1094-1096.
17. Goodman, P. C., Daily, C., and Minagi, H. (1986). Spontaneous pneumothorax in AIDS patients with *Pneumocystis carinii* pneumonia. *AJR 147*:29-31.
18. Medina, I., Mills, J., and Wofsy, C. (1987). Serum lactate dehydrogenase levels (LDH) in *Pneumocystis carinii* pneumonia in AIDS: Possible indicator and predictor of disease activity. *Proc. III Int. Conf. AIDS*. Washington, D.C., p. 109.
19. Bigby, D., Margolskee, D., Curtis, J. L., Michael, P. F., Sheppard, D., Hadley, W. K., and Hopewell, P. C. (1986). The usefulness of induced sputum in the

diagnosis of *Pneumocystis carinii* pneumonia in patients with the acquired immunodeficiency syndrome. *Am. Rev. Respir. Dis. 133*:515-518.

20. Suffredini, A. F., Ognibene, F. P., Lack, E. E., Simmons, J. T., Brenner, M., Gill, V. J., Lane, H. C., Fauci, A. S., Parrillo, J. E., Masur, H., and Shelhamer, J. H. (1987). Nonspecific interstitial pneumonitis: A common cause of pulmonary disease in the acquired immunodeficiency syndrome. *Ann. Intern. Med. 107*:7-13.

21. Fitzgerald, W., Bevelaque, F. A., Garay, S. M., and Aranda, C. P. (1987). The role of open lung biopsy in patients with the acquired immunodeficiency syndrome. *Chest 91*:659-662.

22. Stulbarg, M. S. and Golden, J. A. (1987). Open lung biopsy in the acquired immunodeficiency syndrome (AIDS). *Chest 91*:639-640.

23. Barrio, J. L., Narcup, C., Baier, H. J., and Pitchenik, A. E. (1987). Value of repeat fiberoptic bronchoscopies and significance of nondiagnostic bronchoscopic results in patients with the acquired immunodeficiency syndrome. *Am. Rev. Respir. Dis. 135*:422-425.

24. CDC (1987). Revision of the Centers for Disease Control surveillance case definition for acquired immunodeficiency syndrome. *MMWR 14*:36-155.

25. Gordin, F. M., Simon, G. L., Wofsy, C. B., and Mills, J. (1984). Adverse reactions to trimethoprim-sulfamethoxazole in patients with the acquired immunodeficiency syndrome. *Ann. Intern. Med. 100*:495-499.

26. Wharton, B. M., Coleman, D. L., Wofsy, C. B., Luce, J. M., Blumenfeld, W., Hadley, W. K., Ingram-Drake, L., and Volberding, P. A. (1986). Prospective randomized trial of trimethoprim-sulfamethoxazole versus pentamidine for *Pneumocystis carinii* pneumonia in the acquired immunodeficiency syndrome. *Ann. Intern. Med. 105*:37-44.

27. Medina, I., Leoung, G., Mills, I., Hopewell, P., Feigel, D., and Wofsy, C. (1987). Oral therapy for *Pneumocystis carinii* pneumonia (PCP) in AIDS. A randomized double blind trial of trimethoprim-sulfamethoxazole (S) versus dapsone-trimethoprim (D) for first episode *Pneumocystis carinii* pneumonia in AIDS. *Abstr. 27th Intersci. Conf. Antibiot. Agents Chemother.*, New York.

28. Cowan, R., Nielsen, D., Ruskin, J., and Sattler, F. (1987). TMP-SMX (T/S) vs. pentamidine (pent) for pneumocystis (PCP): Prospective non-crossover study. *Abstr. 27th Intersci. Conf. Antimicrob. Agents Chemother.* New York.

29. Outwater, E. and McCutcheon, J. A. (1985). Neutrophil-associated antibodies and granulocytopenia in AIDS. *Abstr. Int. Conf. AIDS*, Atlanta, Ga, p. 23.

30. Winston, D. J., Lau, W. K., Gale, R. P., and Young, L. S. (1980). Trimethoprim-sulfamethoxazole for the treatment of *Pneumocystis carinii* pneumonia. *Ann. Intern. Med. 92*:762.

31. Western, K. A., Perera, D. R., and Schultz, M. G. (1970). Pentamidine isethionate in the treatment of *Pneumocystis carinii* pneumonia. *Ann. Intern. Med. 73*:695.

32. Conte, J. E. and Lin, E. T. (1987). Pentamidine (P) pharmokinetics (PK) in AIDS patients with impaired renal function. *Abstr. 27th Intersci. Conf. Antimicrob. Agents Chemother.* New York.

33. Hughes, W. T. and Smith, B. L. (1984). Efficacy of diaminodiphenylsulfone and other drugs in murine *Pneumocystis carinii* pneumonia. *Antimicrob. Agents Chemother. 26*:436.
34. Leoung, G. S., Mills, J., Hopewell, P. C., Hughes, W., and Wofsy, C. (1986). Dapsone-trimethoprim for *Pneumocystis carinii* pneumonia in the acquired immunodeficiency syndrome. *Ann. Intern. Med. 105*:45-48.
35. Mills, J., Leoung, G., Medina, I., Hopewell, P., Hughes, W., and Wofsy, C. (1988). Dapsone treatment of *Pneumocystis carinii* pneumonia in the acquired immunodeficiency syndrome. *Antimicrob. Agents Chemother. 32*:1057-1060.
36. Ranier, C., Geigal, D., Clement, M., and Wofsy, C. (1987). Prognosis and natural history of *Pneumocystis carinii* pneumonia: Indicators for early and later survival. *Proc. III Int. Conf. AIDS*, Washington, D.C., p. 189.
37. Allegra, C. J., Chabner, B. A., Tuazon, C. U., Ogata-Arakaki, D., Baird, B., Drake, J. C., Simmons, J. T., Lack, E. E., Shelhamer, J. H., Balis, F., Walker, R., Kovacs, J. A., Lane, H. C., and Masur, H. (1987). Trimetrexate for the treatment of *Pneumocystis carinii* pneumonia in patients with the acquired immunodeficiency syndrome. *N. Engl. J. Med. 317*:978-985.
38. Golden, J. A., Sjoerdsma, A., and Santi, D. V. (1984). *Pneumocystis carinii* pneumonia treated with alpha-difluromethylornithine: A prospective study among patients with the acquired immunodeficiency syndrome. *West. J. Med. 141*: 613-623.
39. McLees, B. D., Barlow, J. L. R., Kuzma, R. J., Baringtang, D. C., Schechter, P. J., and Sjoerdsma, A. (1987). Studies on successful eflornithine treatment of *Pneumocystis carinii* pneumonia (PCP) in AIDS patients failing conventional therapy. *Proc. III Int. Conf. AIDS.* Washington, D.C., Abstr. Th4.2 p. 155.
40. Queener, S. F., Barlett, M. S., Durkin, M. M., Jay, M. A., and Smith, J. W. (1987). Activity of clindamycin with primaquine toward *Pneumocystis carinii* in vitro and in vivo. *Program 27th Intersci. Conf. Antimicrob. Agents Chemother.* New York.
41. Debs, R. J., Blumenfeld, W., Brunette, E. N., Straubinger, R. N., Montgomery, A. B., Lin, E., Agabian, N., and Papahadjopoulos, D. (1987). Successful treatment with aerosolized pentamidine of *Pneumocystis carinii* pneumonia in rats. *Antimicrobial. Agents Chemother. 31*:37-41.
42. Montgomery, A. B., Debs, R. J., Luce, J. M., Corkery, K. J., Turner, J., Brunette, E. N., Lin, E. T., and Hopewell, P. C. (1987). Aerosolized pentamidine as sole therapy for *Pneumocystis carinii* pneumonia in patients with acquired immunodeficiency syndrome. *Lancet 1*:480-483.
43. Conte, J. E., Hollander, H., and Golden, J. A. (1987). Inhaled or reduced-dose intravenous pentamidine for *Pneumocystis carinii* pneumonia. *Ann. Intern. Med. 107*:495-498.
44. Bernard, E., Schmitt, H., Pagel, L., Seltzer, M., and Armstrong, D. (1987). Safety and effectiveness of aerosol pentamidine for prevention of *P. carinii* in patients with AIDS. *Program Abstr. 27th Intersci. Conf. Antimicrob. Agents Chemother.* Abstr. 944.

45. MacFadden, D. K., Edelson, J. D., Hyland, R. H., Rodrigues, C. H., Inouye, T., and Rebuck, A. S. (1987). Corticosteroids as adjunctive therapy in treatment of *Pneumocystis carinii* pneumonia in patients with acquired immunodeficiency syndrome. *Lancet 1*:1477-1479.

46. Mottin, D., Denis, M., Dombret, H., Rossert, J., Mayaud, C., and Akoun, G. (1987). Role for steroids in treatment of *Pneumocystis carinii* pneumonia in AIDS [Letter]. *Lancet 2*:519.

47. Wachter, R. M., Luce, J. M., Turner, J., Volberding, P. A., and Hopewell, P. C. (1986). Intensive care of patients with acquired immunodeficiency syndrome. *Am. Rev. Respir. Dis. 134*:891-896.

48. Medina, I., Feigel, D., and Wofsy, C. (1987). Cross-allergy to sulfonamides/ sulfones (sulfa), and folic antagonists in AIDS. *Proc. III Int. Conf. AIDS.* Washington, D.C., p. 208.

49. Silvestri, R. C., Jensen, W. A., Zibrak, J. D., Alexander, R. C., and Rose, R. M. (1987). Pulmonary infiltrates and hypoxemia in patients with the acquired immunodeficiency syndrome re-exposed to trimethoprim-sulfamethoxazole. *Am. Rev. Respir. Dis. 136*:1003-1004.

50. Hughes, W. T., Rivera, G. K., Schell, M. J., Thornton, D., and Lott, L. (1987). Successful intermittent chemoprophylaxis for *Pneumocystis carinii* pneumonitis. *N. Engl. J. Med. 316*:1627-1632.

51. Fischl, M. A., Dickinson, G. M., and La Voie, L. (1985). Safety and efficacy of sulfamethoxazole and trimethoprim chemoprophylaxis for *Pneumocystis carinii* pneumonia in AIDS. *Program Abstr. 25th Intersci. Conf. Antimicrob. Agents Chemother.* Minneapolis, Minn.

52. Kaplan, L. D., Abrams, D. I., Wofsy, C. B., and Volberding, P. A. (1986). Trimethoprim-sulfamethoxazole prophylaxis against *Pneumocystis carinii* pneumonia in acquired immunodeficiency syndrome (AIDS) [Abstract]. *Clin. Res. 33*:406A.

53. Busch, D. F. and Follansbee, S. E. (1986). Continuation therapy with pentamidine isethionate for prevention of relapse of *Pneumocystis carinii* pneumonia in AIDS. *Proc. Int. Conf. AIDS*, Paris, France.

54. Gottlieb, M. S., Knight, S., Mitsuyasu, R., Weisman, J., Roth, M., and Young, L. S. (1984). Prophylaxis of *Pneumocystis carinii* infection in acquired immunodeficiency syndrome (AIDS) with pyrimethamine-sulfadoxine. *Lancet 2*:398-399.

55. Zitelli, B. J., Alexander, J., Taylor, S., Miller, K. D., Howrie, D. L., Kuritsky, J. N., Perez, T. H., and Van Thiel, D. H. (1987). Fatal hepatic necrosis due to pyrimethamine-sulfadoxine (Fansidar). *Ann. Intern. Med. 106*:393-395.

56. Metroka, C. E., Lange, M., Braun, N., O'Sullivan, M., Josefberg, H., and Jacobus, D. (1987). Successful chemoprophylaxis for *Pneumocystis carinii* pneumonia with dapsone in patients with AIDS and ARC. *Proc. III Int. Conf. AIDS.* Washington, D.C., p. 202.

18
Toxoplasmosis in Patients with the Acquired Immunodeficiency Syndrome

Joseph A. Kovacs *National Institutes of Health, Bethesda, Maryland*

Toxoplasma gondii is a major pathogen of patients with the acquired immunodeficiency syndrome (AIDS) (1-3). In this patient population *T. gondii* can cause severe morbidity and mortality, usually from focal encephalitis, but occasionally from more widely disseminated disease. The diagnosis may be difficult to establish, because standard serologic assays are not useful, and therapy, although effective, needs to be continued for prolonged periods because of the high frequency of relapse following discontinuation of therapy (4,5). This chapter will briefly review the life cycle of *T. gondii*, and clinical manifestations of infection in nonimmunocompromised patients; it will then review the clinical presentation and management of disease in patients with AIDS.

LIFE CYCLE

Toxoplasma gondii is an obligate intracellular protozoan of the order Coccidia that exists in three separate forms: tachyzoite, tissue cyst with internal bradyzoites, and oocyst (6). The organism can proliferate in a variety of mammals, including humans, but cats are the definitive host. After ingestion of tissue cysts or oocysts by the cat, organisms excyst, invade intestinal epithelial cells, and undergo asexual and sexual reproduction, resulting in the release of oocysts that subsequently sporulate and become infectious.

Tachyzoites are the easily recognized crescentic form of the organisms that actively invade host cells during acute disease. Once in the cells they replicate by endogeny and eventually burst from the cell and spread to nearby cells, continuing the replicative process. Eventually, tissue cysts with a true cyst wall and many internal organisms develop. Once the infection is controlled by the immune system of the host organism, the tissue cysts appear to remain viable, and allow reactivation of disease in the setting of an impaired immune system. If the cysts are ingested by mammals, the internal organisms are liberated, and the cycle begins again.

EPIDEMIOLOGY AND CLINICAL MANIFESTATIONS IN IMMUNOCOMPETENT HOST

Humans usually acquire infection by ingesting either infectious occysts, through contact with cats or cat feces, or by eating meat that contains tissue cysts. Based on serologic studies, 20% to 90% of healthy adults have been infected with *T. gondii*, with some variation based on geographic location (7). In the United States, for example, 15% to 68% of adults have been infected, whereas in Paris, 87% of adults have been infected by 40 years of age (8,9).

After infection, most immunocompetent individuals remain asymptomatic, although it has been estimated that 10% to 20% go on to develop an infectious mononucleosislike syndrome, characterized by lymphadenopathy, fever, malaise, and hepatosplenomegaly (10). Symptoms may persist for weeks to months, but will eventually resolve without long-term sequelae. At this point, the organism has encysted and remains inactive, but viable. If the individual subsequently develops an immunodeficiency, caused by either drugs or by an underlying disease, the infection can reactivate and cause morbidity and mortality. *Toxoplasma gondii* can also be transmitted congenitally and can cause severe congenital disease, including hydrocephalus and retinochoroiditis. Retinochoroiditis can also be a late sequela of congenital infection.

EPIDEMIOLOGY AND CLINICAL MANIFESTATIONS IN PATIENTS WITH AIDS

The specific prevalence of toxoplasmosis in patients with AIDS is unknown. On the basis of reports to the Centers for Disease Control (CDC), a minimum of 3% of patients with CDC-defined AIDS have active toxoplasmosis (11). This figure is almost certainly an underestimate because patients are reported at the time of diagnosis of AIDS, and undoubtedly additional patients developed toxoplasmosis during the course of their illness.

Toxoplasmosis in most AIDS patients appears to represent reactivation of latent infection, rather than primary infection. Such a conclusion is based on serologic studies as well as on manifestations of disease. For example, in one study (1) antitoxoplasma IgG antibodies were detected in all 15 patients for whom sera were available a few months before development of clinical disease.

It is unclear why toxoplasmosis reactivates in some AIDS patients but not in others. Given the serologic data, a much larger proportion of AIDS patients have been previously infected with *T. gondii* than develop clinical disease. Thirty-five (31%) of 113 patients with AIDS or lymphadenopathy syndrome, but without clinical toxoplasmosis who were evaluated in New York City, had detectable antitoxoplasma antibodies in their sera (3). In a French study (12), 62% of AIDS patients, compared with 69% of patients with lymphadenopathy and 64% of healthy controls had detectable antibodies in their sera. Only a small proportion of those at risk for reactivation of latent disease (based on the presence of antitoxoplasma IgG antibodies) go on to develop symptoms. It is possible that a latent infection was not established in all patients after an acute infection. Alternatively, a specific immune defect that is not present in all AIDS patients may be necessary for reactivation of latent disease.

The clinical manifestations of active toxoplasmosis in AIDS patients are varied, but the overwhelming majority of patients have symptoms referable to a focal process in the central nervous system (1-3,5; Tables 1 and 2). Symptoms usually develop subacutely, over the course of a few weeks. The most common presenting symptoms include focal neurologic abnormalities, most often mild to severe hemiparesis, confusion, and lethargy. Twenty-nine percent to 89% of patients have focal signs, and 14% to 63% have symptoms suggesting a diffuse encephalopathy (1,2,5). Encephalopathy and focal abnormalities will frequently occur in the same patient. Focal or generalized seizures are present in 15% to 43% of patients. Headaches, which are often

TABLE 1   Organ System Involvement in AIDS Patients with Toxoplasmosis

Frequent
  brain (focal encephalitis)
Rare
  eyes (retinochoroiditis)
  lungs
  testicles
Rare, of uncertain clinical significance
  heart
  stomach
  adrenals
  pancreas
  striated muscle

TABLE 2 Clinical Manifestations of Toxoplasma Encephalitis

Manifestation	Frequency (%)
Focal neurologic abnormalities (e.g., hemiparesis)	29-89
Diffuse encephalopathy	14-63
Seizure	15-43
Headache	50
Fever	60
Meningismus	< 10

severe, bilateral, and unremitting, occur in approximately half the patients. Fevers are common, but by no means invariable, occurring in only about 60% of patients. Signs of meningeal irritation are rare, having been reported in less than 10% of patients.

Other clinically significant sites of *T. gondii* infection in AIDS patients are rare. Retinochoroiditis, documented histopathologically or by culture, has been reported on occasion, and may appear prior to, associated with, or independent of focal encephalitis (13,14). Pulmonary toxoplasmosis has been documented in a few patients, and testicular toxoplasmosis has been reported in two patients (15,16). In autopsy studies toxoplasma have been detected in the heart, stomach, adrenals, pancreas, and striated muscle in addition to the brain, eyes, and lungs (17). The specific symptoms attributable to *T. gondii* infection of many of these organs have not been well established.

HISTOPATHOLOGY

In biopsy and autopsy brain specimens from patients infected with *T. gondii*, the primary process is a focal necrotizing encephalitis that is characterized by a central area of necrosis surrounded by acute and chronic inflammatory cells (1,4). There may be an associated arteritis and thrombosis. Edema and a mild astrocytosis can be seen nearby. In one study (4), the inflammatory cells seen in AIDS patients were primarily neutrophils, whereas in non-AIDS patients they were primarily mononuclear cells. At autopsy, multiple necrotic lesions, usually in the cerebral and cerebellar cortex, are invariably seen. In patients that have been partially treated, organizing and chronic abscesses are seen at autopsy (1).

Confirmation that the necrotic process is caused by *T. gondii* requires demonstration of the organisms in the involved area. Organisms are usually found in the periphery, not in the central necrotic area (1,4,18). Identification of tachyzoites, which may be difficult to see with hematoxylin and eosin (H and E) stains, is necessary for establishing the diagnosis. Cysts, which are recognized more easily on H and E stains, do not, by themselves, indicate active infection, although their presence certainly strongly suggests the diagnosis of toxoplasmosis. Special techniques, such as immunoperoxidase stains, appear to be more efficient in demonstrating the tachyzoites in histopathologic specimens (4).

LABORATORY EVALUATION

Routine blood tests in AIDS patients with toxoplasmosis are unrevealing (see Chap. 21). Patients may have an anemia or leukopenia and lymphopenia; these are not specific for toxoplasmosis, but are only manifestations of the underlying disease. Cerebrospinal fluid analysis usually will be abnormal, but nondiagnostic. In one study (1), 18 of 21 patients had an elevated protein value (mean, 96 mg/dl), 9 patients had a mononuclear pleocytosis (4 to 67 cells/mm^3), and 3 patients had a minimally depressed glucose value (38 to 43 mg/dl).

The most useful noninvasive diagnostic study for evaluating a patient with suspected CNS toxoplasmosis is computed tomography (CT). The CT scans will usually demonstrate one or more focal abnormalities, often associated with edema, that will show enhancement after administration of contrast. In one study, all 58 scans obtained at the time of clinical presentation demonstrated abnormalities (5). However, in two other studies, 1 of 13 and 3 of 26 scans were negative initially (1,2). In one patient, three scans were negative over a 6-week period before a mass lesion was documented (2). Multiple lesions are common, occurring in 5 of 13 and 12 of 22 patients in two series (1,2).

Contrast enhancement of lesions is seen in most patients, although 3 of 26 patients in one study (1) had only hypodense lesions demonstrable by CT. Ring enhancement is most commonly seen; occasionally enhancement will be in a homogeneous pattern (1,18). The sensitivity of CT scanning can be improved by using a double dose of contrast and delaying the scan for 45 min to 1 hr (18). This procedure enables the detection of more lesions, which may be important for determining the optimal lesion to biopsy. The role of magnetic resonance imaging (MRI) has not yet been defined, although there is a suggestion that it may be superior to CT scanning. In one patient in whom CT demonstrated only one lesion after a double-dose, delayed-view scan, multiple lesions were demonstrated by MRI (1).

DIAGNOSIS

The optimal method for diagnosing toxoplasmosis in any patient is by the demonstration of tachyzoites in clinical or pathologic specimens or by culturing the organism from clinical specimens. Because these methods may require an invasive procedure, and tachyzoites cannot always be easily demonstrated or cultured, the diagnosis of toxoplasmosis in a nonimmunocompromised host has traditionally been made on the basis of serologic studies. A variety of serologic assays for detecting IgG are available and include the Sabin-Feldman dye test, indirect immunofluorescence, and IgG enzyme-linked immunosorbent assays (ELISA; 10). Although a high titer in one of these assays or a fourfold change in titer has been used for diagnosis, variability in techniques, as well as the persistence in some individuals of high titers for prolonged periods, has made these assays less than ideal. Assays to measure IgM, especially a double-sandwich ELISA technique, appear to be much more accurate in diagnosing acute toxoplasmosis in immunocompetent individuals (19).

Unfortunately, in immunocompromised individuals, especially patients with AIDS, serologic studies play a very limited role in diagnosing toxoplasmosis (4,17). Immunoglobulin G antibodies to *T. gondii* are virtually always present in AIDS patients with toxoplasmosis, but very high titers, which suggest active infection, are found in only a small proportion of patients. For example, in one study evaluating sera from 37 AIDS patients with toxoplasmosis, all had positive Sabin-Feldman dye tests, but only eight (22%) had titers above 1:1024, as opposed to nonimmunocompromised patients with acute lymphadenopathic toxoplasmosis, among whom 94% had titers above 1:1024 (4). Given the high proportion of AIDS patients without toxoplasmosis who have antitoxoplasma IgG detectable in serum, diagnosis based on IgG serology is unreliable. However, absence of IgG antibodies is strong evidence against *T. gondii* infection, although rare AIDS patients with documented toxoplasmosis may have undetectable IgG antibodies (2). Fourfold increases in titer are also unusual and unreliable for diagnosis (1,4). Equally unreliable are IgM assays. In the previously described study (4), only 1 of 37 patients had detectable IgM by ELISA, a finding again confirmed by other studies.

Because of the lack of reliability of serologic studies, diagnosis must be made by alternative means. The most common method currently used is histopathologic detection of organisms in biopsy specimens. Because the brain is the organ most frequently affected, obtaining a biopsy specimen is somewhat more complicated than at other sites. The development of newer techniques for brain biopsy, specifically the use of CT scan-directed stereotactic needle biopsy, has improved the safety of such procedures (2). Although arguments have been made for initial empiric therapy in patients with AIDS and a compatible clinical and radiographic picture, the risk of biopsy is warranted in patients who have an easily accessible site for biopsy.

Toxoplasma gondii can be detected in biopsy specimens by a number of techniques. The organism, specifically the cyst form, may be recognized in H and E stained specimens, although the tachyzoite may be much more difficult to discern clearly. However, because of necrosis and other factors, the organism may not be seen in routine H and E sections in over 50% of cases (4). To improve diagnosis, immunoperoxidase and immunofluorescent stains have also been used. With use of the immunoperoxidase technique, all specimens were positive for *T. gondii* organisms or antigen in fixed tissue specimens in one study, whereas in another study only about half the specimens were positive (2,4). Immunofluorescence, using monoclonal antibodies against *T. gondii* to detect the organism in impression smears made from biopsy specimens, has also been reported to be useful in establishing the diagnosis (20). At NIH the diagnosis was rapidly established by immunofluorescence with polyclonal antiserum in one patient in whom the standard H and E sections were negative for organisms.

Homogenates of biopsy specimens can also be inoculated into the peritoneum of mice to establish the diagnosis. Because encysted organisms can also be cultivated in this manner, this may not distinguish latent infection from active disease. This method, which is not routinely available other than in research laboratories, requires a number of weeks to establish the diagnosis. *Toxoplasma gondii* can also be cultured from clinical specimens, such as blood and pulmonary bronchoalveolar lavage fluid, but positive cultures have been reported only rarely (21). For cultures, the specimen can be placed into tissue culture or be injected into the peritoneum of mice. Other techniques for diagnosing toxoplasmosis in AIDS patients are being investigated, but they are not now clinically applicable. For example, studies have suggested that *T. gondii* antigens can be detected in the blood of acutely infected animals using techniques such as ELISA (22).

DIFFERENTIAL DIAGNOSIS

Although the radiographic picture of focal encephalitis caused by *T. gondii* is characteristic, it is not diagnostic, and a similar pattern can be seen with other diseases. Central nervous system lymphoma is probably the most common disease having a similar presentation and with a similar CT pattern. Although central nervous system lymphoma will enhance with contrast, it will usually give a homogeneous pattern, not the ring enhancement commonly seen with toxoplasmosis (23). A CNS lymphoma can occur in the setting of disseminated lymphoma; however, especially in patients with AIDS, it may be limited to the CNS. See Chapter 6 for further details.

Progressive multifocal leukoencephalopathy (PML) presents as a focal CNS process with hypodense lesions on CT scan that do not contrast-enhance (24). Because not all lesions caused by *T. gondii* will have contrast enhancement, both processes must be considered in patients with such a presentation.

A number of other processes can present with focal CNS lesions, although they are seen less frequently. Kaposi's sarcoma has rarely been seen in the brain. Other infections, such as *Cryptococcus, Aspergillus, Mycobacterium tuberculosis,* and *Candida* species, have also been seen (25).

THERAPY

The only regimen that has been clearly documented to be effective in the treatment of active toxoplasmosis is the synergistic combination of pyrimethamine, a semiselective inhibitor of dihydrofolate reductase, and a sulfonamide, which inhibits the incorporation of *p*-aminobenzoic acid into dihydrofolate (Table 3, Fig. 1; 26). Although no well-controlled clinical studies with this combination have been published, it is clear from large uncontrolled studies, that in immunocompromised patients, especially patients with AIDS, this combination will lead to a rapid improvement in symptoms and in the CT scans in most patients, usually within a few weeks (1-3). Over 80% of

TABLE 3   Drug Regimens for Treatment of Toxoplasmosis

Drug	Effective dose
Definitely effective	
pyrimethamine plus	25-75 mg/d
sulfadiazine	4 to 8 g/d in four doses
Commonly used alternative regimens of poorly documented clinical efficacy	
pyrimethamine	25-50 mg/d
or	
pyrimethamine plus	25-50 mg/d
clindamycin	1200-2400 mg/d in four doses
Other alternative regimens of undocumented efficacy	
spiramicin	Unknown
trimethoprim plus	Unknown
sulfamethoxazole	
trimetrexate	Unknown
trimetrexate plus	Unknown
a sulfonamide	

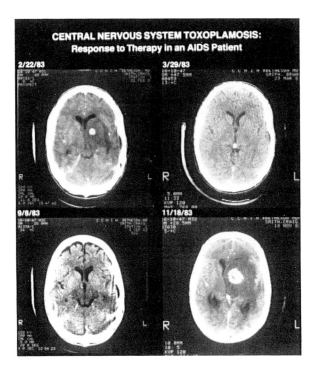

FIGURE 1 Radiographic improvement is seen following initiation of therapy (top). Following discontinuation of therapy, the lesion recurs rapidly (bottom).

AIDS patients in two reports (1,2) responded clinically and radiographically to this combination. Pyrimethamine is usually given at a dosage of 25-75 mg/day. The sulfonamide usually administered is sulfadiazine, given at a dosage of 1 to 2 g four times a day. Because pyrimethamine can cause bone marrow suppression that is reversible by leucovorin, patients are also usually given leucovorin (5-formyl tetrahydrofolic acid) at a dosage of 5 to 10 mg/day, although higher dosages can be given. Leucovorin has no effect on the therapeutic efficacy of pyrimethamine (26,27).

The optimal duration of therapy for toxoplasmosis in AIDS patients has not been determined. When therapy has been stopped, either because of adverse reactions or because it was felt that an adequate course of therapy had been given, the frequency of relapse is very high. In one study, the prevalence of relapse after discontinuation of pyrimethamine plus sulfadiazine was nearly 50%, whereas in another study it approached 100% (2,5). Clinical or radiologic relapse will usually occur within 2 to 12 weeks (Figure 1).

Because of the high frequency of relapse, antitoxoplasma therapy should be continued for prolonged periods, probably for life. As no studies have been conducted to evaluate the efficacy of specific regimens in maintaining a therapeutic response, no firm recommendations for maintenance or suppressive regimens can be made. Standard doses of pyrimethamine plus sulfadiazine should probably be used pending additional data, although alternative regimens (e.g., 25 mg pyrimethamine plus 2 g sulfadiazine three to five times per week) are currently being used in some centers (28).

The prevalence of adverse reactions associated with pyrimethamine plus sulfadiazine is high, approaching 60%; in 30% to 40% of patients, standard therapy must be discontinued because of these reactions (2,5). The most common reactions include neutropenia, fever, and rash, and appear to be related to the sulfonamide component. A similar prevalence of adverse reactions has been seen during the treatment of *Pneumocystis carinii* pneumonia with trimethoprim plus sulfamethoxazole (29).

For patients who develop adverse reactions to pyrimethamine plus sulfadiazine, no alternative regimen has been shown to be consistently effective in preventing a relapse. Pyrimethamine alone was effective in only three of seven patients in one report (1). Other drugs that have been reported to have antitoxoplasma activity, based on in vitro studies, animal studies, or anecdotal reports, include clindamycin, spiramycin, trimethoprim-sulfamethoxazole, and trimetrexate (27,30-32). None of these agents have been as effective as pyrimethamine plus a sulfonamide. For example, spiramycin, a macrolide antibiotic widely used in Europe, has been reported to be ineffective in treating or preventing relapse in four AIDS patients (33). Clindamycin plus pyrimethamine has been used to treat three patients who showed clinical deterioration during therapy (2). Trimethoprim-sulfamethoxazole appears to offer no advantage over pyrimethamine plus sulfadiazine, especially since trimethoprim-sulfamethoxazole therapy is associated with a high frequency of adverse reactions in AIDS patients. At least three patients have been reported to have developed clinical toxoplasmosis while receiving trimethoprim-sulfamethoxazole. Trimetrexate is a dihydrofolate reductase (DHFR) inhibitor like pyrimethamine and is approximately 500 times more potent than pyrimethamine in inhibiting *T. gondii* DHFR (27). It is a lipid-soluble analogue of methotrexate that enters cells and organisms by passive diffusion. Although trimetrexate can inhibit the DHFR of mammalian cells, concurrent administration of leucovorin will bypass the toxicity to mammalian cells, although not affecting antitoxoplasma activity (27). Tissue culture and animal studies have confirmed that trimetrexate is very active against *T. gondii* (34). Preliminary studies in humans with AIDS have shown that trimetrexate does have antitoxoplasma activity, although with prolonged therapy, clinical deterioration was eventually seen in all patients (35).

Given the currently available data, no firm recommendations can be made for alternative therapy for patients who develop adverse reactions, or for those who are not responding to pyrimethamine plus sulfadiazine. Pyrimethamine (25-75 mg/day) plus clindamycin (300 to 600 mg four times a day orally or intravenously) or pyrimethamine alone, perhaps at higher dosages than are currently being used (with a concomitant increase in leucovorin dosing to minimize toxicity) are reasonable regimens that require further evaluation.

Corticosteroids are frequently used in conjunction with pyrimethamine plus sulfadiazine, primarily to manage cerebral edema associated with toxoplasmosis. The beneficial role of corticosteroids in relieving edema must be weighed against the potential harm that can be caused by using an agent that may lead to further immunosuppression. In a retrospective study, no beneficial or harmful effect was associated with the use of corticosteroids in this setting (5). It would seem prudent to reserve corticosteroids for those patients in whom clinically evident cerebral edema develops.

Anticonvulsants are also frequently used in treating patients with CNS toxoplasmosis. Although they are clearly indicated in patients with seizures, their role in other patients is less clear, especially because the frequency of seizures after initiation of antitoxoplasma therapy is unknown. Because of the morbidity of seizures, it seems prudent to routinely administer anticonvulsant therapy and to continue it, if tolerated, until there has been clinical and radiologic improvement. Because the prevalence of toxoplasmosis in AIDS patients is low, and the prevalence of adverse reactions to pyrimethamine plus sulfadiazine is high, at present one should not attempt to prevent T. gondii encephalitis in seropositive patients without clinical disease.

As noted previously, some physicians will not attempt to obtain a histopathologic diagnosis of toxoplasmosis, but will initiate empiric therapy in a patient with a typical history and CT observations, especially if antitoxoplasma IgG antibodies are present in the serum, even at low titers (1). Because a rapid clinical and radiographic response can be seen following initiation of specific therapy, a biopsy is reserved for those patients in whom no response is seen within 1 to 2 weeks. Although this approach can be used successfully, a number of potential pitfalls exist. As steroids are frequently used in conjunction with specific antimicrobial therapy, primarily when edema is present, the apparently specific response may be due to the nonspecific anti-inflammatory response caused by the steroids (1). Additionally, delay in obtaining the correct diagnosis, if in fact it is not toxoplasmosis, may result in delay of appropriate therapy for other treatable processes.

Lack of a histopathologic diagnosis can also make subsequent therapeutic decisions more difficult. In a patient with toxoplasmosis who does not appear to be responding to therapy, the diagnosis may be obscured on subsequent biopsy specimens because of partial treatment. In patients in whom an adverse reaction develops, a histopathologic diagnosis makes assessment of alternative, less reliable therapies simpler. For all of these reasons, at the NIH a stereotactic CT-guided needle biopsy is obtained if lesions are easily accessible. Empiric therapy is reserved for those patients in whom lesions are inaccessible or are located in critical areas. Empiric therapy is also warranted when a biopsy is nondiagnostic, especially if the histopathologic as well as the clinical picture is suggestive of toxoplasmosis.

If empiric therapy is instituted, the patient must be followed closely both clinically and radiographically. If the patient does not respond to empiric therapy after 2 to 3 weeks, a biopsy should be obtained to establish the diagnosis. Steroids should be avoided, if possible, because of the nonspecific clinical improvement that may be seen with these drugs.

In summary, toxoplasmosis in patients with AIDS is similar to other opportunistic infections seen in this patient population. The diagnosis may be difficult to establish, and available therapy is limited and is associated with a high prevalence of adverse reactions. Following cessation of therapy, relapse is very common, and can occur within a few weeks. The ultimate prognosis of patients with toxoplasmosis, even those who respond to therapy, is poor. The median survival for 56 of 61 patients who have died in one study (5) was 4 months (range, 7 days to 18 months). Improved methods of diagnosis, and improved therapeutic regimens are clearly needed for this disease. However, without reversal of the immunosuppression associated with AIDS, the prognosis of toxoplasmosis will almost certainly remain grim in this population.

REFERENCES

1. Navia, B. A., Petito, C. K., Gold, J. W. M., Cho, E.-S., Jordan, B. D., and Price, R. W. (1986). Cerebral toxoplasmosis complicating the acquired immune deficiency syndrome: Clinical and neuropathological findings in 27 patients. *Ann. Neurol. 19*:224-238.
2. Wanke, C., Tuazon, C. U., Kovacs, A., Dina, T., Davis, D. O., Barton, N., Katz, D., Lunde, M., Levy, C., Conley, F. K., Lane, H. C., Fauci, A. S., and Masur, H. (1987). Toxoplasma encephalitis in patients with acquired immune deficiency syndrome: Diagnosis and response to therapy. *Am. J. Trop. Med. Hyg. 36*:509-516.
3. Wong, B., Gold, J. W. M., Brown, A. E., Lange, M., Fried, R., Grieco, M., Mildvan, D., Giron, J., Tapper, M. L., Lerner, C. W., and Armstrong, D. (1984). Central-nervous-system toxoplasmosis in homosexual men and parenteral drug abusers. *Ann. Intern. Med. 100*:36-42.
4. Luft, B. J., Brooks, R. G., Conley, F. K., McCabe, R. E., and Remington, J. S. (1984). Toxoplasmic encephalitis in patients with acquired immune deficiency syndrome. *JAMA 252*:913-917.

5. Haverkos, H. W. (1987). Assessment of therapy for toxoplasma encephalitis. *Am. J. Med. 82*:907-914.

6. Frenkel, J. K. (1973). Toxoplasmosis: Parasite life cycle, pathology, and immunology. In *The Coccidia*. (Hammond, D. M., ed.). Baltimore, University Park Press, pp. 343-410.

7. Remington, J. S. and Desmonts, G. (1983). Toxoplasmosis. In *Infectious Diseases of the Fetus and Newborn*, 2nd ed. (Remington, J. S. and Klein, J. O., eds.). Philadelphia, W.B. Saunders, pp. 143-263.

8. Feldman, H. A. and Miller, L. T. (1956). Serologic study of toxoplasmosis prevalence. *Am. J. Hyg. 64*:320-335.

9. Desmonts, G. (1960). Diagnostic serologique de la toxoplasmose. *Pathol. Biol. 8*:109-125.

10. McCabe, R. E. and Remington, J. S. (1985). *Toxoplasma gondii*. In *Principles and Practice of Infectious Diseases*, 2nd ed. (Mandell, G. L., Douglas, R. G., Jr., and Bennett, J. E., eds.). New York, John Wiley & Sons, pp. 1540-1549.

11. CDC (1986). Update: Acquired immunodeficiency syndrome—United States. *MMWR 35*:542.

12. Derouin, F., Beauvais, B., and Lariviere, M. (1986). Serologic study of the prevalence of toxoplasmosis in 167 patients with acquired immunodeficiency syndrome (AIDS) or chronic lymphadenopathy syndrome (LAS). *Biomed. Pharmacother. 40*:231-232.

13. Weiss, A., Margo, C. E., Ledford, D. K., Lockey, R. F., and Brinser, J. H. (1986). Toxoplasmic retinochoroiditis as an initial manifestation of the acquired immune deficiency syndrome. *J. Ophthalmol. 101*:248-249.

14. Parke, D. W. and Font, R. L. (1986). Diffuse toxoplasmic retinochoroiditis in a patient with AIDS. *Arch. Ophthalmol. 104*:571-575.

15. Catterall, J. R., Hofflin, J. M., and Remington, J. S. (1986). Pulmonary toxoplasmosis. *Am. Rev. Respir. Dis. 133*:704-705.

16. Nistal, M., Santan, A., Paniaqua, R., and Palacios, J. (1986). Testicular toxoplasmosis in two men with the acquired immunodeficiency syndrome. *Arch. Pathol. Lab. Med. 110*:744-746.

17. Luft, B. J., Conley, F., Remington, J. S., Laverdiere, M., Wagner, K. F., Levine, J. F., Craven, P. C., Strandberg, D. A., File, T. M., Rice, N., and Meunier-Carpentier, F. (1983). Outbreak of central-nervous-system toxoplasmosis in western Europe and North America. *Lancet 1*:781-783.

18. Post, M. J. D., Chan, J. C., Hensley, G. T., Hoffman, T. A., Moskowitz, L. B., and Lippmann, S. (1983). Toxoplasma encephalitis in Haitian adults with acquired immunodeficiency syndrome: A clinical-pathological-CT correlation. *Am. J. Neuroradiol. 4*:155-162.

19. Naot, Y. and Remingtin, J. S. (1980). An enzyme-linked immunosorbent assay for the detection of IgM antibodies of *Toxoplasma gondii*: Use for diagnosis of acute acquired infection. *J. Infect. Dis. 142*:757-766.

20. Sun, T., Greenspan, J., Tenenbaum, M., Farmer, P., Jones, T., Kaplan, M., and Peacock, J. (1986). Diagnosis of cerebral toxoplasmosis using fluorescein-labeled antitoxoplasma monoclonal antibodies. *Am. J. Surg. Pathol. 10*:312-316.

21. Hofflin, J. M. and Remington, J. S. (1985). Tissue culture isolation of *Toxoplasma* from blood of a patient with AIDS. *Arch. Intern. Med. 145*:925-926.
22. Ise, Y., Iida, T., Sato, K., Suzuki, T., Shimada, K., and Nishioka, K. (1985). Detection of circulating antigens in sera of rabbits infected with *Toxoplasma gondii. Infect. Immun. 48*:269-272.
23. Gill, P. S., Levine, A. M., Meyer, P. R., Boswell, W. D., Burkes, R. L., Parker, J. W., Hofman, F. M., Dworsky, R. L., and Lukes, R. J. (1985). Primary central nervous system lymphoma in homosexual men: Clinical, immunologic, and pathologic features. *Am. J. Med. 78*:742-748.
24. Berger, J. R., Kaszovitz, B., Post, M. J. D., and Dickinson, G. (1987). Progressive multifocal leukoencephalopathy associated with human immunodeficiency virus infection: A review of the literature with a report of sixteen cases. *Ann. Intern. Med. 107*:78-87.
25. Levy, R. M., Bredesen, D. E., and Rosenblum, M. L. (1985). Neurological manifestations of the acquired immunodeficiency syndrome (AIDS): Experience at U.C.S.F. and review of the literature. *J. Neurosurg. 62*:475-495.
26. Frenkel, J. K. and Hitchings, G. H. (1957). Relative reversal by vitamins (*p*-aminobenzoic, folic, and folinic acids) of the effects of sulfadiazine and pyrimethamine on *Toxoplasma*, mouse and man. *Antibiot. Chemother. 7*:630-638.
27. Allegra, C. J., Kovacs, J. A., Drake, J. C., Swan, J. C., Chabner, B. A., and Masur, H. (1987). Potent in vitro and in vivo antitoxoplasma activity of the lipid-soluble antifolate trimetrexate. *J. Clin. Invest. 79*:478-482.
28. Mills, J. (1986). *Pneumocystis carinii* and *Toxoplasma gondii* infections in patients with AIDS. *Rev. Infect. Dis. 8*:1001-1011.
29. Kovacs, J. A., Hiemenz, J. W., Macher, A. M., Stover, D., Murray, H. W., Shelhamer, J., Lane, H. C., Urmacher, U., Honig, C., Longo, D. L., Parker, M. M., Natanson, C., Parrillo, J. E., Fauci, A. S., Pizzo, P. A., and Masur, H. (1984). *Pneumocystis carinii* pneumonia: A comparison between patients with the acquired immunodeficiency syndrome and patients with other immunodeficiencies. *Ann. Intern. Med. 100*:663-671.
30. Araujo, F. G. and Remington, J. S. (1974). Effect of clindamycin on acute and chronic toxoplasmosis in mice. *Antimicrob. Agents Chemother. 5*:647-651.
31. Garin, J. P. and Eyles, D. E. (1958). Le traitement de la toxoplasmose experimentale de la souris par la spiramycine. *Presse Med. 66*:957-958.
32. Norrby, R., Eilard, T., Svedhem, A., and Lycke, E. (1975). Treatment of toxoplasmosis with trimethoprim-sulfamethoxazole. *Scand. J. Infect. Dis. 7*:72-75.
33. Leport, C., Vilde, J. L., Katlama, C., Regnier, B., Matheron, S., and Saimot, A. G. (1986). Failure of spiramycin to prevent neurotoxoplasmosis in immunosuppressed patients. *JAMA 255*:2290.
34. Kovacs, J. A., Allegra, C. J., Chabner, B. A., Swan, J. C., Drake, J., Lunde, M., Parrillo, J. E., and Masur, H. (1987). Potent effect of trimetrexate, a lipid-soluble antifolate, on *Toxoplasma gondii. J. Infect. Dis. 155*:1027-1032.
35. Chabner, B. A. (1987). Improved therapy for pneumocystis pneumonia and toxoplasmosis, pp. 578-579. In Developmental Therapeutics and the Acquired Immunodeficiency Syndrome. (DeVita, V. T. Jr., moderator). *Ann. Intern. Med. 106*:568-581.

19
Cryptosporidium spp. and *Isospora belli*

Pearl Ma *St. Vincent's Hospital and Medical Center of New York, New York, New York*

CRYPTOSPORIDIUM

Introduction

In 1907, Professor Tyzzer, chairman of the Department of Pathology, Harvard Medical School, discovered numerous tiny parasites in a gastric tumor of a mouse. He classified them as coccidial protozoans under the phylum apicomplexa, genus *Cryptospodium* (Fig. 1). Most of the early work on cryptosporidiosis focused on animals, particularly farm animals (1) and cryptosporidial infection was formerly believed to be a zoonosis. *Cryptosporidium* species were known to be the causative agents of diarrhea in mammals, birds, fish, and reptiles. In birds, respiratory infection had been reported with or without intestinal involvement.

Human cryptosporidiosis was unheard of until 1976, when two cases were reported in the setting of contact with farm animals. One was a healthy 3-year-old farm girl with self-limited diarrhea; the other was a man receiving high-dose corticosteroids for bullous pemphigoid, whose diarrhea stopped when the corticosteroids were discontinued. In 1979 and 1980, five cases of human cryptosporidiosis were reported; two patients had hypogammaglobulinemia, and one patient was an immunosuppressed renal transplant recipient. The fifth case was a 27-year-old immunocompetent man, who had 5 days of vomiting and watery diarrhea with severe abdominal cramplike pain which spontaneously resolved. Seven days before, his 8-year-old daughter had similar symptoms, as well as the children in her school and in the neighborhood.

355

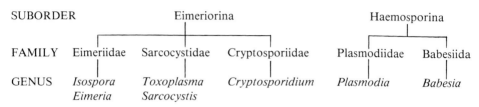

FIGURE 1   Classification of *Cryptosporidium* and *Isospora belli* as related to other members of the Coccidia [from Soulsby, E. J. L. (1982). *Helminths, Arthropods, and Protozoa of Domesticated Animals*, 7th ed. Lea & Febiger, and Levine, N. D. Taxonomy and review of the coccidian genus Cryptosporidium (Protozoa, Ampicomplexa). J Protozool 31:94, 1984].

This was the first case of cryptosporidiosis diagnosed by stool examination (all of the previous cases were diagnosed by intestinal or rectal biopsies with electron microscopy). These cases represented a spectrum of infections (1-5) with or without animal contacts in a presumably heterosexual population. The importance of *Cryptosporidium* was not fully appreciated until it was rediscovered as the causative agent of intractable watery diarrhea in homosexual men during the epidemic of acquired immunodeficiency syndrome (AIDS) (2). In 1981, cryptosporidiosis was diagnosed in a 48-year-old homosexual man from Boston, who suffered persistent diarrhea caused by combined cryptosporidiosis and cytomegalovirus (CMV) infections. Although AIDS was not recognized at that time, it is highly probable that the patient had AIDS. The first case of AIDS-associated cryptosporidiosis diagnosed at St. Vincent's Hospital, in August 1981, was in a homosexual man, also from Boston, who had *Pneumocystis carinii* pneumonia, candidiasis, intestinal cryptosporidiosis, and Kaposi's sarcoma.

Epidemiology

The genus *Cryptosporidium*, although ubiquitous and globally distributed, was largely an unknown parasite until a few years ago. It has now gained worldwide recognition as an important pathogen in immunocompromised hosts, especially in patients with AIDS and AIDS-related complex (ARC), whereas it causes self-limited infections in immunocompetent individuals. A review of the literature from 1976 to 1986 (2) reveals a large number of outbreaks involving children in day care centers and in small communities. Although the number of cases is low in the immunocompetent individuals, it is 10-fold higher in the AIDS-associated group. The clusters of cases in children in day care centers and in homosexual men support the idea that the mode of transmission is by fecal-oral contamination. From 1981 to 1986, 869 cases of cryptosporidiosis in AIDS patients were reported to the Centers for Disease Control (CDC; T. Peterman, personal communication). In a study conducted at St. Vincent's Hospital from 1981 to 1987, 58.9% of 147 cases of diarrhea caused by cryptosporidia occurred in homosexual or bisexual men (6). Another study showed a prevalence rate of 35% of AIDS patients in Haiti (2). Consequently, a diarrheal illness caused by cryptosporidia persisting for more than 1 month has been designated as an AIDS diagnosis by the CDC.

A partial list of the incidence of cryptosporidiosis in patients with diarrhea is shown in Table 1.

TABLE 1 Geographic Distribution of Cryptosporidiosis in Patients with Diarrhea

Location	Study dates	Patients tested	Number with cryptosporidia	Positive rate (%)
British Columbia	10/81-10/84	7300	46	0.6
Liverpool	6/83-4/84	1967	27	1.4[a]
Wales	8/84-3/85	500	7	1.4
Denmark	Spring 83	800	16	2.0
France	8/84-3/85	190	4	2.1[a]
London	9/83-2/84	213	7	3.2[a]
Thailand	1/85-6/85	410	13	3.2[a]
Australia	12/84-3/85	884	36	4.1
Costa Rica	1/82-12/82	278	12	4.3[a]
Bangladesh	1/84-5/84	578	25	4.3
Rwanda	10/83-1/84	293	23	7.8
Liberia		278	22	7.9[a]
Venezuela	3/84-4/83 & 5/84-9/84	120	13	10.8[a]
India	8/83-2/85	682	89	13.1[a]
New York City	4/81-5/87	1012	147	14.5[b]
New Zealand	12/84-3/85	36	8	22.0[a]
Spain		107	25	23.0
Haiti				35.0[c]

[a]In children. Refs. 1,5,6.
[b]58.9% in AIDS patients (all subjects were homosexual or bisexual men). 12.9% in non-AIDS patients.
[c]35% in AIDS patients.

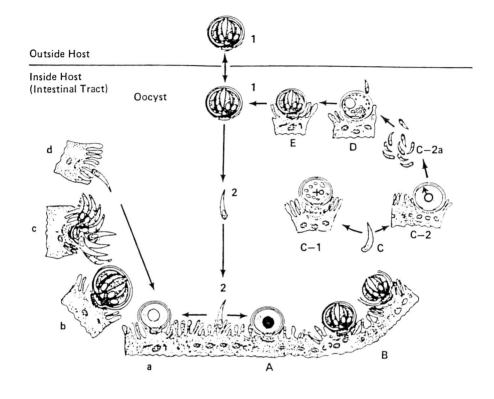

Outside Host

Inside Host
(Intestinal Tract)

Oocyst

	ASEXUAL		SEXUAL
1 —	Infective Oocyst	1 —	Infective Oocyst
2 —	Sporozoite	2 —	Sporozoite
a —	Trophozoite	A —	Trophozoite
b —	1st generation Meront	B —	2nd generation Meront
c —	1st generation Merozoite	C —	2nd generation Merozoite
d —	1st generation Merozoite	1 —	Macrogamont
	attached to microvill	2 —	Microgamont
		a —	Microgamete
		D —	Zygote
		E —	Sporulated Oocyst

FIGURE 2   Schematic life cycle of *Cryptosporidium* sp. [from Ma, P. (1987). In *Current Clinical Topics in Infectious Diseases*, Vol. 8. (Remington, J. S. and Swartz, M. N., eds.). McGraw-Hill Book Co., reproduced with permission of publisher].

The Causative Agent

The causative agent is *Cryptosporidium*; at least 20 species have been named (3) based on the assumption that *Cryptosporidium* is host-specific. Tzipori (1) postulated that the success of cross transmission of cryptosporidial oocysts between different mammals, including humans, is a strong evidence that there is only one species. Levine suggests that there are four species representing those for mammals, birds, reptiles, and fish. Recent cross-transmission studies suggest that isolates from mammals are generally infective for mammals and, similarly, isolates from avians are infective for avians, whereas avian-to-mammalian transmission has not been successful (1-3). The taxonomy of *Cryptosporidium* as related to other protozoans can be seen in Figure 1.

Life Cycle

The life cycle of cryptosporidia consists of alternating sexual and asexual reproduction, similar to that of *Plasmodium* (Fig. 2), with the following exception: the *Plasmodium* life cycle involves two hosts, man and mosquito, whereas in *Cryptosporidium* both cycles are completed within *one* host (monoxenous). Plasmodia parasitize erythrocytes; cryptosporidia infect the mucosal cells of the intestine, paraintestinal organs, such as the biliary tree (1-4, 7-9), the respiratory tract (10,11), the esophagus (12), and even the genital tract (13).

Asexual life cycle   The ingested oocyst (oval-spherical, double-walled structure, measuring 4 to 5 μm) contains four banana-shaped sporozoites, the *infective* stage. The sporozoites are liberated in the presence of trypsin and bile in the stomach and attach themselves by means of an electron-dense band (Fig. 3a) to the microvilli of the intestinal tract (Fig. 3b), preferably in

---

FIGURE 3   Endogenous stages of *Cryptosporidium* sp. in AIDS patients. (a) Histologic section of an autopsied duodenal section of an AIDS patient with intestinal cryptosporidiosis, showing numerous endogenous stages lining the microvilli of the host enterocytes. (b) Open lung biopsy specimen touch preparation showing four cryptosporidial oocysts (3 to 4 μm) inside macrophage. Minute red granules are visible in cytoplasm (Hemacolor, oil immersion lens, original mangification $\times$ 400) [from Ma, P. et al. *JAMA 252*:1298-1301, Sept. 1984. Copyright 1984, American Medical Association, with permission]. (c) Two type I meronts (ME-I) with eight merozoites. Cross-sectional view. Note the large size of this meront in comparison with the type II meronts shown in (d). [MV, microvilli (original magnification $\times$ 5400) EMU-3G RCA EM, Transmission EM]. (d) Two type II meronts (ME-II) with four merozoites. Both showed dense band (DB) attachment of the parasite to the enterocyte mucous membrane of the microvilli of the host [(original magnification $\times$ 5400), EMU-3G RCA EM, Transmission EM].

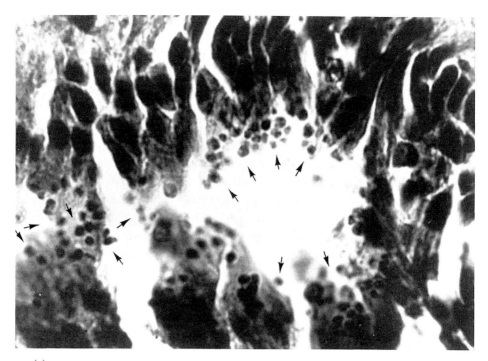

(a)

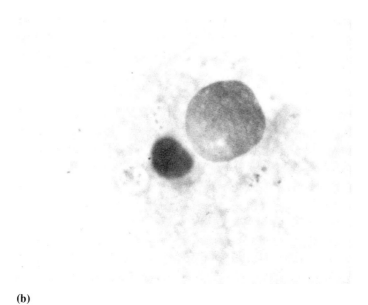

(b)
FIGURE 3

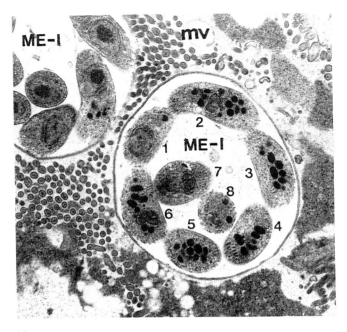

(c)

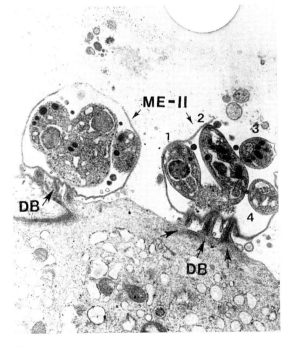

(d)

the small intestine. The surrounding microvilli remain uninfected. The parasite is regarded as intracellular, but extracytoplasmic, enclosed in a parasitophorus vacuole attached to the mucous membrane of the enterocytes and is not visible in the cytoplasm. All reproductive processes occur within the vacuole.

Asexual reproduction   In **merogony**, the *sporozoite* rounds up to become a *trophozoite* and undergoes asexual reproduction to produce a maximum

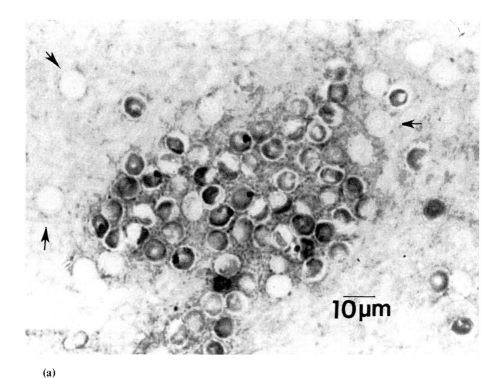

(a)

FIGURE 4   Various staining preparations of *Cryptosporidium* sp. from AIDS patients. (a) Direct stool preparation showing a large cluster of oocysts which stained red (acid-fast). Arrow, some are colorless because of over decolorization or they are young endogenous stages extruded in a case of explosive diarrhea [(original magnification ×250; bar = 10 μm) modified cold Kinyoun (MCK)-stained prep]. (b) Indirect immunofluorescent preparation of fecal oocysts showing green fluorescences [oil immersion lens (original magnification ×500; bar = 5 μm) Nikon Labophot with epifluorescent attachment]. (c) Sucrose flotation preparation showing numerous oocysts with a pink hue examined with a AO scope [high dry objective (original magnification ×500); bar = 5 μm).

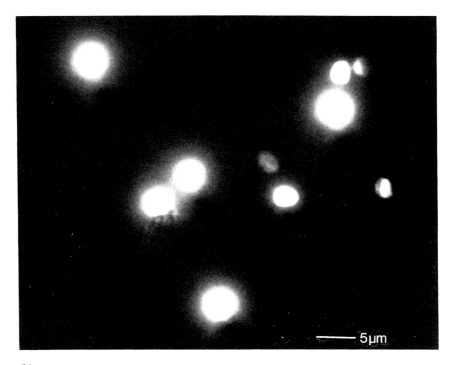

(b)

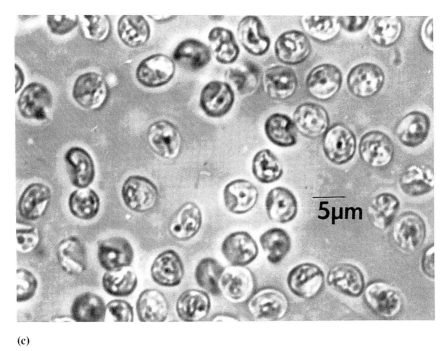

(c)

of eight first-generation (type 1) *merozoites* in the first-generation (type-1) *meront* (Fig. 3c). At maturity, the merozoites are liberated, and each of them attaches to an uninfected microvillus, and the cycle repeats itself. This may occur repeatedly in chronic infections.

Sexual reproduction   At some point in the life cycle, the trophozoite undergoes reproductions to form a maximum of four second-generation (type-2) *merozoites* inside a second-generation (type-2) *meront* that is *smaller* (Fig. 3d) than the type-1 meront (Fig. 3c). At maturity, these merozoites undergo **gametogony** and differentiate into *microgamonts* (male) and *macrogamonts* (female). The microgamont matures into a *microgametocyte* that gives rise to 14 *microgametes*, whereas the macrogamont develops into a *macrogamete*. Fertilization takes place between a microgamete and a macrogamete to form a *zygote*. When matured, a cyst wall is developed around the zygote and an *oocyst* is formed. This is the end of the sexual life cycle.

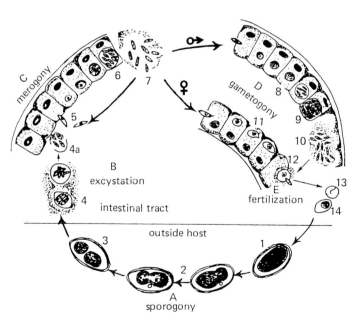

FIGURE 5   Schematic life cycle of *Isospora belli* [from: Ma, P. and Armstrong, D. (eds.) (1989). *AIDS and Infections of Homosexual Men*, 2nd ed. Boston, Butterworth Publishing, with permission].

Sporogony, the production of four sporozoites (sporulation) in the oocysts takes place inside the host. Unlike *Isospora*, there is no sporocyst surrounding the sporozoites. At maturity, the oocyst is extruded into the lumen of the intestine and is excreted, already in the *infective* stage, in stool specimens (Fig. 4). This differs from the *Isospora belli* oocyst, which is *not* infective until after the oocyst has been exposed in the environment for a short time (Figs. 5, and 6a,b) (14). This may explain why the incidence of cryptosporidiosis is so much higher than that of isosporiasis (15). The complete life cycle, from the ingestion of oocyst to the production of a new oocyst, takes approximately 3 to 5 days. In active infection, the number of oocysts detected in

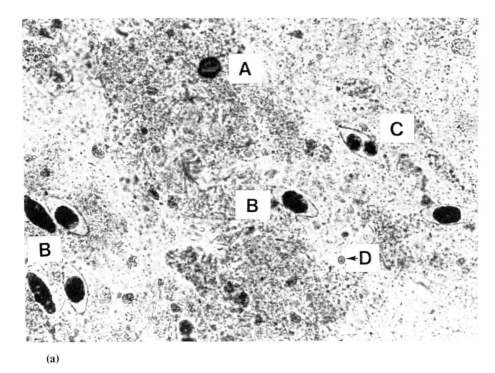

(a)

FIGURE 6 *Isospora belli*: Histologic section and stool preparations from AIDS patient. (a) Iodine preparation: *I. belli* oocyst: A. sporont, B. sporoblast, C. sporocyst, D. *Cryptosporidium* oocyst (unstained) (High-power objective). (b) Sucrose flotation preparation: Three *I. belli* oocysts (oil immersion lens; original magnification ×500). (c) Histologic preparation of jejunum showing endogenous stage of *I. belli* in the cytoplasm of the host enterocytes. (Hematoxylin and eosin; original magnification ×500).

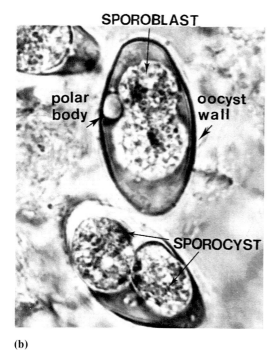

(b)

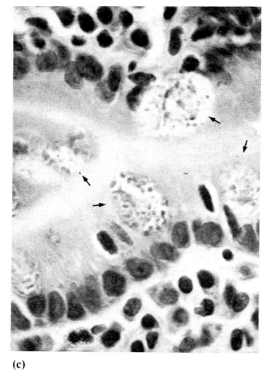

(c)

watery diarrheal stool can exceed 10^6/ml. In semisolid stool specimens, the number is much lower, and concentration procedures may be needed to detect them. However, even in active infection, the excretion of oocysts waxes and wanes. The oocysts are quite hardy and remain viable for weeks and months, especially when stored in 2.5% potassium dichromate at 4 °C. It is conceivable that they can easily be airborne in the environment.

Pathogenesis

The clinical presentation of active cryptosporidial infection, especially in AIDS-associated cryptosporidiosis, is voluminous watery diarrhea resembling cholera. This suggests that toxin may be the mechanism of pathogenesis. However, tests of stool filtrate have failed to demonstrate any enterotoxin. It appears that disruption of the physical barrier of the host intestinal mucous membrane by the endogenous stages of this parasite may be the cause of the tremendous fluid loss, as in secretory diarrhea.

Efforts to look at antibody response showed that individuals with AIDS-associated cryptosporidiosis lacked IgM and IgA, but they had low levels of IgG, whereas in the non-AIDS immunocompetent individuals, all three immunoglobulins were present (6). This leads to speculation that the lack of IgM, and especially IgA, may be related to the failure of the host to clear occysts. It is well known that secretory IgA plays a vital role in defensive mechanism of mucous membranes. Further evidence is noted in the low frequency of cryptosporidiosis in breastfed versus nonbreastfed infants in Haiti (15). Successful treatment of a child with AIDS-associated cryptosporidiosis, with hyperimmune bovine colostrum containing high concentration of IgA, was reported by Tzipori and associates in Australia (16). Leukocytes and erythrocytes are seldom detected in stool from patients with cryptosporidiosis. However, in respiratory cryptosporidiosis, the organisms have been found inside macrophages (10). Similarly, cryptosporidia are found in vaginal macrophages in experimental intrauterine infections of adult BALB/c mice (17). Whether or not the dissemination of the organism from the intestinal tract occurs via macrophage is of interest, but unknown.

Clinical Manifestations

Incubation times vary from 4 to 12 days in immunocompetent individuals (2). However, in immunocompromised patients, it is difficult to determine the incubation period. The major clinical manifestation of cryptosporidiosis, as in cholera, is watery nonbloody diarrhea, with fluid loss as high as 10 to 17 L/day documented in AIDS patients. Other symptoms may include abdominal pain, nausea, vomiting, bloating, anorexia, some fever, and headache (1-5). Cryptosporidiosis lacks any distinguishing features that would lead one to suspect the diagnosis. Manifestations of respiratory cryptosporidiosis include copious white sputum, sore throat, cough, and shortness of breath. A hoarse cry has been recently reported in a case of an infant with AIDS-associated laryngotracheitis caused by cryptosporidia (18). Involvement of the liver and a calculous cholecystitis may be manifested by right-upper quadrant pain and elevation in the liver function tests, particularly the alkaline phosphatase values (7,9). Disseminated cryptosporidiosis has been reported in a newborn with double immune deficiency (19) and in an AIDS patient with simultaneous multiple-systems involvement of the pancreatic-biliary, respiratory, and gastrointestinal tracts (8). Mixed infections of cryptosporidiosis with CMV and other opportunists are frequently seen in AIDS patients.

Diagnosis

Diagnostic Procedures

Before the AIDS epidemic, stool examination for oocyst to diagnose cryptosporidiosis was known; hence, radiographic evaluation followed by intestinal biopsy, was the standard procedure for diarrhea of unknown origin. Inflammatory changes in the mucosa of the small bowel, ranging from subtle to marked, and narrowing and irregularity of the gastric antrum with possible ulceration, were noted in patients with cryptosporidiosis on barium study and computed tomography (20). Endoscopy may prove useful in diagnosing the disease in cases of esophageal, laryngotrachael cryptosporidiosis (12). Rarely is an intestinal biopsy necessary to establish a diagnosis since the introduction of stool examination for oocysts.

Laboratory Diagnosis

Cryptosporidial oocysts have been demonstrated in specimens other than stool, including duodenal aspirates, bile, sputum, and biopsy specimens of gallbladder, lung, common bile duct, pancreas, liver, esophagus, pharynx, and rectum. In patients with intestinal cryptosporidiosis, possible involvement of these sites should be considered if there are symptoms of pneumonia, hepatitis, cholecystitis, or biliary tract disease.

Stool examination The three-step stool examination (21,22) was initiated primarily to incorporate the acid-fast stain and sucrose flotation tests into the iodine smear examination. The latter is normally performed in the clinical parasitology laboratory to detect amebic trophozoites and cysts. Other tests available include the auramine rhodamine stain (a fluorochrome stain) routinely used in detecting acid-fast bacilli; 21,22), and recently, the indirect fluorescent antibody method using a monoclonal antibody (23). The acid-fast stain procedure is easily available in most clinical mycobacteriology laboratories. Many versions of the methods have been published. St. Vincent's Hospital used the modified cold kinyoun (MCK) method (21,22), simple because it is rapid, requiring only 1 min with the Kinyoun stain incorporated with a surface-acting agent (Tergitol). Because numerous materials in a stool smear will take up the stain, a strong decolorizer (10% H_2SO_4) is then used to provide a clean background for the counterstain. One must be careful not to over decolorize the smear because the oocysts can lose their acid-fast character. For those who have worked with cryptosporidia, it is not difficult to detect the minute protozoan, even in an iodine-stained preparation, because it remains unstained, whereas yeast, although morphologically similar, will stain brown. The oocysts also present a greenish, glassy appearance. Another rapid way to identify the oocysts is to prepare a sucrose smear with 1 drop of the liquid stool and 1 drop of sucrose solution on a slide and examine it under a coverslip under a bright-field microscope (40 × objective). With the AO microscope (Nikon microscope), the oocysts are easily detected as pink structures, immediately below the coverslip, as they tend to float to the top of the sucrose, whereas yeasts do not appear pink (22). Although the auramine rhodamine stain is used by some laboratories, some oocysts fail to be stained and will not be visible on the preparation. The advantage of the MCK technique is the ability to keep a permanent record of smears for future reference in treatment. Even though some oocysts fail to pick up the stain, they are still visible whether the unstained structures (see Fig. 4a) are decolorized oocysts or immature endogenous stages that normally are not acid-fast. When the volume of specimens is high, an automated system using the MIDAS II (EM Diagnostic, Inc.) can be programmed to stain 20 slides simultaneously. The results are consistent and provide a clean, green background to allow easy detection of the red (acid-fast) oocysts. An indirect immunofluorescent monoclonal antibody test has been used to screen suspected population in outbreaks of cryptosporidiosis; however, it does cross-react with some other coccidia. Other drawbacks are the requirement for a fluorescent scope and that permanent smears will not be available for future reference.

Biopsy Presently, a biopsy is rarely required because the diagnosis can be made so easily and rapidly with stool examination. The exception will be in complications involving specific organs, such as the gallbladder (7), the common bile duct (8), the liver (9), or the esophagus (12). Very rarely, the stool examination is negative and the biopsy is positive; more often, the opposite is true because lesions can be focal, and the biopsy may not be representative. By using a hematoxylin and eosin preparation of intestinal biopsy specimens, blunting, shortening and fusion of microvilli are commonly observed, along with reduction of the crypt/villi height ratio. Minute amphophilic organisms (2 to 3 μm), representing various endogenous stages of the parasite, are usually seen embedded along the microvillous surface of the small-intestinal villous epithelia or within the glycocalyx overlying the intestinal epithelial surface and lining the glands (19).

No special stain is needed for identification of the minute endogenous stage that lines the mucous membrane, even though stains such as toluidine blue and the indirect fluorescent antibody test have been used. Acid-fast staining is not helpful in detecting the oocysts in histologic section. Because only matured oocysts are acid-fast, and most of them would already have been extruded into the lumen of the intestine and lost during processing, it is crucial to make touch preparation of tissue to secure the oocysts before they are lost during histologic processing.

Respiratory cryptosporidiosis (10,11,19) has been reported as complications of intestinal cryptosporidiosis. The endogenous stages of cryptosporidia have been demonstrated lining the bronchiolar epithelial mucosal cells (11,19), and oocysts have been seen in open-lung biopsy (10; see Fig. 3b), sputum (10), and tracheal aspirates (18). Biliary involvement usually presents with right upper-quadrant pain (7). The organism can be demonstrated using the Enterotest to obtain duodenal aspirate or by biopsy (2,21,22). Disseminated infection with gallbladder and liver involvement has been recently reported. Examination of the gallbladder reveals luminal exudates, focal mucosal ulceration, and diffuse mucosal edema with marked subacute and chronic inflammation. Organisms are visible lining the gallbladder mucosa. The liver biopsy reveals subacute pericholangitis, and numerous cryptosporidia can be seen attached to the epithelium of the large bile duct (8,9,19).

Serology Cryptosporidial serology can be carried out using indirect fluorescent antibody test (6) or the enzyme-linked immunoassay (ELISA) (3) to demonstrate a fourfold rise in titer in active infection. Both procedures used fecal oocysts as the antigen. A 4-year study of patients with AIDS-associated cryptosporidiosis at St. Vincent's Hospital in New York City shows that the AIDS patients generate low IgG antibody response. A fourfold rise is usually not demonstrated, except in some ARC patients with smaller degrees of immunodeficiency. For the indirect fluorescent antibody test, a 1:10 is the low level of positivity. The IgM titer appears within 7 days after the onset of symptoms and disappears within 1 to 2 months, whereas the IgG titer usually rises to high levels within 3 to 4 months. Serologic tests can be helpful in diagnosing active infection by demonstrating a change of titers in immunocompetent individuals. Unfortunately, none of these tests are now commercially available.

Modes of Transmission

Before the AIDS epidemic, it was believed that cryptosporidiosis was primarily a zoonosis. However, there are now numerous reports of cryptosporidiosis without any animal contact. The most common mode of transmission is probably person to person by the oral-fecal route (including fecal-oral contamination occurring during sexual activity), as one sees in outbreaks in day care centers, within families, and among homosexual and bisexual men. The number of AIDS-associated cryptosporidiosis cases has declined recently along with cases of other sexually transmitted diseases such as gonorrhea. They may have reversed the prevalence trend of this parasitic infection because no case was detected in a small study conducted in healthy homosexual men last year in New York Blood Center (24). On the other hand, one may conclude that the prevalence is high in homosexual men simply because they are exposed to fecal environment in bath houses or in group activities. A 4-year study at St. Vincent's Hospital indicated that travel to tropical endemic areas by this group was highly associated with contracting cryptosporidiosis (25). Adequate indirect evidence in outbreaks involving large communities indicates that water or milk may be the common source.

Cases of respiratory cryptosporidiosis have been reported as a complication of intestinal cryptosporidiosis. It is difficult to determine if the pulmonary infection is an extension of the primary intestinal source through macrophages, because the organism is not invasive. On the other hand, in turkeys, respiratory infections occur without intestinal involvement. It is conceivable that inhalation of the oocysts is the mode of transmission. The recent report of a perinatal infection of a newborn infant with cryptosporidia (13) simulates experimental perinatal transmission in mice. Finally, contact with animal feces is also an important mode of transmission.

Treatment

In immunocompetent individuals, the diarrhea usually lasts from 1 to 2 weeks, never more than 4 weeks. In immunocompromised persons, such as those with hypogammaglobulinemia, transplantation patients, and AIDS, the infection is devastating and may be fatal. A total of 79 antimicrobials or immunomodulators have been used with unfavorable results (2,26). In some patients with leukemia, there has been a favorable response to spiramycin (27). A recent report of three cases of AIDS treated with hyperimmune bovine colostrum containing high levels of IgG is the most encouraging report in the realm of treatment (17; S. Tzipori, personal communication). St. Vincent's Hospital is currently offering this mode of treatment now (28).

Prevention

As with all other enteric pathogens, infection may be prevented simply by practicing good hygiene with enteric precautions such as handwashing and proper disposal of contaminated material in the hospital setting. The practice of safe sex is probably important in preventing infections in homosexual and bisexual individuals. For the immunocompromised person visiting endemic tropical countries, contact with infected animals or humans should be avoided. Formalin, ammonia, and full-strength sodium hypocholorite have been used to disinfect contaminated materials in the clinical laboratory (1-3).

ISOSPORA BELLI

Isospora belli is another coccidial protozoan (see Fig. 1) that is very rare in the United States. Unlike the genus *Cryptosporidium*, *I. belli* has been known for many years as a parasite acquired from endemic tropical countries, although a few sporadic cases had been detected in institutional populations. With the advent of the AIDS epidemic, the infection has been diagnosed in an increasing number of AIDS patients. However, it still remains as an unusual, rare parasitic infection. Isosporiasis, persistent for more than a month, is regarded by CDC as diagnostic of AIDS.

Epidemiology

Unlike *Cryptosporidium*, the geographic and species distributions of *I. belli* are not known. There is an increased prevalence of this parasite in AIDS patients (15,29,30). We first diagnosed this infection in two homosexual men within the same week in 1981 (14). One had a travel history to endemic areas, and the other probably acquired it in a bath house (both patients frequented bath houses in New York City). The incidence of this parasitic infection is much lower than cryptosporidiosis. In our study, the diagnosis was made in only eight cases compared with 147 cases of cryptosporidiosis in the same period (2). The highest prevalence is from Haiti: among patients with diarrhea, 80 (61%) had *I. belli*, 60 (46%) had cryptosporidiosis, and an additional five (4%) had both infections (27%). In contrast, only 20 cases of isospora infection in 14,519 AIDS patients (< 0.2%) were reported to CDC by November 1985. Part of this low incidence probably resulted from underreporting and underdiagnosing. In AIDS patients, it can be diagnosed as a single infection (15,30) or in combination with cryptosporidial infection (12,29). It has been reported in other immunocompromised hosts (31) such as patients with T-cell lymphoma.

Even though *Isospora* oocysts are 10 times as large as the cryptosporidial oocysts, the former are not easily detected in stool specimens unless specific concentration procedures, such as sugar flotation, are carried out.

Causative Agent

There is only one species of *Isospora*, *I. belli*, that is pathogenic for humans. The life cycle is depicted in Figure 5. It is essentially the same as shown for

Cryptosporidium (see Fig. 2) with the following exceptions: the I. belli oocyst is ellipsoidal measuring 22 to 33 μm by 10 to 19 μm (Fig. 6b). The mature oocyst is characterized by two spherical sporocysts within which are four sporozoites. Oocysts excreted in the stool are unsporulated and, hence, not infectious until sporulation takes place outside of the host (16,312). The life cycle also consists of alternating asexual and sexual life cycles that are completed in one host, as with Cryptosporidium. The oocyst with enclosed sporocysts is the infective form. The life cycle starts with ingestion of oocysts, followed by excystation, merogony, gametogony, fertilization, zygote formation, and oocyst excretion, followed by sporogony outside the host (Fig. 5).

Asexual Reproduction

Sporogony   The immature oocyst is represented by the sporont, which consists of a mass of granules. The mass of granules increases in size, and undergoes sporulation to form the sporoblast, which undergoes several additional divisions to form two sporocysts each of which produces four sporozoites, the infectious stage (Figs. 6a,b). Excystation occurs in the stomach in the presence of bile and trypsin. The liberated sporozoites infect gastrointestinal epithelial cells by penetrating the cytoplasm; all of the reproductive processes take place within the parasitophorus vacuole. The parasite is intracytoplasmic; hence, it is different from Cryptosporidium which is extracytoplasmic.

Merogony   The sporozoite transforms into a trophozoite, which undergoes several asexual divisions to give rise to merozoites in the meront. The number of divisions is unknown. At maturity, the merozoites are liberated and each invades other uninfected cells, and the cycle repeats itself as in chronic infections.

Sexual Reproduction

Gametogony   At some time, the merozoites differentiate into microgamont (male) and macrogamont (female). The microgamont develops into a microgametocyte which produces microgametes, whereas the macrogamont develops into a macrogamete. Fertilization takes place between a microgamete and macrogamete to form a zygote. A cyst wall is formed around the zygote to become the oocyst. At maturity, the oocyst is extruded into the lumen of the intestine and finds its way in the stool as the sporont, the unsporulated oocyst. Sporogony takes place and the cycle repeats itself.

Pathogenesis

Nothing is known about the diarrhea associated with I. belli. It causes diarrhea and malabsorption similar to cryptosporidia, and chronic infection lasting for years has been reported.

Clinical Manifestations

Patients with isospora infection usually have severe diarrhea and steator-rhea. Nausea, vomiting, colicky abdominal pain, fever, headache, anorexia, flatulence, and weight loss may also be seen. The stool varies from watery to semisolid and from light clay to light brown. It is characterized by a high fat content, and numerous Charcot-Leyden crystals are detected in some cases. In humans, the latency period (ingestion of oocyst to the appearance of unsporulated oocyst in the stool) is known to be 7 to 10 days, and the clinical illness (oocyst excretion) lasts from a few days to several weeks. In AIDS patients, the diarrhea persists as with cryptosporidiosis.

Modes of Transmission

Like cryptosporidia, the most common mode of transmission is oral-fecal. *Isospora belli* is a human pathogen, and there are no reports of transmission of the oocysts from humans to other mammals. There are multiple *Isospora* species associated with animal diseases; however, there is no report of a human acquiring the illness by animal contact, as with cryptosporidiosis.

Laboratory Diagnosis

Before the AIDS epidemic, the frequency of a positive stool examination for *I. belli* was very low. Careful examination of serially sectioned suction biopsies of small-bowel mucosa and of intestinal contents gave excellent results in 19 patients (33). The pathology of the small-bowel mucosa varied; none had a normal mucosa. Some showed flat mucosa, others revealed tall villi. Various endogenous stages could be identified in the H and E preparation (Fig. 6c) but colophonium Giemsa stain offered improved staining characteristics. The periodic acid-Schiff (PAS)-positive schizonts may be mistaken for goblet cells. All endogenous stages were located within the parasitophorus vacuole located within the cytoplasm of the host cell. *Isospora belli* oocysts can be detected with the three-step stool examination used for detecting cryptosporidia (21,22). The stool is usually greasy with undigested foods. Mucus and Charcot-Leyden crystals may be present, whereas fecal leukocytes are usually absent. The ellipsoidal oocysts measure 22 to 33 μm by 10 to 19 μm. In freshly passed stool specimens, the immature stage, sporoblast should predominate (see Figs. 6a,b). If the specimen is allowed to stand at room temperature, one will encounter other stages such as the sporoblast, and the matured sporoblast undergoing divisions to form two sporocysts (see Figs. 6a,b). It is important to examine the specimen while it is fresh because one may ingest animal *Isospora* species in the sporocyst stage resulting in a spurious diagnosis. The contents of the oocyst stain brown with D'Antoni iodine;

red to pink (acid-fast) with MCK (32), and have a pink hue with sucrose flotation technique. Although the oocysts can be concentrated by the standard formalin-ether procedure, sucrose flotation not only gives a better yield but a better morphologic definition. Periodically, the oocysts appear distorted when stained with iodine or acid-fast stain and are difficult to identify. No serologic test is available.

Treatment

Immunocompetent patients with isosporaisis usually respond well to treatment. The first two homosexual men treated at St. Vincent's Hospital had a good response to quinacrine, 100 mg three times a day (15). One patient showed dramatic response within 8 days, and the consecutive stool examinations showed drastic reduction of oocysts over a period of 10 days. On the other hand, the second patient failed to have negative stool specimens until he was treated for 2-½ weeks (21). Trimethoprim-sulfamethoxazole given to 15 Haitian patients resulted in cessation of diarrhea in 2 days (29). In AIDS patients, recurrence is frequent. Cholecystectomy in one AIDS patient led to cessation of diarrhea, indicating that the gallbladder may have been the reservoir of the infection. Other antimicrobial agents that have been used successfully are metronidazole and pyrimethamine-sulfadiazine, whereas treatment with tetracycline, ampicillin, nitrofurantoin, and quinacrine are reported to be unsatisfactory (34).

REFERENCES

1. Tzipori, S. (1983). Cryptosporidiosis in animals and humans. *Microbiol. Rev. 47*: 84-96.
2. Ma, P. (1987). Cryptosporidiosis and immune enteropathy: A review. In *Current Clinical Topics in Infectious Diseases*, Vol. 8. (Remington, J. S. and Swartz, M. N., eds.). New York, McGraw-Hill, pp. 99-153.
3. Fayer, R. and Ungar, B. L. P. (1986). *Cryptosporidium* spp. and cryptosporidiosis. *Microbiol. Rev. 50*:458-483.
4. Janoff, E. N. and Reller, L. B. (1987). *Cryptosporidium* species, a protean protozoan. *J. Clin. Microbiol. 25*:967-975.
5. Navin, T. R. (1985). Cryptosporidiosis in humans; review of recent epidemiologic studies. *Eur. J. Epidemiol. 1*:77-83.
6. Ma, P. and Tsaihong, J. Immune response of AIDS and non-AIDS individuals to *Cryptosporidium*. Session 72. Abstr. 822. *Proc. 27th Intersci. Conf. Antimicrob. Agents Chemother.* October 1987. New York, New York.
7. Blumberg, R. S., Kelsey, P., Perrone, T., Perrone, R., Dickersin, R., Laquaglia, M., and Ferruci, J. (1984). Cytomegalovirus- and *Cryptosporidium*-associated acalculous gangrenous cholecystitis. *Am. J. Med. 76*:1118-1123.

8. Gross, T. L., Wheat, J., Bartlett, M., and O'Connor, W. (1986). AIDS and multiple system involvement with *Cryptosporidium. Am. J. Gastroenterol. 81*: 456-458.

9. Kahn, D. G., Garfinkle, J. M., Klonoff, D. C., Pembrook, L. J., and Morrow, D. F. (1987). Cryptosporidial and cytomegaloviral hepatitis and cholecystitis. *Arch. Pathol. Lab. Med. 111* (in press).

10. Ma, P., Villanueva, G., Kaufman, D., and Gillooley, J. F. (1984). Respiratory cryptosporidiosis in the acquired immune deficiency syndrome. Use of modified cold Kinyoun and Hemacolor stains for rapid diagnoses. *JAMA 252*:1298-1301.

11. Forgacs, P., Tarshis, A., Ma, P., Federman, M., Mele, L., Silverman, M. L., and Shea, J. A. (1983). Intestinal and bronchial cryptosporidiosis in an immunodeficient homosexual man. *Ann. Intern. Med. 99*:793-794.

12. Kazlow, P. G., Kumudini, S., Benkov, K. J., Dische, R., and LeLeiko, N. S. (1986). Esophageal cryptosporidiosis in a child with acquired immune deficiency syndrome. *Gastroenterology 91*:1301-1303.

13. Lahdevirta, J., Jokipii, A. M., Sammalkorpi, L., and Jokipii, L. (1987). Perinatal infection with *Cryptosporidium* and failure to thrive [Letter]. *Lancet 1*: 48-49.

14. Ma, P., Kaufman, D., and Montana, J. (1984). *Isospora belli* diarrheal infection in homosexual men. *AIDS Res. 1*:327-338.

15. Pape, J. W., Levine, E., Beaulieu, M. E., Marshall, F., Verdier, R., and Johnson, W. D., Jr. (1987). Cryptosporidiosis in Haitian children. *Am. J. Trop. Med. Hyg. 36*:333-337.

16. Tzipori, S., Robertson, D., and Chapman, C. (1980). Remission of diarrhea due to *Cryptosporidiosis* in an immunodeficient child treated with hyperimmune bovine colostrum. *Br. Med. J. 293*:1276-1277.

17. Liebler, E. M., Pohlenz, J. F., and Woodmansee, D. B. (1986). Experimental intrauterine infection of adult BALB/c mice with *Cryptosporidium* sp. *Infect. Immun. 54*:25-259.

18. Harari, M. D., West, B., and Dwyer, B. (1986). *Cryptosporidium* as cause of laryngotracheitis in an infant. *Lancet 1*:1207-1986.

19. Kocoshis, S. A. (1986). Diagnosis and treatment of cryptosporidiosis in children. *Compr. Ther. 12*:56-61.

20. Soulen, M. C., Fishman, E. K., Scatarige, J. C., Huchins, D., and Zerhouni, E. A. (1986). Cryptosporidiosis of the gastric antrum: Detection using CT. *Radiology 159*:705-706.

21. Ma, P. and Soave, R. (1983). Three-step stool examination for cryptosporidiosis in 10 homosexual men with protracted watery diarrhea. *J. Infect. Dis. 147*: 824-828.

22. Ma, P. (1986). *Cryptosporidium*—biology and diagnosis. In *Infections in the Immunocompromised Host.* (Actor, P., Evangelista, A., Poupard, J., and Hinks, E., eds.). New York, Plenum, pp. 135-152.

23. Garcia, L. S., Brewer, T. C., and Bruckner, D. A. (1987). Fluorescence detection of *Cryptosporidium* oocysts in human fecal specimens by using monoclonal antibodies. *J. Clin. Microbiol. 25*:119-121.

24. Chaissom, M. A., Vermund, S. H., Ma, P., Guigli, P. E., and Stevens, C. E. (1985). A prevalence survey for *Cryptosporidium* and other parasites in healthy homosexual men in New York City. In *Abstr. 33rd Annu. Meet. Am. Soc. Trop. Med. Hyg.* Abstr. 203.

25. Ma, P., Vermund, S., Tsaihong, J., Bunin, J. R., Lehman, S., and Kaufman, D. A prospective study of cryptosporidiosis in the greater New York area. Travel to warm climate countries as a risk factor for *Cryptosporidium* in men with AIDS. (submitted for publication).

26. Rolston, K. V. I. and Fainstein, V. (1986). Cryptosporidiosis [Editorial]. *Eur. J. Clin. Microbiol.* *5*:135-137.

27. CDC (1982). Cryptosporidiosis. Assessment of chemotherapy of males with acquired immune deficiency syndrome (AIDS). *MMWR 31*:598.

28. Nord, J., Ma, P., Tacket, C. O., Dijohn, D., Tzipori, S., Sahner, D., and Shieb, G. Treatment of AIDS associated cryptosporidiosis with hyperimmune colostrum from cows vaccinated with *Cryptosporidium.* Submitted to VI International Congress on AIDS, Montreal, 1989.

29. DeHovitz, J. A., Pape, J. W., Boncy, M., and Johnson, W., Jr. (1986). Clinical manifestations and therapy of *Isospora belli* infection in patients with the acquired immunodeficiency syndrome. *N. Engl. J. Med. 315*:87-90.

30. Forthal, D. N. and Guest, S. S. (1984). *Isospora belli* enteritis in three homosexual men. *Am. J. Trop. Med. Hyg. 33*:1060-1064.

31. Kitsukawa, K., Kamihira, S., Kinoshita, K. et al. (1981). An autopsy case T-cell lymphoma associated with disseminated varicella and malabsorption syndrome due to *Isospora belli* infection. *Rinsho Ketsueki 22*:258-265.

32. Ma, P., and Marsden, P. Cryptosporidiosis, isosporidia and microsporidia. In Ma, P., and Armstrong, D. (eds). *AIDS and Infections of Homosexual Men*, 2nd ed. Boston, Butterworths Inc.

33. Brandborg, L. L., Goldberg, S. B., and Breidenbach, W. C. (1970). Human coccidiosis—a possible cause of malabsorption: The life cycle in small-bowel mucosal biopsies as a diagnostic feature. *N. Engl. J. Med. 283*:1306-1313.

34. Trier, J. S., Moxey, P. C., Schimmel, E. M., and Robles, E. (1976). Chronic intestinal coccidiosis in man: Intestinal morphology and response to treatment. *Gastroenterology 66*:923-935.

20
Ameba and Giardia Infections

Carolyn Petersen, *University of California and San Francisco General Hospital, San Francisco, California*

Sexual transmission of enteric protozoa among homosexual men was reported in 1967 in New York City (1). Since then an epidemic of amebiasis and giardiasis has been amply documented in this population (2-10). A similar epidemic has not occurred in other AIDS risk groups. The prevalence of enteric infection in homosexual men has been correlated with a history of oral-anal contact and multiple sexual partners (11).

In studies from Sweden, Germany, Canada, England, and the United States, stool samples from symptomatic and asymptomatic homosexual men have revealed *Entamoeba histolytica* prevalence rates of 21% to 36% (12-14). Over half of infected individuals are asymptomatic. Some authors have stressed the benign course of amebiasis in the homosexual male and have questioned the need for treatment of the asymptomatic patient (12). Others have urged caution because of unsettled questions in our understanding of this disease (15) or have argued that subtle symptoms may indeed be due to *E. histolytica* and may respond to treatment (16). Still others suggest that untreated amebiasis may stimulate the immune system and may accelerate progression of human immunodeficiency virus (HIV) infection (17-19).

The prevalence of giardiasis in homosexual males has been reported as 4% to 18% (2,7-11,20). As in amebiasis, a large proportion of infected persons are asymptomatic. Unsuspected giardiasis, especially at extremes of age, may cause malnutrition and diarrhea and be very difficult to diagnose (21). However, the presence of unsuspected giardiasis in patients with the acquired immunodeficiency syndrome (AIDS) has not been reported and is probably very unusual. Indeed, there are no published series of amebiasis or giardiasis in AIDS or in HIV-positive patients and no indications that their clinical course or treatment varies from that in the general population. Experience at San Francisco General Hospital is in agreement with this observation.

Entamoeba histolytica and *Giardia lamblia* exist in two stages in the host, the motile and infectious trophozoite and the environmentally resistant cyst. The cyst is ingested, excysts in the upper gastrointestinal tract and forms trophozoites. Trophozoites of giardia localize mainly in the duodenum and upper small intestine; those of ameba in the colon.

In considering enteric protozoal infection in AIDS patients and homosexual men, as well as the general population, three points must be considered.

1. Pathogenic protozoa do not always produce symptoms in infected persons.
2. Asymptomatic persons may serve as reservoirs for protozoal infection.
3. Finding a pathogenic protozoan is not proof that it is causing the patient's symptoms.

AMEBIASIS

Pathophysiology

Worldwide, E. histolytica prevalence has been estimated at 500 million; however, only about 10% of these cases, predominantly in the tropics, are associated with invasive disease (22,23). Geographic differences in invasiveness (i.e., the propensity to penetrate the gastrointestinal mucosa or to metastasize to other organs) are marked; in Mexico one of five infections is estimated to be invasive, compared with only 1 of 100 to 1000 infections in temperate areas (22). Although host factors may modify invasiveness somewhat, current research indicates that the virulent parasite has special adherence properties, is capable of contact-dependent cytolysis and erythrophagocytosis, and elaborates proteolytic and toxic products (22).

The virulence of *E. histolytica* has also been correlated with isoenzyme patterns (zymodemes). The electromobility of several isoenzymes, hexokinase, and phosphoglucomutase, differ between isolates of *E. histolytica* from asymptomatic carriers with negative serology and symptomatic patients with positive serology, and these enzymes have been used as markers to differentiate pathogenic (virulent) and nonpathogenic (nonvirulent) strains (24,25). Using zymodemes defined in this way, Peter Sargeaunt and his co-workers (12) have never found a nonpathogen and pathogen together in any single host. In long-term in vitro culture studies, they saw no switch in isoenzyme pattern. Pathogenic zymodemes have been isolated from patients with mild or no clinical disease (26), and these individuals may be an important reservoir, or they may go on to develop clinical disease. In one large study from South Africa, 10% of the population had *E. histolytica* infection, but only 1% of asymptomatic individuals had amebas with pathogenic zymodemes (27). The World Health Organization has recommended that asymptomatic cyst passers in endemic areas not be treated because of the large numbers of infected persons and the generally benign course of infection in this group (28). In the male homosexual population, venereal transmission by the fecal-oral route also leads to a high prevalence of this organism, with many asymptomatic infections. However, many health authorities in the United States, including the Centers for Disease Control (CDC), recommend treatment of homosexuals because of the unsettled questions of conversion of nonpathogenic ameba to virulent forms and the large reservoir of infected individuals (29,30). Sargeaunt has suggested that zymodeme patterns are stable markers and could be used to determine which patients with ameba in their stools require treatment (31); however, this is currently impractical, as the test is still considered a research procedure.

Recently, Mirelman has reported (23,32) that a cloned culture of a nonpathogenic strain, when grown under axenic conditions, could switch to a pathogenic isoenzyme pattern with an associated increase in virulence of the ameba as assayed by their ability to induce hepatic abscesses in hamsters. When the newly converted pathogenic trophozoites were reassociated and cultured with the bacterial flora that accompanied trophozoites in the original xenic culture, reconversion to a nonpathogenic zymodeme occurred. Mirelman's observations that culture conditions and associated bacterial flora can cause changes in the zymodeme and virulence of a cloned ameba isolate raise the possibility of such changes occurring in vivo. This possibility has not yet been documented, and the clinical relevance of zymodeme typing remains uncertain. Further knowledge of the frequency of these conversions, what regulates them, and whether they are phenotypic or genotypic may allow us to more rationally decide which patients harboring ameba are at risk for disease and are likely to benefit from pharmacologic intervention.

Sargeaunt et al. (33) analyzed the zymodemes of 52 strains of ameba isolated from homosexual men from England and found no invasive isoenzyme patterns. In the United States, a further 18 isolates from homosexual men with gastrointestinal symptoms were analyzed by the CDC (30) and were found to be nonpathogenic. A serologic survey in Los Angeles (34) revealed an indirect hemagglutination (IHA) titer > 1:128 in 5.7% of asymptomatic homosexual men, although the prevalence of *E. histolytica* infection was 27.1%. Thus, the prevalence of virulent amebiasis in homosexual men in the developed Western world is very low. However, the introduction of a pathogenic zymodeme into an urban homosexual population could be clinically significant in the future (30). Serologic data from Italy suggests that potentially invasive strains do infect asymptomatic homosexual men in areas where invasive disease is more common than in England or the United States. Twenty-one percent of 138 asymptomatic homosexual men were serologically positive compared with 1% to 2% of controls (35). Occasional sexual transmission of virulent amebiasis has been documented (13).

Clinical Presentation

Most ameba-infected persons experience no symptoms. Some have mild symptoms consisting of loose diarrheal stools and abdominal discomfort. Because rates of cyst excretion in symptomatic and asymptomatic homosexual men may be similar (3), it is difficult to ascribe mild gastrointestinal symptoms in a given homosexual man to intestinal amebiasis with certainty. Trophozoites may be seen in both of these populations, but typically they are not numerous. A much smaller number of patients have more severe colonic disease with bloody diarrhea, volume depletion, and fever. Presence of motile hematophagous trophozoites on stool examination is a hallmark of this group. Bowel perforation, peritonitis, and ameboma formation may complicate severe intestinal disease. Uncommonly, fistula formation from the rectocolon to the perineum or a chronic irritable bowel syndrome, called postdysenteric ulcerative colitis, develops (36). Extragastrointestinal disease, particularly hepatic abscess, with or without pleural or pericardial disease, may occur (37).

Severe amebiasis (hepatic abscess or severe colitis with perforation) has been reported in only a few homosexual men (13,38-40) and has not been reported in AIDS patients. Amebiasis of the penis may be acquired through homosexual contact with an infected male (41). This lesion is rare and may be mistaken for a penile carcinoma.

Diagnosis

The diagnosis of amebic infection requires demonstration of ameba in the stools or of antibody in serum samples. Examination of fresh stool or an endoscopically obtained sample diluted with saline may demonstrate amebic cysts in patients with asymptomatic carriage, mildly symptomatic or severe gastrointestinal disease, but motile hematophagous (containing RBCs) trophozoites are a feature of severe disease (42) and are considered to be a characteristic of virulent, highly invasive strains of ameba (22). Trophozoites that are not hematophagous may be found whenever there is infection, even in the patient who in the literature has been designated as an asymptomatic cyst passer. This term has little clinical significance and is better replaced with the category of asymptomatic infection.

A high degree of observer skill is required to detect and speciate ameba in stool samples. Yield is maximized when a fresh (voided within 20 min), rather than refrigerated or preserved, specimen is examined and when multiple samples are obtained on separate days. The fresh specimen is examined by direct saline wet mount, as well as by iron hematoxylin- or trichrome-stained smear. Increased sensitivity can be achieved by using stool concentration techniques such as merthiolate-iodine-formalin (42). A large number of substances in stool, including tetracycline, sulfonamides, antiprotozoal drugs, castor and mineral oils, magnesium hydroxide, barium sulfate, enemas, and bismuth and kaolin compounds may interfere with stool examination for parasites (42).

Serologic diagnosis is routinely employed in invasive extragastrointestinal disease, most notably amebic hepatic abscess. It may also be of benefit in symptomatic gastrointestinal disease when stool examination has not been helpful because of interfering substances (14). Commonly available serologic tests include indirect hemagglutination (IHA), counterimmunoelectrophoresis (CIE), and agar gel diffusion (AGD) tests. The IHA test is considered the reference standard. If a titer of 1:256 or greater is considered positive, this test is the most sensitive (43). High titers can persist for a long period; therefore, its usefulness in the diagnosis of acute amebiasis is diminished, particularly in persons from an endemic area. Agar gel diffusion tests become negative in more than 65% of patients within 6 months of infection, whereas the IHA may remain positive up to 20 years in invasive disease (43). The presence of reactive bands in the CIE and AGD tests correlates with an IHA higher than 1:256 (43). Patients with right upper-quadrant or pleuropulmonary disease with intestinal amebiasis, or at risk for amebiasis, should have computed tomography (CT) or ultrasonographic imaging of the liver to look for an hepatic abscess.

Treatment

Therapy for amebic infection (Table 1) is dictated by the patient's signs and symptoms, the stool examination, and the epidemiologic circumstances of infection. Understanding of the pathophysiologic basis for therapeutic decisions has lagged behind empirically determined regimens. As discussed in sections on pathophysiology and diagnosis, a number of questions remain unanswered. It appears that characteristics of the infecting ameba strain confer virulence and the ability to invade the mucosa with distant spread. Whether or not these characteristic are stable characteristics of the organism is currently an area of major study. The contribution of the luminal amebic life cycle to the generation of mild symptoms in patients with nonvirulent strains has not been studied. The degree to which negligible or mild symptoms are caused by virulent strains has not been extensively documented, but appears low (27). However, the presence of antibody to E. histolytica in certain patients with mild symptoms indicates that some hosts have a low-

TABLE 1   Drugs for Treatment of Amebiasis and Giardiasis

Infection	Drug	Adult dosage
Amebiasis (*Entamoeba histolytica*)		
asymptomatic	Paromomycin	25-30 mg/kg/d in three doses × 7 d
	or	
	Iodoquinol	650 mg t.i.d. × 20 d
	or	
	Diloxanide furoate	500 mg t.i.d. × 10 d
mild to moderate intestinal disease		
drugs of choice	Metronidazole plus	750 mg t.i.d. × 10 d
	Paromomycin	As above
	or	
	Iodoquinol	
	or	
	Diloxanide furoate	
alternative	Paromomycin	25-30 mg/kg/d in three doses × 7 d
severe intestinal and extraintestinal disease		
drugs of choice	Metronidazole plus	750 mg t.i.d. × 10 d
	Paromomycin	As above
	or	
	Iodoquinol	
	or	
	Diloxanide furoate	
Giardiasis (*Giardia lamblia*)		
drugs of choice	Quinacrine HCl	100 mg t.i.d. × 5 d
	or	
	Metronidazole	250 mg t.i.d. × 5-7 d
alternative	Furazolidone	100 mg q.i.d. × 7-10 d

grade invasion that may be endogenously controlled. In addition, the development of hepatic abscess in the absence of a history of previous gastrointestinal symptoms, particularly in the tropics, indicates that virulent ameba may invade the gastrointestinal mucosa in the absence of symptoms (37).

Many useful drugs are available and allow considerable leeway in the treatment of patients who cannot tolerate the first-line regimen or who fail initial therapy. Drugs used in the treatment of amebiasis may act locally in the gut (luminal agent) or through the systemic circulation (tissue amebicide). Persons with asymptomatic intraluminal infection are treated with a luminally active agent such as paromomycin, diloxanide or iodoquinol (see Table 1).

Iodoquinol is an halogenated 8-hydroxyquinoline that eradicates parasites in approximately 75% of asymptomatic infected persons when given in the standard 20-day regimen (44). Significant neurotoxicity, especially subacute myelooptic neuropathy leading to blindness, can be caused by iodochlorhydroxyquin, a congener of iodoquinol (45). Occasional optic atrophy and loss of visual acuity has been reported with iodoquinol, but only when the drug was taken for excessive periods (46). Because of this serious side effect, some authorities have recommended that alternative luminal agents be substituted (47). However, iodoquinol is still widely used. Other adverse reactions include peripheral neuropathy, nausea, vomiting, diarrhea and headache.

Iodoquinol is contraindicated in patients with hepatic damage or iodine sensitivity. Similarly to other iodinated compounds, it may interfere with thyroid function tests for months after therapy is completed.

Diloxanide furoate, a dichloroacetamide derivative, is effective in asymptomatic patients and in those with mild diarrhea; cure rates of 85% to 95% are reported (48,49). Side effects are mild and include flatulence, vomiting, pruritus and uritcaria (49). Diloxanide reportedly has a cure rate of 70% in patients with dysentery, but use of this drug alone is not recommended in these patients because higher cure rates can be achieved when a systemic amebicide is added (48,50-52). Unfortunately, this drug can only be obtained in the United States from the CDC on a case-by-case basis because the FDA has not approved it for this indication.

Paromomycin, a nonabsorbable aminoglycoside, is effective in the treatment of patients with asymptomatic or mild intestinal amebiasis. A 5-day course of 25 to 30 mg/kg per day results in an 84% to 90% cure rate (53-55). Paromomycin has also been quite effective in the treatment of mild disease in male homosexuals in the United States (56). Mild intestinal disease may also be treated with systemic amebicide-containing regimens used for severe gastrointestinal disease. Serious consideration of such a regimen is required in a homosexual patient who has marked gastrointestinal symptoms or who may have contracted disease in an area where virulent organisms are more common than in the United States. For example, one might treat a mildly symptomatic urban homosexual man who had cysts and a few nonhematophageous trophozoites on stool examination with paromomycin alone, but add metronidazole if the same person gave a history of recent travel to Mexico. Advantages of paromomycin, compared with available multidrug therapy, include low toxicity, brief duration of therapy, and a high rate of patient compliance (56). Side effects most commonly associated with paromomycin include diarrhea, nausea, and headache (54).

Severe intestinal amebiasis and extraintestinal amebiasis should be treated with a tissue amebicide and a luminal agent to eradicate all cysts. Metronidazole, the most frequently used tissue amebicide, is about 85% effective in effecting cure when used alone in patients with severe diarrhea including dysentery (57,58). Metronidazole is even more effective in the treatment of hepatic amebiasis (57,59). The drug is also about 90% effective in eradicating luminal cysts (58,60) when given for the usual course (10 days at a dosage of 750 mg three times a day), but a second luminal agent is recommended in the setting of severe disease to eradicate all cysts.

Metronidazole is associated with dose-related disulfiramlike activity (61). Patients treated with the drug should be cautioned not to drink alcohol during, and for 48 to 72 hr before and after, administration.

In patients treated with metronidazole for protracted lengths of time, significant neurotoxicity, including paresthesias, peripheral neuropathy, and seizures, has been reported (62-64). At usual dosages, adverse symptoms include nausea, metallic taste, gastrointestinal symptoms, headache, dizziness, depression, reversible leukopenia, and rashes (65,66).

Tinidazole, which is not available in the United States, is reportedly effective for dysentery and hepatic abscess when given for shorter courses than metronidazole (67,68).

Tetracycline in a dosage of 250 to 500 mg four times a day for 5 to 10 days may be a useful adjunct to therapy of patients with acute dysentery. Although tetracycline promotes rapid resolution of symptoms, incomplete healing of ulcers and relapse at 1 month are common if no other amebicide is used concurrently (69).

Emetine and dehydroemetine, once mainstays of therapy, are now rarely used unless the nitroimidazoles fail or are contraindicated. They may be effective for the treatment of liver abscess, but should not be used alone in the treatment of bowel disease. Parenteral administration is required. Serious cardiotoxicity can complicate their use. Current indications include use as an adjunct in life-threatening, unstable disease, with metronidazole administered as the first-line drug (70). Chloroquine can be used alone for protracted periods or combined with another agent to cure liver abscess, but it has no indication in the treatment of intestinal disease (71).

Unanswered Questions

Major questions concerning host determinants of susceptibility to amebic disease remain inadequately answered. It is unclear whether or not effective immunity develops and, if it does, what arm of the immune system is most important. Increased susceptibility to disease has been noted in pregnancy, malnutrition, and steroid therapy (22). Thus far, it has not been observed that nonpathogenic zymodemes are capable of causing serious disease in immunocompromised hosts (12).

Petri and Ravdin (18) have suggested that enteric infection with *E. histolytica* may accelerate progression to AIDS in HIV-infected patients by stimulating replication of infected T cells with parasite proteins such as the amebic lectin. They postulate that treatment of amebic infections in HIV-infected patients without clinical signs of AIDS might decrease mitogenic stimulation and slow progression to AIDS. This hypothesis has not yet been corroborated by clinical data.

GIARDIASIS

Pathophysiology

The mechanism by which *Giardia lamblia* causes human disease has not been firmly established. Toxin secretion, competition for nutrients, physical alteration of the epithelium, and induction of an inflammatory response, all have been considered as possible pathogenetic events. Evidence for the latter two mechanisms is strongest (72). Disaccharidase deficiency and fat and vitamin B_{12} malabsorption have been documented (73,74) and are consistent with the frequent presence of malabsorption-type stools in giardiasis. Mucosal invasion by giardia is not common and is not generally felt to be a factor in the functional abnormalities of the disease (75).

Mice infected with *G. muris* provide an animal model for human giardiasis. Immunocompetent mice clear organisms from the gut in a few weeks by, as yet, unidentified mechanisms; nude mice, deficient in T lymphocytes, are unable to clear giardia infection at a normal rate. In the nude mouse model, a profound deficiency of Peyer's patch helper/inducer T lymphocytes has been identified. It has been suggested that this deficiency may be responsible for defective initiation of intestinal immune responses and subsequent impairment of the capacity to clear organisms through immunologic means (76). Both experimental and clinical evidence suggest that antibody is important in limiting giardia infections. Rats develop biliary IgA to giardia after instillation of trophozoites in the duodenum; persons with congenital hypogammaglobulinemia experience protracted infection; infants of mothers with high titers of specific secretory IgA in their milk have significantly lower infection rates (77-81).

Clinical Presentation

The most frequent symptoms of giardiasis are abdominal distress, watery diarrhea, and weight loss. Anorexia, nausea, flatulence, and foul-smelling stools are also common. Fever and chills may occur. Symptoms may mimic peptic ulcer or gallbladder disease. The usual duration of symptomatic disease is 1 to several weeks. By definition, acute giardiasis lasts less than 6 months and is characterized by spontaneous recovery. Historically, protracted or severe diarrhea has been noted in patients with achlorhydria, malnutrition, and immunodeficiency. Recently, however, chronic giardiasis, defined as symptomatic disease lasting more than 6 months, has been reported to be more common than previously suspected in otherwise healthy persons (82).

Diagnosis

Diagnosis may be made by finding either cysts or trophozoites on stool examination for parasites. Because *Giardia* organisms may be inconsistently present in stools, three specimens, collected several days apart, are indicated. Specimens should be examined by direct wet mount and by a concentration method. If organisms are not identified by either of these methods, permanent stains may be helpful (83). If stool examination is consistently negative, the string test (Enterotest, Hedeco, Palo Alto, California) (84), duodenal aspiration, or small-bowel biopsy may yield trophozoites. String test or aspirated materials can be examined by wet mount. In processing biopsy tissue, it is best to make impression smears as well as sections because giardia are found in the mucus or attached to epithelium, not in the tissue. Impression smears may be stained with trichrome or Giemsa. Recently, several groups have develops ELISA tests for the diagnosis of giardia in stool (85, 86). One of these is FDA approved. It appears to be considerably more sensitive than stool O and P and can be used on specimens treated with 10% neutral formalin, SAF fixative, and Cary-Blair transport medium, as well as on untreated specimens (86). Fecal counterimmunoelectrophoresis correlates well with current infection, but reported methods require untreated stool (87,88).

Treatment

Asymptomatic as well as symptomatic persons are treated (see Table 1) to prevent spread of the disease. Assessment of efficacy of drugs is complicated because the organism, when present, cannot be reliably detected in stool.

Quinacrine hydrochloride, 100 mg t.i.d. for 7 days, reportedly results in about a 90% to 95% cure rate (89-91). Cure rates in immunocompromised individuals are not available, but eradication of the parasite may be impossible and lifelong therapy may be necessary. Headache, altered consciousness, including frank psychosis, gastrointestinal disturbances, hematologic abnormalities, and rashes may complicate quinacrine therapy. Toxic symptoms of long-term use of quinacrine were documented in World War II when it was used for malaria prophylaxis. Yellow skin discoloration may occur, but the most serious side effect is toxic psychosis, which may occur in up to 1.5% of patients (90). Patients with psoriasis frequently develop exacerbation of their skin lesions when given quinicrine, and it is relatively contraindicated in this setting.

Metronidazole, although not yet approved by the FDA for giardiasis, is 60% to 95% effective in curing the disease when given for 7 days at a dosage of 250 mg three times a day (92-94). The mode of action and side effects of metronidazole are discussed in the section on amebiasis.

Furazolidone appears to be less efficacious than quinacrine, with a reported cure rate of 80% when given in a dosage of 100 mg four times a day to adults for 7 days (92). Better cure rates have been reported in children (95). Serious side effects include a disulfiramlike reaction to alcohol and hemolytic anemia in glucose-6-phosphate dehydrogenase (G6PD)-deficient patients. Nausea, vomiting, rash, and brown discoloration of urine may occur (90).

Unresponsive cases of giardiasis may resolve with combined therapy (96) using established drugs. Some agents that have not been clinically assessed, including mefloquine, doxycycline, and possibly rifampin, have in vitro activity against *Giardia* (97). Avoidance of fat and milk products during and immediately after giardia treatment may help alleviate symptoms of malabsorption.

OTHER PROTOZOANS

The presence of nonpathogenic protozoa or those of low pathogenicity in a patient has, to most clinicians, implied that ingestion of feces (either directly or by contamination of food or water) has occurred. In this setting, repeated stool examinations often yield a conventional pathogen (2). However, several intestinal protozoa in addition to *E. histolytica* and *G. lamblia* may be pathogenic under some circumstances. Suspected pathogens include *Balantidium coli, Dientamoeba fragilis,* and *Blastocystis hominis.* No systemic studies of these organisms in homosexual men or AIDS patients has been reported. Nonetheless, *D. fragilis* and *B. hominis* have been catalogued in studies of homosexual men examined for enteric protozoa (8,9,98).

Balantidium coli is a large ciliated protozoan, generally acquired through direct or indirect contact with pigs, although many other animals may harbor the organism (99). Several outbreaks have occurred in mental hospitals, suggesting that human fecal-oral spread occurs (99). Clinical manifestations of infection range from the asymptomatic carrier state to chronic constipation alternating with diarrhea to acute dysentery (100). Perforation of the bowel and trophozoite invasion of the lungs has been reported rarely (101). Metronidazole therapy was evaluated in Venezuela and found to be effective

TABLE 2 Drugs for Treatment of Other Intestinal Protozoa

Infection	Drug	Adult dosage
Balantidium coli		
drug of choice	Tetracycline	500 mg t.i.d. × 10 d
alternatives	Iodoquinol	650 mg t.i.d. × 20 d
	Metronidazole	750 mg t.i.d. × 5 d
Blastocystis hominis		
drug of choice	Iodoquinol	650 mg t.i.d. × 20 d
	or	
	Metronidazole	750 mg t.i.d. × 10 d
Dientamoeba fragilis		
drug of choice	Iodoquinol	650 mg t.i.d. × 20 d
	or	
	Tetracycline	500 mg q.i.d. × 20 d
	or	
	Paromomycin	25-30 mg/kg/d in three doses × 7 d

Source: Modified with permission from *Med. Lett.* 28:9-18, 1986.

(102), but reports of failure with this drug in the South Pacific have appeared (99), and tetracycline at a dosage of 500 mg four times a day for 10 days is currently the drug of choice (Table 2).

Dientamoeba fragilis is a flagellate related to the trichomonads. Pathogenicity of the organism has been controversial for years, but improvement in gastrointestinal symptoms after treatment has been reported (103-105). In one study of a semicommunal group, 56% of adults carried the parasite and 85% of the infected had gastrointestinal symptoms, especially pain and flatus, infrequently diarrhea. Iodoquinol in a dosage of 650 mg three times a day for 20 days eliminated the parasite in 83% of those treated, but the number treated was small and no control group was reported. Tetracycline and paromomycin are also effective (see Table 2).

Blastocystis hominis may be found in up to 25% of stool specimens and, only occasionally, causes symptoms when found in large numbers (106,107). In the absence of other known pathogens, finding more than five organisms per high-power field is evidence supporting *B. hominis* as the cause of gastrointestinal symptoms (108). Diarrhea and abdominal pain are the most commonly reported findings. It has been suggested that *B. hominis* infection is more common in immunocompromised patients (109), but this has not been rigorously investigated. Metronidazole or iodoquinol are the drugs of choice (110; see Table 2).

A report that nonpathogenic protozoa, such as *Entamoeba coli, Entamoeba hartmanni, Endolimax nana,* and *Iodamoeba buetschlli,* produce diarrheal disease in patients with AIDS has appeared. Rolston et al. (98) reported 11 patients with severe diarrhea (10 to 15 bowel movements daily) and nonpathogenic ameba; six had concomitant cryptosporidia. All patients responded to a 10-day course of metronidazole. No placebo group was studied. The number of stool samples examined was not indicated; duodenal aspirates or biopsies for *Giardia lamblia* were not obtained. Most patients had a relapse of diarrhea from 1 week to 9 months after therapy; although three patients with nonpathogenic amebae had no further diarrhea. On the basis of this limited data, Rolston et al. suggest that moderate to severe diarrhea can be caused by nonpathogenic ameba in AIDS patients and that symptoms generally respond to metronidazole, although relapses occur. They further speculate that *Cryptosporidium* may act as a copathogen. In the absence of controls and studies to rule out known pathogens, and given the prevalence of idiopathic diarrhea in AIDS patients, the data in this report do not support the conclusions promulgated.

Because of our current inability to rule out pathogenic protozoan disease definitively in AIDS patients with diarrhea and parasites of only low or unreported pathogenicity in their stool, some physicians empirically treat these patients with a course of antiparasitic drugs (e.g., metronidazole, quinacrine). Unpublished experience at San Francisco General Hospital indicates that such therapy rarely results in an improvement of symptoms or signs, perhaps because these patients are suffering from diarrhea caused by HIV or an as yet unrecognized pathogens.

REFERENCES

1. Most, H. (1968). Manhattan: A tropical isle? *Am. J. Trop. Med. Hyg. 17*:333-354.
2. William, D. C., Shookoff, H. B., Felman, Y. M., and DeRamos, S. W. (1978). High rates of enteric protozoal infection in selected homosexual men attending a venereal disease clinic. *Sex. Transm. Dis. 5*:155-157.
3. Keystone, J. S., Keystone, D. L., and Proctor, E. M. (1980). Intestinal parasitic infections in homosexual men: Prevalence, symptoms and factors in transmission. *Can. Med. Assoc. J. 123*:512-514.
4. Hakansson, C., Thoren, K., Norkrans, G., and Johannisson, G. (1984). Intestinal parasitic infection and other sexually transmitted diseases in asymptomatic homosexual men. *Scand. J. Infect. Dis. 16*:199-202.
5. Schmerin, M. J., Gelston, A., and Jones, T. C. (1977). Amebiasis: An increasing problem among homosexuals in New York City. *JAMA 238*:1386-1387.
6. Medical Staff Conference, University of California, San Francisco (1979). Venereal aspects of gastroenterology. *West. J. Med. 130*:236-246.
7. Phillips, S. C., Mildvan, D., William, D. C., Gelb, A. M., and White, M. C. (1981). Sexual transmission of enteric protozoa and helminths in a venereal disease clinic population. *N. Engl. J. Med. 305*:603-606.

8. Ortega, H. B., Borchardt, K. A., Hamilton, R., Ortega, P., and Mahood, J. (1984). Enteric pathogenic protozoa in homosexual men from San Francisco. *Sex. Transm. Dis. 11*:59-63.

9. Markell, E. K., Havens, R. F., Kuritsubo, R. A., and Wingerd, J. (1984). Intestinal protozoa in homosexual men of the San Francisco Bay area; prevalence and correlates of infection. *Am. J. Trop. Med. Hyg. 33*:239-245.

10. Quinn, T. C., Stamm, W. E., Goodell, S. E., Mkrtichian, E., Benedetti, J., Corey, L., Schuffler, M. D., and Holmes, K. K. (1983). The polymicrobial origin of intestinal infections in homosexual men. *N. Engl. J. Med. 309*:576-582.

11. Bienzle, U., Coester, C. H., Knobloch, J., and Guggenmoos-Holzmann, I. (1984). Protozoal enteric infections in homosexual men. *Klin. Wochenschr. 62*: 323-327.

12. Allason-Jones, E., Mindel, A., Sargeaunt, P., and Williams, P. (1986). *Entamoeba histolytica* as a commensal intestinal parasite in homosexual men. *N. Engl. J. Med. 315*:353-356.

13. Saltzberg, D. M. and Hall-Craggs, M. (1986). Fulminant amebic colitis in a homosexual man. *Am. J. Gastroenterol. 81*:209-212.

14. Healy, G. R. (1986). Immunologic tools in the diagnosis of amebiasis: Epidemiology in the United States. *Rev. Infect. Dis. 8*:239-246.

15. Krogstad, D. J. (1986). Isoenzyme patterns and pathogenicity in amebic infections. *N. Engl. J. Med. 315*:390-391.

16. Sullam, P. M. (1987). *Entamoeba histolytica* in homosexual men [Letter]. *N. Engl. J. Med. 316*:690.

17. Pearce, R. B. (1983). Intestinal protozoal infections and AIDS [Letter]. *Lancet 2*:51.

18. Petri, W. A., Jr. and Ravdin, J. I. (1986). Treatment of homosexual men infected with *Entamoeba histolytica* [Letter]. *N. Engl. J. Med. 315*:393.

19. Pearce, R. B. and Abrams, D. I. (1987). *Entamoeba histolytica* in homosexual men [Letter]. *N. Engl. J. Med. 316*:690-691.

20. Kean, B. H., William, D. C., and Luinais, S. K. (1979). Epidemic of amebiasis and giardiasis in a biased population. *Br. J. Vener. Dis. 55*:375-378.

21. Beaumont, D. M. and James, O. F. W. (1986). Unsuspected giardiasis as a cause of malnutrition and diarrhoea in the elderly. *Br. Med. J. 293*:554-555.

22. Guerrant, R. (1986). Amebiasis: Introduction, current status, and research questions. *Rev. Infect. Dis. 8*:218-227.

23. Mirelman, D. (1987). Effect of culture conditions and bacterial associates on the zymodemes of *Entamoeba histolytica*. *Parasitol. Today 3*:37-40.

24. Sargeaunt, P. G. and Williams, J. E. (1979). Electrophoretic isoenzyme patterns of the pathogenic and nonpathogenic intestinal amoebae of man. *Trans. R. Soc. Trop. Med. Hyg. 73*:225-227.

25. Sargeaunt, P. G. (1987). The reliability of *Entamoeba histolytica* zymodemes in clinical diagnosis. *Parasitol. Today 3*:40-43.

26. Goldmeier, D., Price, A. B., Billington, O., Borriello, P., Shaw, A., Sargeaunt, P. G., Munday, P. E., Dixon, I., Cardner, J. M., Hilton, J., and Jeffries, D. J. (1986). Is *Entamoeba histolytica* in homosexual men a pathogen? *Lancet 1*:641-644.

27. Gathiram, V. and Jackson, T. F. G. (1985). Frequency of distribution of *Entamoeba histolytica* zymodemes in a rural South African population. *Lancet 1*: 719-721.
28. Allason-Jones, E., Mindel, A., and Sargeaunt, P. (1987). *Entamoeba histolytica* in homosexual men [Letter]. *N. Engl. J. Med. 316*:691-692.
29. H. Washburn, CDC, personal communication.
30. Mathews, H. M., Moss, D. M., Healy, G. R., and Mildvan, D. (1986). Isoenzyme analysis of *Entamoeba histolytica* isolated from homosexual men. *J. Infect. Dis. 153*:793-795.
31. Editorial. (1985). Is that amoeba harmful or not? *Lancet 1*:732-734.
32. Mirelman, D., Bracha, R., Wexler, A., and Chayen, A. (1986). Changes in isoenzyme patterns of a cloned culture of nonpathogenic *Entamoeba histolytica* during axenization. *Infect. Immun. 54*:827-832.
33. Sargeaunt, P. G., Oates, J. K., MacLennan, I., Oriel, J. D., and Goldmeier, D. (1983). *Entamoeba histolytica* in male homosexuals. *Br. J. Vener. Dis. 59*:193-195.
34. Sorvillo, F. J., Strassburg, M. A., Seidel, J., Visvesvara, G. S., Mori, K., Todd, A., Portigal, L., Finn, M., and Agee, B. A. (1986). Amebic infections in asymptomatic homosexual men, lack of evidence of invasive disease. *Am. J. Public Health 76*:1137-1139.
35. Aceti, A., Pennica, A., Ippolito, G., Moretto, D., Rezza, G., Titti, F., and Pevucci, C. A. (1987). Antiamebic antibodies in homosexual men. *N. Engl. J. Med. 316*:692.
36. Adams, E. B. and MacLeod, I. N. (1977). Invasive amebiasis. I. Amebic dysentery and its complications. *Medicine 56*:315-323.
37. Adams, E. B. and MacLeod, I. N. (1977). Invasive amebiasis. II. Amebic liver abscess and its complications. *Medicine 56*:325-334.
38. Burnham, W. R., Reeve, R. S., and Finch, R. (1980). Case Report. *Entamoeba histolytica* infection in male homosexuals. *Gut 21*:1097-1099.
39. Ylvisaker, J. T. and McDonald, G. B. (1980). Sexually acquired amebic colitis and liver abscess. *West. J. Med. 132*:153-157.
40. Thompson, J. E., Jr., Freischlag, J., and Thomas, D. S. (1983). Amebic liver abscess in a homosexual man. *Sex. Transm. Dis. 10*:153-155.
41. Thomas, J. A. and Antony, A. J. (1976). Amoebiasis of the penis. *Br. J. Urol. 48*:269-273.
42. Walsh, J. A. (1986). Problems in recognition and diagnosis of amebiasis: Estimation of the global magnitude of morbidity and mortality. *Rev. Infect. Dis. 8*: 228-238.
43. Patterson, M., Healy, G. R., and Shabot, J. M. (1980). Serologic testing for amoebiasis. *Gastroenterology 78*:136-141.
44. Most, H. (1960). Treatment of amebiasis. *N. Engl. J. Med. 262*:513-514.
45. Oakley, G. P. Jr. (1973). The neurotoxicity of the halogenated hydroxyquinolines; a commentary. *JAMA 225*:395-397.
46. Fleisher, D. I., Hepler, R. S., and Landau, J. W. (1974). Blindness during diodohydroxyquin (Diodoquin) therapy: A case report. *Pediatrics 54*:106-108.
47. Krogstad, D. J., Spenser, H. C., Jr., and Healy, G. R. (1978). Amebiasis. *N. Engl. J. Med. 298*:262-265.

48. Woodruff, A. W., and Powell, S. (1967). The evaluation of amoebicides. *Trans. R. Soc. Trop. Med. Hyg. 61*:435-439.

49. Wolfe, M. S. (1973). Nondysenteric intestinal amebiasis. Treatment with diloxanide furoate. *JAMA 224*:1601-1604.

50. Boteo, D. (1964). Treatment of acute and chronic intestinal amoebiasis with entamide furoate. *Trans. R. Soc. Trop. Med. Hyg. 58*:419-421.

51. Wilmot, A. J., Powell, S. J., McLeod, I., and Elsdon-Dew, R. (1962). Some newer amoebicides in acute amoebic dysentery. *Trans. R. Soc. Trop. Med. Hyg. 56*:85-86.

52. Suchak, N. G., Satoskar, R. S., and Sheth, U. K. (1962). Entamide furoate in the treatment of intestinal amebiasis. *Am. J. Trop. Med. Hyg. 11*:330-332.

53. Forsyth, D. M. (1962). The treatment of amebiasis. A field study of various methods. *Trans. R. Soc. Trop. Med. Hyg. 56*:400-403.

54. Simon, M., Shookhoff, H. B., Terner, H., Weingarten, B., and Parker, J. G. (1967). Paromomycin in the treatment of intestinal amebiasis; a short course of therapy. *Am. J. Gastroenterol. 48*:504-511.

55. Wilmot, A. J., Powell, S. J., MacLeod, I., Elsdon-Dew, R. (1962). Paromomycin in acute amoebic dysentery. *Ann. J. Trop. Med. Parasitol. 56*:383-386.

56. Sullam, P. M., Slutkin, G., Gottlieb, A. B., and Mills, J. (1986). Paromomycin therapy of endemic amebiasis in homosexual men. *Sex. Transm. Dis. 13*:151-155.

57. Powell, S. J., MacLeod, I., Wilmot, A. J., and Elsdon-Dew, R. (1966). Metronidazole in amoebic dysentery and amoebic liver abscess. *Lancet 2*:1329-1331.

58. Pehrson, P. O. and Bengtsson, E. (1984). A long term follow up study of amoebiasis treated with metronidazole. *Scand. J. Infect. Dis. 16*:195-198.

59. Cohen, H. G. and Reynolds, T. B. (1975). Comparison of metronidazole and chloroquine for the treatment of amoebic liver abscess. *Gastroenterology 69*:35-41.

60. Kanani, S. R. and Knight, R. (1972). Experiences with the use of metronidazole in the treatment of non-dysenteric intestinal amoebiasis. *Trans. R. Soc. Trop. Med. Hyg. 66*:244-249.

61. Semer, J. M., Friedland, P., Vaisberg, M., and Greenbeg, A. (1966). The use of metronidazole in the treatment of alcoholism. *Am. J. Psychiatry 123*:722-724.

62. Ursing, B. and Kamme, C. (1975). Metronidazole for Crohn's disease. *Lancet 1*:775-777.

63. Frytak, S., Moertel, C. G., Childs, D. S., and Albers, J. W. (1978). Neurologic toxicity associated with high-dose metronidazole therapy. *Ann. Intern. Med. 88*:361-362.

64. Coxon, A. and Pallis, C. A. (1976). Metronidazole neuropathy. *J. Neurol. Neurosurg. Psychiatry 39*:403-405.

65. Roe, F. J. C. (1983). Toxicologic evaluation of metronidazole with particular reference to carcinogenic and teratogenic potential. *Surgery 93*:158-164.

66. Lefebvre, I. and Hesseltine, H. C. (1965). The peripheral white blood cells and metronidazole. *JAMA 194*:15-18.

67. Scagg, J. N., Rubige, C. J., and Proctor, E. M. (1976). Tinidazole in the treatment of acute amebic dysentery in children. *Arch. Dis. Child. 51*:385-387.

68. Hatchuel, W. (1975). Tinidazole for the treatment of amoebic liver abscess. *S. Afr. Med. J. 49*:1879-1881.

69. Powell, S. J. (1967). Short term follow-up studies in amoebic dysentery. *Trans. R. Soc. Trop. Med. Hyg. 61*:765-769.
70. Knight, R. (1980). The chemotherapy of amebiasis. *J. Antimicrob. Chemother. 6*:577-593.
71. Cohen, H. G. and Reynolds, T. B. (1975). Comparison of metronidazole and chloroquine for the treatment of amoebic liver abscess. *Gastroenterology 69*:35-41.
72. Stevens, D. P. (1982). Giardiasis: Host-pathogen biology. *Rev. Infect. Dis. 4*: 851-858.
73. Hoskins, L. C., Winawer, S. J., Broitman, S. A., Gottlieb, L. S., and Zamcheck, N. (1967). Clinical giardiasis and intestinal malabsorption. *Gastroenterology 53*: 257-279.
74. Morecki, R. and Parker, J. G. (1967). Ultrastructural studies of the human *Giardia lamblia* and subjacent jejunal mucosa in a subject with steatorrhea. *Gastroenterology 52*:151-164.
75. Saha, T. K. and Ghosh, T. K. (1977). Invasion of small intestinal mucosa by *Giardia lamblia* in man. *Gastroenterology 72*:402-405.
76. Heyworth, M. F., Owen, R. L., and Jones, A. L. (1985). Comparison of leukocytes obtained from the intestinal lumen of *Giardia*-infected immunocompetent mice and nude mice. *Gastroenterology 89*:1360-1365.
77. Loftness, T. J., Erlandsen, S. L., Wilson, I. D., and Meyer, E. A. (1984). Occurrence of specific secretory immunoglobulin A in bile after inoculation of *Giardia lamblia* trophozoites into rat duodenum. *Gastroenterology 87*:1022-1029.
78. Loalbo, P. R., Sampson, H. A., and Buckley, R. H. (1982). Symptomatic giardiasis in three patients with X-linked agammaglobulinemia. *J. Pediatr. 101*: 78-80.
79. Owen, R. L. (1980). The immune response in clinical and experimental giardiasis. *Trans. R. Soc. Trop. Med. Hyg. 74*:443-445.
80. Ament, M. E., Ochs, H. D., and Davis, S. D. (1973). Structure and function of the gastrointestinal tract in primary immunodeficiency syndromes, a study of 39 patients. *Medicine 52*:227-248.
81. Nayak, N., Ganguly, N. K., Walia, N. S., Wahi, V., Kanwar, S. S., and Mahajan, R. C. (1987). Specific secretory IgA in the milk of *Giardia lamblia*-infected and uninfected women. *J. Infect. Dis. 155*:724-727.
82. Chester, A. C., MacMurray, F. G., Restifo, M. D., and Mann, O. (1985). Giardiasis as a chronic disease. *Dig. Dis. Sci. 30*:215-218.
83. Thornton, S. A., West, A. H., DuPont, H. L., and Pickering, L. K. (1983). Comparison of methods for identification of *Giardia lamblia*. *Am. J. Clin. Pathol. 80*:858-860.
84. Beal, C. B., Viens, P., Grant, R. G. L., and Hughes, J. M. (1970). A new technique for sampling duodenal contents. *Am. J. Trop. Med. Hyg. 19*:349-352.
85. Ungar, B. L. P., Yolken, R. H., Nash, T. E., and Quinn, T. C. (1984). Enzyme-linked immunosorbent assay for the detection of *Giardia lamblia* in fecal specimens. *J. Infect. Dis. 149*:90-97.
86. Rosoff, J. D., Sanders, C. A., DeLay, P. R., Hadley, W. K., O'Hanley, P. D., Vincenzi, F. F., and Yajko, D. M. Coprodiagnosis of giardiasis by detection of

Giardia-specific antigen 65 (GSA 65) using a commercially available enzyme-immunoassay. In preparation.

87. Craft, J. D. and Nelson, J. D. (1982). Diagnosis of giardiasis by counterimmu-noelectrophoresis of feces. *J. Infect. Dis. 145*:499-504.

88. Vinayak, V. K. et al. (1985). Detection of *Giardia lamblia* antigen in the feces by counterimmunoelectrophoresis. *Pediatr. Infect. Dis. 4*:383-386.

89. Turner, J. A. (1985). Giardiasis and infections with *Dientamoeba fragilis. Pediatr. Clin. N. Am. 32*:865-880.

90. Wolfe, M. S. (1975). Giardiasis. *JAMA 233*:1362-1365.

91. Wright, G., Tompkins, A. M., and Ridley, D. S. (1977). Giardiasis: Clinical and therapeutic aspects. *Gut 18*:343-350.

92. Bassily, S., Farid, Z., Mikail, J. W., Kent, D. C., and Lehman, J. S., Jr. (1970). The treatment of *Giardia lamblia* infection with mepacrine, metroni-dazole and furazolidone. *J. Trop. Med. Hyg. 73*:15-18.

93. Levi, G. C., deAvila, C. A., and Neto, V. A. (1977). Efficacy of various drugs for treatment of giardiasis. *Am. J. Trop. Med. Hyg. 26*:564-565.

94. Khambatta, R. B. (1971). Metronidazole in giardiasis. *Ann. Trop. Med. Parasitol. 65*:487-489.

95. Craft, C. J., Murphy, T., and Nelson, J. D. (1981). Furazolidine and quina-crine. Comparative study of therapy of giardiasis in children. *Am. J. Dis. Child. 135*:164-166.

96. Smith, P. D., Gillin, F. D., Spira, W. M., and Nash, T. E. (1982). Chronic giardiasis: Studies on drug sensitivity, toxin production, and host immune re-sponse. *Gastroenterology 83*:797-803.

97. Crouch, A. A., Seow, W. K., and Thong, Y. H. (1986). Effect of twenty-three chemotherapeutic agents on the adherence and growth of *Giardia lamblia* in vitro. *Trans. R. Soc. Trop. Med. Hyg. 80*:893-896.

98. Rolston, K. V. I., Hoy, J., and Mansell, P. W. A. (1986). Diarrhea caused by "nonpathogenic amoebae" in patients with AIDS [Letter]. *N. Engl. J. Med. 315*:192.

99. Walzer, P. D., Judson, F. N., Murphy, K. B., Healy, G. R., English, D. K., and Schultz, M. G. (1973). Balantidiasis outbreak in Truk. *Am. J. Trop. Med. Hyg. 22*:33-41.

100. Swartzwelder, J. C. (1950). Balantidiasis. *Am. J. Dig. Dis. 17*:173-179.

101. Dorfman, S., Ragel, O., and Bravo, L. G. (1984). Balantidiasis: Report of a fatal case with appendicular and pulmonary involvement. *Trans. R. Soc. Trop. Med. Hyg. 78*:833-834.

102. Garcia-Laverde, A. and De Bonilla, L. (1975). Clinical trials with metronida-zole in human balantidiasis. *Am. J. Trop. Med. Hyg. 24*:781-783.

103. Kean, B. H. and Malloch, C. L. (1966). The neglected amoeba: *Dientamoeba fragilis*. A report of 100 "pure" infections. *Am. J. Dig. Dis. 11*:735-744.

104. Spencer, M. J., Garcia, L. S., and Chapin, M. R. (1979). *Dientamoeba fragilis*, an intestinal pathogen in children? *Am. J. Dis. Child. 133*:390-393.

105. Millet, V., Spenser, M. J., Chapin, M., Wart, M., Yatabe, J. A., Brewer, T., and Garcia. L. (1983). *Dientamoeba fragilis*, a protozoan parasite in adult mem-bers of a semicommunal group. *Dig. Dis. Sci. 28*:335-339.

106.   Melvin, D. M. and Healy, G. R. (1985). Intestinal and urogenital protozoa. In *Manual of Clinical Microbiology*. 4th ed. (Lennette, E. H., Balows, A., Hausler, W. J., Jr., and Shadomy, H. J., eds.). Washington, D.C., American Society for Microbiology, p. 649.
107.   Ricci, N., Toma, P., Furlani, M., Caselli, M., and Gullini, S. (1984). *Blastocystis hominis*: A neglected cause of diarrhoae [Letter]? *Lancet 1*:966.
108.   Zierdt, C. H. (1983). *Blastocystis hominis*, a protozoan parasite and intestinal pathogen of human beings. *Clin. Microbiol. Newslett. 5*:57-59.
109.   Garcia, L. S., Bruckner, D. A., and Clancy, M. N. (1984). Clinical relevance of *Blastocystis hominis* [Letter]. *Lancet 1*:1233-1234.
110.   Zierdt, C. H., Swan, J. C., and Hosseini, J. (1983). In vitro response of *Blastocystis hominis* to antiprotozoal drugs. *J. Protozool. 30*:332-334.

Part VII
Ancillary Services

21
Optimal Use of Diagnostic Laboratories for Evaluation of Patients with the Acquired Immunodeficiency Syndrome

Valerie L. Ng and W. Keith Hadley, *University of California and San Francisco General Hospital, San Francisco, California*

The destruction of the host immune system after infection with the family of human immunodeficiency viruses (HIV-1 and HIV-2; 1-4) has resulted in a parallel epidemic of unusual cancers and opportunistic infections that collectively constitute the disease spectrum known as the acquired immunodeficiency syndrome (AIDS). The opportunistic pathogens are numerous and are being recovered from body fluids and sites that are infrequently involved in non-AIDS patients.

The diagnosis of AIDS is dependent on the laboratory identification of the opportunistic infecting organism(s), as well as on the detection of HIV antibodies, the presence of which are an essential part of an AIDS diagnosis in a patient infected with a less-common opportunistic pathogen. This demand for the services of the pathology and microbiology laboratories has increased dramatically since the onset of the AIDS epidemic. Thus, the purpose of this chapter will be to direct clinicians to the most efficient and cost-effective strategy for using the pathology and microbiology laboratories to evaluate the patient who is clinically suspected of having AIDS.

BACKGROUND

The human immunodeficiency virus is a lentivirus (a subfamily within the family of retroviruses; 5,6) with a particular tropism for CD4+ (OKT4, Leu3) cells. This population includes T-helper cells, B cells, macrophages, and neural tissue (?neuroglial cells; 7-12).

Once infected with HIV, the host probably remains chronically infected for life. Although infection of T-helper cells rapidly results in cell fusion, lysis, and death, infection of macrophages results in the establishment of a latent persistent infection (13). Thus, the chronically infected macrophage is thought to serve as the reservoir of HIV in the infected host, continually producing low levels of HIV to ultimately infect and deplete the host T-helper cell population.

CULTURE AND HIV DETECTION

The discovery of the family of human immunodeficiency viruses (HIV-1 and HIV-2) was made possible by the development of new tissue culture techniques. These permitted, for the first time, the long-term in vitro culture of human T lymphocytes (the target cells for HIV infection). This new capacity incorporates many recent advances in basic science—including the discovery and isolation of interleukin-2 (T-cell growth factor; 14) which is critical for maintaining T cells in in vitro culture, and the discovery that antibodies to α-interferon enhance production of murine retroviruses from chronically infected cultures (15). These two factors are now integral components of the culture technique for HIV isolation from clinical specimens.

In 1983-1984, three independent laboratories (1-3) reported the successful isolation of a new human retrovirus, now known as HIV-1 (previously designated as HTLV-III, LAV, and ARV). Culture techniques have not improved since that time, and the isolation of HIV from patient specimens remains cumbersome and expensive. Recovery of HIV by culture requires the harvesting of peripheral blood lymphocytes from the patient and placing these cells in culture with T lymphocytes that express high levels of CD4 (the AIDS virus receptor, also known as OKT4 or Leu3, a surface glycoprotein that defines the helper/inducer subset of T cells; 7). Cells from the patient are the ideal specimen for culture, as these cells are the richest source of virus. Because infection of the CD4+ T cells results in cytolysis (16), the cultures must be continuously supplemented with fresh donor peripheral blood lymphocytes (requiring that a steady source of peripheral blood lymphocytes be available). To enhance transmission and virus production from the presumably infected CD4+ T cells, concanavalin A, interleukin-2 and antibodies to α-interferon are added to the culture medium. The culture supernatants are monitored at frequent intervals (for at least 4 weeks) for reverse transcriptase activity or for p24 (the HIV major virion core protein) expression, which is indicative of viral particle release. Production of HIV from cultures can be detected as early as 2 to 3 weeks after infection; however, some cultures may take 4 weeks or longer to produce detectable levels of HIV.

Culture of HIV is expensive (from 200 to 600 dollars per culture), as well as labor-intensive, and it currently remains a research laboratory procedure. More rapid culture techniques, as well as antigen detection systems (e.g., p24), are being investigated (17).

Many research laboratories are willing to accept clinical specimens on a limited basis. Although the ideal specimen contains *cells* (e.g., anticoagulated peripheral blood or fresh nonfixed biopsy tissue), virus can also be isolated from body fluids (e.g., cervical fluids, saliva, and the like; 18-21).

The estimated sensitivity of culture (i.e., the likelihood of obtaining a positive culture from a patient known to have HIV infection) ranges from 80% to 90%. False-negative cultures are attributable to inadequate specimens, contaminated cultures (e.g., bacterial or fungal overgrowth), or a low level of viremia in the patient. The age of the specimen is not as critical as once thought; recovery of HIV from split specimens processed immediately versus from cells stored at −190°C yielded comparable rates of recovery (22). At present, the specificity of culture is thought to be 100%, depending on the detection method used. A few false-positive culture results have been observed when recovery of HIV was detected by measuring reverse transcriptase activity in culture supernatants (21). These were determined to be false-positive results when subsequent assays of supernatants from the same cultures failed to demonstrate reverse transcriptase activity.

Reverse Transcriptase Activity Assays

Reverse transcriptase, an unusual enzyme found in HIV, synthesizes a DNA molecule complementary to an RNA template. The RT assay measures the enzyme activity of free virus particles released into the culture supernatant. Briefly, cell culture supernatants are clarified of cellular debris by a low-speed centrifugation step, and free virus is pelleted by ultracentrifugation. The RT activity is detected by incubating samples of this viral pellet in the presence of a synthetic RNA template [commonly poly(rA)-oligo(dT)] and measuring the incorporation of radiolabeled thymidine nucleotides into newly synthesized DNA. Appropriate negative and positive controls are included with each run to establish the appropriate cutoff points.

Reverse transcriptase assays simply detect the presence or absence of free virus particles; quantitation of released virus may be possible (23).

Detection of HIV p24 Antigen

Antigen-capture assay systems have been developed to detect the expression of the HIV major HIV virion core protein, p24, in culture supernatants or body fluids. The antigen-capture assay uses anti-p24-specific antibodies bound to a solid phase to selectively capture the viral p24 antigen. After washing to remove all nonspecifically bound material, a second anti-p24-specific anti-body, coupled to an enzyme, is then added. This second antibody, with enzyme attached, will bind any p24 captured by the first antibody. After adequate incubation and washing, the enzyme substrate is added, and the enzyme activity is measured. With the inclusion of high-affinity monoclonal anti-p24 antibodies (24,25), the amount of enzyme activity can be directly related to the amount of antigen present, allowing quantitation of virus production.

The antigen-capture assay appears to be as sensitive as the RT assay for evaluating HIV cultures (24). It may supplant RT assays in the future as the method of choice because of its ease of performance, lower cost, and nondependence on radioactive substrates.

Cell Fusion Detection Methods

Cellular infection by HIV rapidly results in cell fusion, lysis, and death (16). A new generation of culture techniques is being developed to take advantage of the characteristic syncytia formation induced by HIV infection (26). The definition of a positive culture would be the observation of multinucleated giant cells. To adapt this technique to routine clinical viral cultures, it must first be demonstrated that HIV is the only clinical virus isolate capable of inducing such syncytia.

Another novel method of detection involves recording viability (by trypan blue exclusion) of inoculated cultured cells (27). If the inoculated cell culture appears to contain fewer cells than that of a control uninoculated culture, then it is interpreted as loss of cells because of infection and subsequent cell lysis. Once again, the specificity of such a culture methodology for HIV must be demonstrated before it can be used for clinical specimens. The present use of such a culture technique is to screen potential antiviral chemotherapeutic agents for anti-HIV activity.

Detection Methods for HIV Antibodies

Because HIV is constantly present in the infected host, anti-HIV antibodies are continuously produced for the lifetime of the host. The antibody response after infection with HIV has been fairly well studied. Documented seroconversion with production of anti-HIV IgM antibodies occurs as early as 5 days, and anti-HIV IgG antibodies are detectable within 11 days, after the onset of clinical symptoms of the acute HIV infection syndrome (28,29).

In the four reported cases of nosocomially acquired HIV infection, seroconversion was observed as early as 12 weeks, and documented in all within 9 months, of the incidents implicated in HIV transmission (30,31). These health care workers probably had seroconverted within weeks after the exposure; however, infrequent monitoring did not permit earlier detection. It is generally expected that if seroconversion occurs, it will occur within 6 weeks after accidental contact with infected specimens.

The anti-HIV antibodies produced after infection are directed against several of the viral proteins. In a few well-studied patients, the first antibodies to appear are directed against the major core protein, p24, and the envelope proteins p41 and gp120/160. Antibodies directed against the reverse transcriptase, p66, and p31, appear later in the course of infection. One universal finding was that antibodies against the envelope proteins persisted, even after the patient had progressed to AIDS, whereas the persistence of antibodies against the core proteins was not similarly observed (32-35).

Enzyme-Linked Immunosorbent Assay Methodology

Screening the Blood Supply

The development of the current antibody screening assays was dictated by the necessity of screening the donor blood supply to prevent further cases of transfusion-associated AIDS. The tests were developed to be highly sensitive to identify all possibly contaminated units of blood; specificity (to some extent) was sacrificed for sensitivity.

Enzyme-linked immunosorbent assays (ELISA), by virtue of the ease of performance and of processing many samples, the relatively low cost (as opposed to Western blot, radioimmunoprecipitation, or indirect immunofluorescence assays), and the nondependence on radioisotopes, were developed for screening donor blood (36-39). The current test systems use whole disrupted HIV-1 as the antigen source; the disrupted HIV-1, bound to a solid phase (96-well plastic plate), is incubated with serum from the donor units. In theory, anti-HIV-1 antibodies will remain bound to the solid phase after thorough washing (to remove nonspecifically bound material). Bound antibody from the donor is then detected with a second antihuman antibody coupled to an enzyme. Incubation of this resultant complex with the enzyme substrate allows detection of enzyme activity and, indirectly, the presence of anti-HIV antibodies.

The ELISA results are reported as a ratio of optical density (O.D.; representing the amount of substrate converted by enzyme activity) between a negative control sample and the patient/donor serum being tested. Initial characterization of the various ELISA kits involved establishing an absolute cutoff value of 2.0 for the O.D. ratios to maximize the sensitivity and specificity (32). Any ratio above 2.0 would be considered a positive result, and any ratio below 2.0 a negative result. It was recognized that values between 2.0 and 5.0, also known as "low-positives," were often false-positives (when tested by an alternative method) because of cross-reacting antibodies (see later discussion); whereas "high-positive" values were usually true-positives, although exceptions to this rule have also been found (40).

Most of the ELISA kits on the market have comparable sensitivity and specificity (37), although they vary in their ease of performance. However, some kits are more sensitive than others for detecting antibodies to specific viral proteins. Ideally, kits should be maximally sensitive to antienvelope (i.e., gp120/160) antibodies, because these antibodies appear to be the most persistent during the entire course of HIV infection. However, an inherent problem with such an assay is the marked variation in envelope proteins between different types of HIV, such that antienvelope antibodies from a patient infected with HIV-1 may not react with the envelope proteins of HIV-2. A new generation of ELISA kits that contain genetically engineered recombinant viral proteins, that is, they include antigenic envelope epitopes from different HIV types as the antigen source, may solve this problem (41,42).

At present, the only FDA-approved use of the ELISA HIV-1 antibody detection systems is for *screening* the blood supply. Because the sensitivity and specificity (both estimated at 99.8%) of these assays are excellent, it is an ideal test for detecting potentially contaminated units of blood. However, because of the low prevalence of HIV infection in the donor population, most of the positive results obtained are false-positives (as predicted by Baye's theorem; 43). Testing at multiple blood donor centers has shown that 0.3% of the donor units test repeatedly positive by ELISA (44,45). However, when these same units are tested by an alternative and more specific method (e.g., Western blot, radioimmunoprecipitation, or indirect immunofluorescence), only 0.03% will test positive (46). In other words, for every 10 donor units that test positive, only 1 of the 10 will truly contain HIV antibodies. (Remember, one has to test 3333 units to find these 10 positive units.) The positive ELISA results of the remaining nine units will be "false-positive" results.

False-positive results have been observed in a variety of conditions, most of which are linked by the presence of autoimmunity. These conditions include alcoholic hepatitis (47), intravenous drug abuse (48), cancer/leukemia, and systemic lupus erythematosus (39). (The two former conditions are also associated with a polyclonal hypergammaglobulinemia.) In addition, anti-HLA-DR antibodies (e.g., those induced by a previous pregnancy) will react in the assay to give positive results (49-51). This phenomenon is caused by the anti-HLA-DR antibodies reacting with cellular HLA-DR antigens contributed by the cells in which HIV is grown. (The cellular antigens are incorporated into the HIV envelope when the virus buds from the cell surface.) An important feature of these assays would be to include a negative control. (e.g., the uninfected cell line, alone) with each run. Alternatively, virus isolated from a cell line (e.g., CEM) which does not express HLA class II antigens may be a preferable source of antigen (52). Again, the development of kits containing only recombinant viral proteins that are free from cellular protein contamination, may eliminate a substantial proportion of these false-positive results.

Although the sensitivity of these assays is high, a few false-negative results are expected (53-55). These are partially attributable to the *biologic* "window" period—the interval between infection and the development of antibodies to HIV. This false-negative result does *not* usually reflect deficiencies in the assay itself. Currently, only one such documented case of transfusion-associated AIDS from a seronegative donor has occurred. This patient had detectable anti-HIV antibodies when tested 6 months after donating the contaminated unit (56). In a recent study of 780,000 units of blood drawn since March 1985 (57), 15 donors were identified who had antibodies to HIV, but who had tested negative when donating 3 to 6 months earlier. In addition, accounting for first-time donors who may be in the infective stage, but who are HIV antibody-negative, the present risk of being infected by an anti-HIV antibody-negative unit is estimated to be 1:48,000 (range: 1:36,000 to 1:72,000).

Other potential false-negative results have been estimated from the known sensitivity of the ELISA kits. If the kits have an overall sensitivity of 99.8%, and assuming a prevalence of HIV antibodies of 1:5000 donors, a false-negative rate of 1:500,000 units would be expected. The American Red Cross collects 12 million units of blood each year, meaning there is a possibility for 5 units of potentially infectious units to be transfused a year owing to the technical limitations of the assay itself.

Diagnosing HIV Infection

The FDA has not approved any tests for use in *diagnosing* HIV infection. Although the ELISA kits are currently being used and seem to be fairly reliable, it should be emphasized that the kits were designed for *screening* blood of unknown risk for the presence of HIV antibody and not for diagnosis of HIV infection in persons suspected of being infected.

Because the kits were developed for screening purposes, they were designed to have a high sensitivity, at the sacrifice of specificity. We will assume an overall ELISA kit sensitivity of 99% and specificity of 99% for the following examples. The interpretation of a positive result is directly linked to the prevalence of disease in the population being tested (Baye's theorem; 43). The individual being tested should be assessed for risk factors, and placed into a high-risk or low-risk group. If such a person is in a high-risk group, the prevalence of HIV infection is sufficiently high that a positive ELISA result probably represents HIV infection (a "true-positive" test result). For example, if we estimate an 80% infection rate in a high-risk group, then a positive test will have a positive predictive value (i.e., probability of being infected with HIV) of 100%. If the patient belongs to a low-risk group in which HIV infection is not prevalent, then a positive result most probably represents a false-positive result. For example, if we estimate a 0.1% infection rate in a low-risk group, a positive test will have a positive predictive value of 20%. This means for every 1000 people in this population tested, 5 will test positive; 4 of these will have false-positive results, and only 1 will have a true-positive result. In any event, if the test result is discrepant with the clinical situation, an alternative and more specific HIV antibody test (e.g., Western blot, radioimmunoprecipitation, or indirect immunofluorescent) should be requested.

"Confirmatory" Tests

The FDA has not approved all of the following tests for use by blood banks for *confirming* repeatedly reactive ELISA results; however, the FDA cannot regulate the way these tests are used by laboratories other than blood banks. These supplemental tests appear to be fairly reliable as alternative and more specific tests for diagnosing HIV infection by detecting HIV antibodies. They are usually performed in a reference research laboratory because they are dependent on technology usually not available in the standard clinical laboratory setting.

Western Blot

The Western blot technique (58), in principle, detects an antigen-antibody reaction occurring on a solid phase. The technique involves initial electrophoresis of HIV viral proteins on a sodium dodecyl sulfate-containing polyacrylamide gel (SDS-PAGE) matrix, which separates viral proteins on the basis of molecular weight. The separated viral proteins are then electrophoretically transferred to a nitrocellulose membrane to provide a sturdier matrix for further handling. Nonspecific antibody-binding sites are blocked by prior incubation of the nitrocellulose in a buffered solution of irrelevant protein (e.g., casein, bovine serum albumin, or gelatin), after which the membrane is washed and incubated with the serum to be tested. If specific anti-HIV antibodies are present in the serum, they will bind to specific viral proteins on the membrane. After adequate washing to remove nonspecifically bound material, the membrane is incubated with a second antihuman antibody, to which has been coupled an enzyme. The membrane is washed again, and then incubated in the presence of the enzyme substrate. A dark band (representative of enzyme degradation of substrate) will appear wherever an anti-HIV antibody has bound to the membrane. In this manner, one can detect the presence of antibodies to HIV in serum as well as determining the specific viral proteins to which they bind.

There are currently many problems with the Western blot technique, not the least of which is lack of standardization of the procedure. Every laboratory performs the test differently. Although other immunologic assays have shown that low serum dilutions can give rise to many artifacts (e.g., false-positive results), the dilution of serum to be tested varies from undiluted to 1:200. The choice of agents as well as the concentration at which they should be used for blocking nonspecific protein-binding sites also varies from laboratory to laboratory. The CDC procedure (59) does not include a blocking step, and instead relies on the presence of detergent [0.3% (v/v) Tween 20] in all of the buffers to prevent nonspecific protein binding. The choice of blocking agents was critically evaluated, and it was found that blocking with casein, compared with the use of gelatin, allowed greater sensitivity of anti-HIV antibody detection (60). The choice of which enzyme to couple to the second antibody also varies. Another study (61) demonstrated that alkaline phosphatase, when compared with horseradish peroxidase or a radioiodinated second antibody, allowed greater sensitivity of detection. Yet, this latter study did not use the same procedure as the study comparing blocking agents. It is thus impossible to correlate the two studies to determine optimum reagents and procedures. The choice of washing buffers also varies; although most laboratories will use nonionic detergents (e.g., Tween 20) in the buffers to prevent nonspecific binding, the concentration ranges from 0.3% to 0.05% (v/v). To draw any meaningful conclusions about the utility of Western blot analysis in detecting anti-HIV antibodies, a single, standardized procedure should be adopted, only after which interlaboratory variability can be assessed.

A currently commercially available FDA-approved Western blot system from a single manufacturer (E. I. du Pont de Nemours & Co. Inc., Wilmington, Delaware 19898) may alleviate most of the aforementioned problems by forcing laboratories to use the same reagents and procedure. The test is expensive; a single nitrocellulose strip (to test a single patient serum sample) costs 45 dollars. Each sample must have parallel positive and negative controls run (at least two additional strips). After factoring in technologist time and reagent costs, the cost of this test is considerable.

Aside from the technical and labor-intensive aspects of performing a Western blot analysis, interpretation can also be difficult. A national consensus panel established guidelines (62) for the interpretation of Western blot results as follows: the detection of at least two different antibody specificities, one directed against at least one of the HIV envelope proteins (gp120/160, gp41) and the other against the major HIV core protein (p24), is diagnostic of HIV exposure. Ironically, the presence of antibody against only the major core protein, p24, is *not* sufficient evidence for diagnosing HIV exposure. On one hand, there have been reports of early HIV infection in patients whose only serologic manifestation was an anti-p24 antibody (32), who then later went on to develop antibodies against the remaining viral proteins, and from whom virus could be isolated. On the other hand, anti-p24 antibodies appear as a nonspecific reactivity seen in a variety of patients with different diseases. In one study (63), 7 of 124 patients with other viral illnesses had anti-p24 antibodies.

The criteria for determining a positive Western blot test using the Dupont system (63) differs from that of the national consensus panel (62). Dupont states that the serum must show reactivity against *all* the HIV viral proteins (p17, p24, p31, gp41, p51, p55, p66, gp120, and gp160) before a test is considered positive. Reactivity against only a subset of these proteins (in any combination) is considered an indeterminate result. In theory, then, this system will be 100% specific, albeit much less sensitive than other currently existing anti-HIV antibody-screening tests.

The Western blot technique should be highly specific, in that only those antibodies specifically recognizing HIV proteins should react. In practice, false-positive as well as false-negative results have occurred. The former occur rarely, and they are attributable to the same underlying autoimmune processes occurring in those patients who have false-positive ELISA results. Many of the false-positive results were detected by reacting the same serum with antigens prepared from the uninfected cell line and showing the same pattern of reactivity (49-51). The absolute rate at which false-negative results occur is not known.

Indirect Immunofluorescence Assay

The indirect immunofluorescence assay (64-66) for detecting anti-HIV antibodies is an adaptation of a familiar laboratory technique. The HIV-infected cells are fixed onto a glass slide and then incubated with the test serum. The cells are washed to remove nonbound material, and then they are incubated with a fluoresceinated antihuman antibody. The slide is viewed with a fluorescent microscope, and specific immunofluorescence noted.

The advantage of this technique is that uninfected cells (a built-in negative control) are also present on the slide. Thus, one is readily able to distinguish a specific reactivity against only HIV antigens ($\leq$ 40% of the cells will fluoresce) versus a nonspecific pattern of reactivity seen in autoimmune disorders (in which $\geq$ 40% but $\leq$ 100% of cells can fluoresce). In addition, this methodology is familiar to most clinical laboratories and can be instituted fairly easily.

Both immunofluorescence and the Western blot technique show similar sensitivity and specificity when used to confirm positive ELISA results (64-66). Thus, either procedure can be used as an alternative and more specific method for testing for anti-HIV antibodies. From the standpoint of ease of performance and familiarity, immunofluorescence is the preferable alternative. The drawback is that substrate slides are not now commercially available; however, many companies are in the process of developing such substrate slides for marketing, and this should soon solve the supply problem.

Radioimmunoprecipitation

Radioimmunoprecipitation (67,68) is another method of testing for the specificity of antibodies detected in the anti-HIV ELISA. This technique uses a radiolabeled cell lysate, prepared from HIV-infected cells, incubated with test serum, and analysis of the resultant antigen-antibody complexes (immunoprecipitate) by PAGE followed by autoradiography.

This procedure has many disadvantages. First, a tissue culture facility is needed to cultivate HIV-infected cells. Second, radioactive substrates must be used to prepare a radiolabeled cell lysate. Third, analysis of the immunoprecipitates involves high-resolution electrophoretic equipment, as well as autoradiography facilities. For all of these technical reasons, radioimmunoprecipitation will probably remain a specialized procedure performed only by reference research laboratories.

In summary, many alternative methods are available for detecting anti-HIV antibodies. For either screening or diagnostic purposes, the ELISA should be the first test performed; positive ELISA results should be confirmed with indirect immunofluorecence, Western blot, or radioimmunoprecipitation.

A word of caution: it should be emphasized that *no* laboratory test is 100% accurate. In fact, correlation between the various confirmatory tests is not 100% (68). If the test results do not agree with the clinical assessment of the patient, clinicians should always trust their own clinical judgment over and above any conflicting laboratory result.

Antigen Detection Assays

The p24 antigen-capture assay was discussed earlier in conjunction with HIV culture detection methods. Another potential use of this assay is to test serum for the presence of HIV antigens. In a small study (69) following HIV-infected patients treated with azidothymidine (AZT) versus placebo, the use of this assay made possible the demonstration of a decrease in p24 antigenemia with continued AZT therapy; similar results were seen with patients treated with foscarnet (70), whereas no change in the level of p24 antigenemia was detected in patients treated with ribavirin (71). Thus, this test may be of use in following any patient receiving antiviral therapy to determine its effect on viremia.

It should be mentioned that one report of a false-positive p24 antigen capture ture assay has already appeared (72). The serum was from a healthy blood donor, who remained healthy for at least 1 year after his false-positive result. This report is not so surprising when one considers that the HIV viral protein most likely to nonspecifically react by Western blot is p24. In other words, many healthy people have anti-p24 antibodies. One study (63) showed that 7 of 124 patients with another viral illness (2, Epstein-Barr virus; 1, varicella-zoster virus; 3, cytomegalovirus; 3, herpes simplex; 2, measles; 1, mumps; 2, coxsackievirus; 2, adenovirus; 2, influenza A) had anti-p24 antibodies in their serum. This would imply that p24 must share some epitopes with one or more fairly common antigens, such that a significant proportion of healthy individuals will have cross-reacting antibodies. By similar reasoning, if this cross-reacting antigen is prevalent in the population and shares epitopes with p24, then it could react with a monoclonal anti-p24 antibody if that monoclonal antibody is directed against the shared epitope.

More experience with this assay will be necessary before it can be used for widespread screening purposes. One report on the use of this assay system to screen plasma of HIV-infected patients for p24 antigenemia, revealed that this assay was, at best, only 75% sensitive (17). However, with further development and refinement, this type of assay may well be incorporated into the HIV test panel, much as screening for hepatitis B surface antigen (HB_sAg) has become commonplace.

DIAGNOSIS OF OTHER VIRAL ILLNESSES

The acute mononucleosislike symptomatology of acute HIV infection (see Chap. 12) as well as the chronic or recurrent fatigue induced by chronic HIV infection are often mistaken for other, more common, viral infections (e.g., cytomegalovirus, herpes simplex virus, Epstein-Barr virus). Attempting to make a serologic diagnosis of these more common viral illnesses is fraught with problems, including that most of the population will have already developed antibodies to these viruses from childhood exposure and that the presence of antiviral IgM is *not* diagnostic of acute infection.

A study of a group of HIV-infected homosexual men in San Francisco revealed that > 95% had antibodies to cytomegalovirus (CMV) (73). When anti-CMV IgM levels were measured at regular intervals in this population, it was observed that, although the anti-CMV IgG titers remained constant, sporadic peaks of IgM production occurred in the absence of viruria. Thus, it is impossible to interpret CMV serologic results in a patient who is already seropositive.

The histopathologic diagnosis of CMV infection is easily made if intranuclear and intracytoplasmic viral inclusions are detected. Culture of tissue may also be of benefit. However, because CMV can be present in tissues or excreted in various bodily fluids in an acute illness caused by a bacterial or parasitic agent, the recovery of CMV in culture does not necessarily mean that CMV is the agent causing the acute disease.

Most of the American population have been infected with herpes simplex virus (HSV) during childhood and have serum antibodies to this virus. Analogous to the CMV situation, it is impossible to interpret a serologic result in an already seropositive individual. Fortunately, a diagnosis of an acute herpetic attack can be made based on the appearance and distribution of the lesions, as well as examination of direct immunofluorescent staining of smears made from material from the base of a vesicular lesion (74) or by a Tzanck smear, or by culture if necessary.

Epstein-Barr virus (EBV) infects most Americans in childhood, with > 95% of the population having antibodies by 30 years of age. The results of EBV serologic studies in any adult are rarely helpful, except for following selected patients with nasopharyngeal carcinoma or Burkitt's lymphoma.

The recently discovered human B-cell lymphotropic virus (HBLV or HHV-6) (75), a member of the herpes virus family, has been isolated from HIV-infected patients, as well as from a few patients suffering from what was called "chronic EBV syndrome." The role of this virus in disease is not clear, and a serologic test for exposure to this virus is not yet available.

In summary, serologic diagnosis of these common viral illnesses in a population in whom there is a high prevalence of prior infection is not possible unless seroconversion can be documented by comparing acute and convalescent serum specimens. Direct visualization of virus-specific cytopathologic changes in tissue sections, possibly supplemented by culture or detection of specific virus antigens in tissue by immunoperoxidase or immunofluorescence techniques, is the only way to ascribe a particular illness to a viral etiology.

BACTERIAL INFECTIONS

The spectrum of bacterial agents, with the exception of the mycobacterioses, causing septicemia in adult HIV-infected patients is similar to those agents causing septicemia in the general adult population (76,77). However, the disease in the HIV-infected patients may have more severe manifestations— for example, there appears to be a higher frequency of bacteremia caused by *Salmonella* species after an episode of gastroenteritis (78), as well as a higher frequency of recurrent pneumococcal bacteremia following pneumococcal pneumonia (79). The explanation for why AIDS patients have a higher frequency of bacteremias is unknown.

There are no special requirements for bacterial culture that should be employed in AIDS patients, over and above trying to obtain the best specimen possible. Only when an unusual pathogen is suspected should special media be inoculated; in this situation, the laboratory should be consulted about the optimal specimen to be submitted for isolation and identification.

Unusual Bacterial Isolates

Our experience at San Francisco General Hospital mirrors that of other hospitals with a high proportion of HIV-infected individuals, in that the most frequent bacterial isolates in this population are no different from those seen in the general adult population. However, we have noticed a few unusual isolates, some of which are unusual in any setting, and others that may occur more frequently in the HIV-infected population.

Although *Legionella* sp. is recognized as a cause of adult pneumonia, we have *not* isolated this organism with increased frequency from the HIV-infected population. In a 1-year study in which all bronchoalveolar lavages from suspected AIDS patients were cultured for *Legionella* using selective media (80), only two isolates were recovered (from approximately 500 specimens). However, the incidence of legionella infections varies with geographic location, the particular institution, and with construction, or other activities that increase exposure to this soil and water organism. *Legionella* sp. is relatively rare in San Francisco, and this may explain our low recovery.

The laboratory is often asked to perform immunofluorescent staining for *Legionella* to provide a rapid diagnosis; however, estimates of the sensitivity of such staining range from 33% to 70% (81-83). The type of specimen has an important influence on this test; a bronchoalveolar lavage will have minimal nonspecific background staining as compared with sputum, which is often contaminated with other bacteria and debris that stain nonspecifically, yielding false-positive results. Performing such an assay with appropriate parallel controls for different serotypes or pools and different species can also be time-consuming and labor-intensive, often occupying a single technologist for 4 hr. Thus, this technique should be reserved for only those patients in whom an immediate diagnosis is imperative and for whom appropriate antibiotic coverage will not be instituted unless the results of the test are positive (remembering the less-than-optimal sensitivity of the assay). Culture is the definitive method for both isolation and identification of *Legionella* sp., and should be used preferentially in diagnosing infection. A culture on a medium selected to enhance recovery of *Legionella* sp. (80) will often show growth within 3 days, at which time a species identification is possible by immunofluorescent staining of cells from a colony. A semiselective antibiotic-containing medium (84) also has been developed which will allow the growth of *Legionella* sp. while suppressing the growth of contaminating oral flora.

In a separate 3-year study (85) to assess the prevalence of chlamydial pneumonia in the AIDS population, bronchoalveolar lavages and transbronchial brush biopsies from AIDS patients, admitted for pneumonia for a total of 658 hospitalizations, were cultured for all suspected bacterial pathogens. Only three isolates of *Chlamydia trachomatis* were obtained; all three patients had concomitant *Pneumocystis carinii* pneumonia. (This study did not attempt to isolate or identify *C. psittaci*. Also, the role of the recently described *C. psittaci* strain called TWAR (86) is unknown; reagents for detecting the presence of TWAR are not now available.) Thus, AIDS patients seem to be no more susceptible to chlamydial pneumonia than the general population. However, if chlamydial pneumonia is suspected, a sample for culture that includes cellular material (chlamydia is an obligate intracellular bacteria) should be obtained. Culture for chlamydia requires access to tissue culture facilities and specialized techniques and reagents that are usually available only at major research institutions.

Another finding of this study was the unexpected isolation of *Bordetella pertussis* from two AIDS patients. One patient had concurrent *P. carinii* pneumonia (as well as cytomegalovirus and *C. trachomatis* isolated from culture of the bronchoalveolar lavage); bacterial cultures of the broncho-alveolar lavage from the other patient, although symptomatic with cough, fever, and dyspnea, grew only *B. pertussis* and normal oral flora. These isolates grew on the charcoal-containing medium specifically formulated (80) for the isolation of *Legionella* sp. and were only suspected of being an organism *other* than *Legionella* when the gram stain revealed coccobacillary gram-negative organisms that failed to react with the legionella-specific immunofluorescent antisera. A review of the literature revealed that a specific medium designed to enhance the growth of bordetella (87) is very similar to the medium designed to enhance the growth of legionella.

Last of all, we have occasionally isolated *Campylobacter cinaedi* and *Campylobacter fennelliae* (88) from blood cultures of HIV-infected individuals. The frequency of these isolates associated with HIV infection is not known; however, the only reported cases of bacteremia with these organisms are in presumed or known HIV-infected patients (89-91). Positive cultures are detected by positive growth indices in an automated blood culturing system (e.g., BACTEC) or by visualization of organisms with darting motility on dark-field examination. More often than not, the Gram stain does not reveal organisms. Final identification of these organisms may take months, and it is usually accomplished only by a reference research laboratory. If these agents are suspected, in vitro susceptibilities to 20 different antimicrobial agents are known and can help guide therapy (92).

In summary, the current workup for bacterial pathogens is adequate for specimens from both the general adult population, as well as from the HIV-infected population. No special procedures need be followed when culturing a specimen from an HIV-infected individual, however, the laboratory should be alerted to the possibility of recovering unusual pathogens from blood or other specimens.

Mycobacteriosis

Mycobacterial infections are common in HIV-infected patients, and there is a special predisposition toward disseminated infection with *Mycobacterium avium* complex (MAC) organisms (93-96). If mycobacterial infection is suspected, blood is the specimen of choice for culture. Although bone marrow cultures showed a slightly higher rate of recovery of MAC in HIV-infected patients (97), the organisms were isolated from concomitant blood cultures in all except 1 of 25 cases (98). Because drawing blood has less morbidity than obtaining bone marrow, blood should be the initial specimen cultured. However, if a bone marrow aspiration is performed for other reasons, then an aliquot should be cultured. In addition, the paraffin-embedded biopsy specimen should be examined for acid-fast organisms. Although an examination for acid-fast organisms does not correlate perfectly with recovery from culture (98), a positively staining specimen will allow a rapid diagnosis, compared with culture (i.e., days versus weeks). There is little need to culture multiple sites in trying to diagnose mycobacteriosis in this population; the load of organisms is thought to be high enough that mycobacteremia is virtually always present in the untreated patient.

Stool and urine cultures for mycobacteria are not helpful. Although *M. avium* complex can be isolated from these sites, the significance of a positive culture is unclear. A positive culture cannot distinguish between colonization or infection. In addition, *M. avium* complex is a soil and water organism that can be isolated from nonsterile sites from nonbacteremic patients.

The experience of the laboratory is crucial to the differentiation of mycobacteria. For example, the first isolates of *M. avium* complex at San Francisco General Hospital were highly pigmented, even though the classic description of this organism was of a buff-colored nonphotochromogenic colony. Biochemical reactions were essential for determining the exact species. Many hospitals lack the expertise needed for definitive identification of *M. avium* complex and should refer cultures to reference laboratories. Our current practice is to select those cultures with the characteristic colonial morphology of the *M. avium* complex and to use three biochemical tests (semiquantitative catalase, urease, and photochromogenicity) and the rate of growth for presumptive identification of MAC. Antibiotic susceptibility is performed by a reference laboratory and often takes many weeks for results. A recently described microdilution antibiotic susceptibility test system may shorten the turnaround time for results (99).

The clinical response to therapy does not correlate well with in vitro antibiotic susceptibility testing of mycobacteria. This lack of correlation may be partially explained by the different methodologies employed for antibiotic susceptibility testing. Traditional methods do not always take into account the concentration of antimicrobials achievable in the patient's serum nor the possible role of antimicrobial synergism. In addition, these methods measure inhibition of growth, not the killing, of the organism. Recent in vitro studies have shown that there is poor killing of MAC by the concentrations of clofazimine and rifabutin that are normally obtained in patient's serum (100). This may explain the poor clinical response to treatment with these two antimicrobials (101).

The use of radiometric blood culture detection systems (e.g., BACTEC; 102) in conjunction with a lysis-centrifugation processing step (103) enables a more rapid detection of mycobacteremia.

There is currently an effort to develop specific gene probes for the various *Mycobacterium* species in the hope of providing a means for more rapid identification (104). Mycobacterial DNA probes are currently commercially available (105,106; Gen-Probe, San Diego, California 92121).

DIAGNOSIS OF FUNGAL INFECTIONS

The diagnosis of fungal infections in the HIV-infected individual relies heavily on culture techniques. Although *Candida* and *Cryptococcus* sp. will grow on routine bacteriologic culture media and can be detected within 7 days, other fungi (e.g., *Histoplasma capsulatum*) require a fungal culture medium and at least 1 to 3 weeks for detectable growth. If disseminated fungal infection is suspected, then fungal blood cultures should be submitted.

In rare situations, fungal infections can be diagnosed by other means. In a few patients with disseminated histoplasma infection, a careful perusal of a Giemsa-stained peripheral blood smear may reveal yeast cells inside polymorphonuclear cells or monocytes. However, this finding is usually present only when the patient is terminal, and may reflect an uncontrolled replication of yeast in the advanced stages of the disease.

On seven occasions we have identified *Cryptococcus neoformans* or *H. capsulatum* on Giemsa-stained smears of bronchoalveolar lavages or bone marrow aspirates. Direct identification of these yeasts on smears is highly dependent on knowledge of the morphology of these fungi. *Cryptococcus neoformans* is usually a budding, spherical cell (Fig. 1a) with wide variation in size (ranging from 4 to 20 μm in diameter) observable within a single microscopic field. A clear region, the capsule, is seen by negative staining in the Giemsa stain but stains positively with mucicarmine or periodic acid-Schiff (PAS). *Histplasma capsulatum* usually is an ellipsoid, budding yeast (Fig. 1b), with some variation in size (2 to 5 μm in diameter), but may appear spherical and have larger diameter cells. They have a thin unstained region around the yeast cell; the nuclei of the yeast cells are well defined by Giemsa staining.

Tissue stains (e.g., PAS, mucicarmine, silver methenamine) are useful for detecting yeasts. Comparisons of the ability of microscopic examination versus culture to detect the presence of yeast have shown that neither procedure is 100% sensitive, and that correlation between the two techniques is

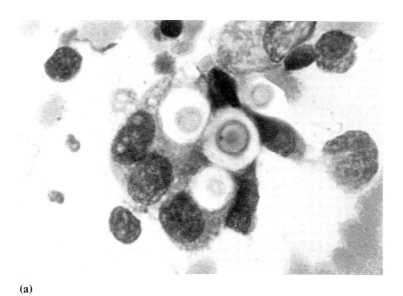

(a)

(b)

FIGURE 1 Giemsa-stained appearance of fungi and of protozoan parasites that commonly infect patients at risk for AIDS. (a) Bone marrow aspirate containing *C. neoformans* yeast cells. Note the prominent capsule that is enhanced by the negative staining. (b) Bronchoalveolar lavage containing an alveolar macrophage that has ingested numerous *H. capsulatum* yeast cells. (c) Touch preparation of a brain biopsy

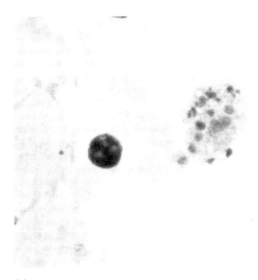

(c)

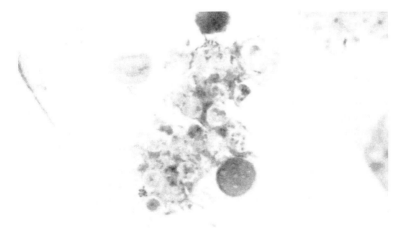

(d)

specimen showing intracellular trophozoites of *T. gondii*. (d) Induced sputum containing a clump of *P. carinii* in various stages of its life cycle. Note the presence of mature cysts (with eight well-defined intracystic bodies) as well as cysts in various stages of development (with a well-defined cyst wall but containing fewer than eight intracystic bodies). Trophozoites are less well defined and scattered throughout the clump.

not 100%. Thus, tissue biopsies should be split and processed for both histologic examination and culture.

Cryptococcus neoformans is unique in that an excellent antigen detection kit is available that is manufactured by Meridien Diagnostics, Inc. (P.O. Box 44216, Cincinnati, Ohio 45244). The kit consists of latex beads, coated with polyclonal specific anticryptococcal antibody, which agglutinate in the presence of cryptococcal antigen. Serum and cerebrospinal fluid can be analyzed rapidly, and the test is highly sensitive (detects 25 ng of antigen per milliliter) and specific. This assay has replaced the old technique of examining fluids with India ink, which was only 50% sensitive, at best. The antigen detection kit is virtually 100% sensitive and specific; the only false-negative results are seen early in the disease when the level of antigenemia is not high enough for detection. False-positive results are usually seen when rheumatoid factor is present (which will agglutinate the latex beads by binding to the antibody coating the bead); however, prior treatment with reducing substances (e.g., dithiotreitol) will remove this interfering factor (107). In addition, all samples are run against a rheumatoid factor control (latex beads coated with a nonspecific immunoglobulin).

There has been one reported case of a prozone phenomenon observed with a cryptococcal latex agglutination test (108). This report has been used as justification to demand that both India ink and cryptococcal antigen tests be done on a specimen from a suspected AIDS patient. However, the authors of this case report (108) did not use a commercial cryptococcal antigen detection kit. By using the Meridien Diagnostics kit, we have observed serum and CSF cryptococcal antigen titers as high as 1:1,000,000 without observing a prozone effect.

The other currently existing tests for antifungal antibodies are generally not useful diagnostically. There are considerable problems with cross-reacting antigens shared between different species of fungus. For example, some patients with histoplasmosis may show antibody responses to *Coccidiodes immitis* or *Blastomyces dermatitidis* (109). In addition, detection of antifungal antibodies cannot distinguish between past versus current infection or reactivation. We, and others (110), have also observed patients with disseminated histoplasmosis who had no evidence of specific antihistoplasma antibodies. Direct examination and culture of tissue or body fluids remain the diagnostic methods of choice for documenting a fungal infection.

DIAGNOSIS OF PARASITIC INFECTIONS

The diagnosis of parasitic infections in HIV-infected individuals relies almost exclusively on microscopic examination of specimens. A variety of concentration methods and stains are used to aid in the identification of these parasites. Currently, serology plays no role in the diagnosis of parasitic infections in this population.

Cryptosporidiosis and Isosporiasis

Cryptosporidium sp. and *Isospora belli*, protozoan parasites in the Coccidia family, are two major causes of severe diarrhea in the HIV-infected host. The diagnosis of infection with these organisms can be made with a stool examination. Although different laboratories will process specimens in different ways (e.g., Sheather sucrose flotation versus formalin-ether sedimentation versus zinc sulfate flotation techniques), all methods are equivalent in their ability to detect these organisms (111). The formalin-ether sedimentation processing, the concentration method most frequently used by clinical parasitology laboratories, has the added advantage of detecting other unrelated parasites that may be missed by the flotation processing (111). For detection of *Cryptosporidium* sp. the Ziehl-Neelsen acid-fast stain or modified Ziehl-Neelsen acid-fast stain is preferable (112). Immunofluorescent antibody stains are also available (113). The most critical factor in identifying the causative organism(s) is the expertise of the laboratory personnel in recognizing the cryptosporidial oocyst with its contained sporozoites and distinguishing them from other components of stool of similar size and shape (e.g., yeasts). Staining reactions must not be used as the sole criterion for identification; morphology must also be a criterion.

   In the rare case of disseminated isosporiasis or cryptosporidiosis present upon respiratory, intestinal, or gallbladder epithelial cells (114-116), diagnosis is made by observing the characteristic morphologic structure of the organism in the affected tissue.

Toxoplasma gondii

Toxoplasmosis in the HIV-infected host usually presents with neurologic symptoms and signs (117-120). This disease is thought to occur by reactivation of a latent infection that was acquired in childhood. Because many urban dwellers have been exposed to and infected with *T. gondii* in childhood, 15% to 25% of the adult population with HIV infection will have antibodies to *T. gondii* (G. Leoung, J. Mills, and J. Remington, unpublished observations). Thus, if reactivation disease is suspected, serology is of little benefit in making the diagnosis (119,121).

   At present, the only way to diagnose CNS toxoplasmosis definitively is by brain biopsy and histologic examination of brain tissue. Bradyzoites and individual tachyzoites are difficult to see in formalin-fixed hematoxylin-eosin-stained tissue sections, although cysts are easily identified. If brain biopsy is performed, *fresh* (*before* fixation) touch preparations on slides must be made and fixed *immediately* with methanol or acetone, Giemsa stained, and examined for cysts and tachyzoites. Tissue for touch preparations must be protected from drying by transport in a sterile Telfa pad barely moistened with sterile saline. (Excess saline will dissolve the natural adhesins that allow cells to stick to a slide.) Tachyzoites are spread out on the surface of the slide (Fig. 1c) and do not have the shrunken appearance seen on histologic sections (caused by processing). Often tachyzoites can be seen adjacent to or within polymorphonuclear leukocytes.

Detection of toxoplasma antigens in tissue sections by immunoperoxidase staining with specific antitoxoplasma antibodies may also be used to diagnose toxoplasma infection (122). This technique is currently available only as a research procedure, but holds great promise for future diagnostic use.

Pneumocystis carinii

Pneumocystis carinii is the most common cause of pneumonia in the HIV-infected patient. Diagnosis relies on the microscopic examination of respiratory secretions or lung tissue, and a variety of different stains are employed to aid in the identification. The choice of specimen type and the stain used will be dependent on the expertise of the individual laboratory. Initial studies at San Francisco General Hospital compared bronchoalveolar lavage (89% sensitive) with transbronchial biopsy (97% sensitive; 123) for diagnosis of *P. carinii* pneumonia. Both procedures combined were 100% sensitive and specific. Since this initial study, our experience has been that bronchoalveolar lavage alone may be sufficient for diagnosis and that an additional biopsy is rarely required. We have recently been able to demonstrate that 74-77% of all diagnoses of *P. carinii* can be made by examining induced sputum which is mucolysed by dithiotreitol and concentrated (124,125), thus sparing a large proportion of patients the discomfort and expense of a bronchoscopic procedure and extra hospitalization. Because of the rapidity of the induced sputum procedure, bronchoscopy and bronchoalveolar lavage can be scheduled the same day if the single, induced sputum examination is found to be negative.

We favor the use of a rapid Giemsa-like stain (Diff-Quik) for the detection of *P. carinii* (126; Fig. 1d); others favor a rapid silver methenamine stain (127) or a toluidine blue-O (128) stain. The latter two stains are cyst wall-specific, whereas the Giemsa stains permit identification of trophozoites as well as cysts. The choice of stain will vary among laboratories depending upon their need for speed of diagnosis and their expertise in recognizing the various stages of *P. carinii*. A new technique being developed uses monoclonal antipneumocystis antibodies in an indirect immunofluorescent assay (129). Preliminary results indicate that this antibody is highly specific *and* more sensitive than any of the current conventional stains.

The decision whether to send a specimen to an anatomic or clinical pathology laboratory will depend on the local expertise. At San Francisco General Hospital, almost all specimens being examined for *P. carinii*, are currently examined in our microbiology laboratory. The services of anatomic pathology are requested only when a transbronchial or open-lung biopsy (a rare event) is obtained. In such cases, the microbiology laboratory will examine Giemsa-stained fresh touch preparations of the tissues; anatomic pathology will examine silver methenamine-stained paraffin embedded specimens. These biopsy preparations have been useful for diagnosing fungal disease (e.g., histoplasmosis or coccidioidomycosis) and usually do not contain *P. carinii*. However, in our recent experience, most histoplasmosis in AIDS have been detected by the microbiology laboratory in Giemsa-stained bronchoalveolar lavage preparations or bone marrow aspirate smears.

NONSPECIFIC LABORATORY TESTS OF QUESTIONABLE UTILITY

General Biochemical Tests

A number of nonspecific laboratory tests have been used as screening tests, as a guide to whether or not a further evaluation for a specific disease is indicated. The decision of whether or not to use a nonspecific screening test must be related to the clinical situation; if a specific infectious agent is suspected, then the specific diagnostic test of choice should be used instead. Although the cost per individual test is small, the overall cost to the laboratory is great because of the large volume of screening tests performed.

The erythrocyte sedimentation rate (ESR) has been used as an indicator of inflammatory processes causing the increased formation of serum globulins and fibrinogen (i.e., acute-phase reactants). Most acutely ill patients will have an elevated ESR; an abnormal result with this test adds nothing to narrowing the differential diagnosis and serves only to increase the suspicion of active disease. A more specific test, depending on the clinical setting, should be ordered instead. However, in very mildly ill patients, an elevated ESR may be a helpful clue indicating that further evaluation and specific testing should be performed.

Total serum lactate dehydrogenase (LDH) levels are notoriously nonspecific. Recently, it was observed that AIDS patients with an acute episode of *P. carinii* pneumonia have elevations of their total serum LDH levels. It was observed that the degree of elevation was roughly correlated to the severity of pneumonia, and that normalization of total LDH values was correlated with clinical improvement in the patient (130). Despite this finding, it must be emphasized that elevation of total serum LDH levels is nonspecific and can be seen in a variety of disorders, including myocardial infarction, progressive muscular dystrophy, delirium tremens, dermatomyositis, neoplastic disease, granulocytic leukemia, megaloblastic anemia, and others (131).

Although it has been shown that patients with *P. carinii* pneumonia have a selective elevation in fraction 3 (130), LDH isoenzyme fractionation in the AIDS population is of questionable value because elevation of LDH fraction 3 has also been observed in patients with granulocytic leukemia, pancreatitis, and extensive carcinomatosis (131).

An elevated total serum alkaline phosphatase (AP) level, in the absence of elevated transaminase levels (e.g., alanine aminotransferase, ALT/SGPT, or aspartate aminotransferase, AST/SGOT) seems to correlate with disseminated *M. avium* complex infection. Macrophages are a source of alkaline phosphatase activity, and an elevated value may reflect increased macrophage activity. However, the sources of AP within the body are many and varied (including bone, intestine, and liver), and an elevated value should be evaluated further, depending on the clinical setting (i.e., blood cultures for mycobacteria and fungi, sonographic examination of the right upper quadrant for possible obstructive hepatobiliary disease or papillary stenosis and sclerosing cholangitis (132).

A polyclonal hypergammaglobulinemia has been one of the earliest abnormalities observed following HIV infection (133). However, this response is fairly nonspecific, and can be seen with many other acute or chronic infections. Thus, an HIV-infected patient with an elevated globulin level may not need further evaluation; however, if a marked elevation is present (i.e., greater than 1.5 times the upper limit of the reference range), a screening serum protein electrophoresis (SPEP) may be warranted to eliminate the possibility of coexistent multiple myeloma. One abnormality frequently seen (estimated to be present in 10% to 15% of hypergammaglobulinemic HIV-infected individuals) is the presence of oligoclonal bands or paraproteins (134-136). The clinical significance of these paraproteins is unclear and may reflect polyclonal B-cell activation following HIV infection. In one well-characterized patient, his paraprotein spike, which was *not* monoclonal in origin, appeared to contain most of the anti-HIV antibody activity present in his plasma (137).

Tests of Immune Function

It was well recognized early in the AIDS epidemic that patients were susceptible to illnesses previously seen only in severely immunodeficient patients. Before the discovery of HIV, immune function tests were performed as part of the routine evaluation. It was recognized that an inverted T-helper/T-suppressor ($T_{H/S}$) ratio (a value < 1.0; normal reference range of 1.1 to 2.4) was commonly seen in AIDS patients. It is now recognized that HIV infection selectively depletes the T-helper subset of lymphocytes (138,139), accounting for the observed inverted $T_{H/S}$ ratio.

While first observed in AIDS patients, inverted $T_{H/S}$ ratios are *not* unique to AIDS. Inverted $T_{H/S}$ ratios have been observed in many other illnesses including systemic lupus erythematosus with renal disease, acute cytomegalovirus infection, burns, graft-versus-host disease, sunburn or ultraviolet-solarium exposure, myelodysplastic syndromes, acute lymphocytic leukemia in remission, recovering marrow transplant, herpes infections, infectious mononucleosis, measles, and even vigorous exercise (140). Many of the aforementioned viral infections may produce clinical symptoms suggestive of HIV infection; currently, the clinical utility of a $T_{H/S}$ ratio is very questionable. At present, the only use of a $T_{H/S}$ ratio, in conjunction with consistent clinical findings and laboratory tests, would be to diagnose AIDS in a child under 15 months of age (141). If HIV infection is suspected, the definitive HIV antibody test should be performed instead.

A more useful test with some prognostic value (142) would be the quantitation of absolute numbers of T-helper cells. It appears that the absolute T-helper cell number correlates inversely with the progression of disease (lower counts mean a higher risk of developing AIDS). Such an indicator may be helpful in counseling HIV-seropositive patients as well as making decisions about therapeutic interventions. An absolute T-helper cell count can also be used, in conjunction with other clinical findings and laboratory tests, to diagnose HIV infection in a patient lacking HIV antibodies (141).

Other tests of immune function (e.g., concanavalin A, pokeweed mitogen, phytohemagglutinin, and other agents used in lymphocyte mitogen stimulation tests) were popular in the early years of the AIDS epidemic to assess immune function. However, the difficulty of finding a laboratory capable of performing such tests, the difficulty of interpreting the test results (143), and the expense of these tests has limited their usefulness. Currently, these tests have little value in the routine evaluation of a patient at risk for the development of AIDS.

CONCLUSIONS

In conclusion, the diagnosis of AIDS relies on the laboratory identification of the numerous opportunistic pathogens causing disease in this immunodeficient population. Table 1 outlines the laboratory methodologies of choice for identification of the various infectious agents. These specific methodologies should be requested when a specific diagnosis is entertained. Otherwise, there should be close communication with the microbiology laboratory to determine the most efficient and cost-effective manner for evaluating the patient.

TABLE 1   Definitive Diagnostic Methods for Diseases Indicative of AIDS

Diseases	Definitive diagnostic methods
Pneumocystosis Toxoplasmosis Cryptosporidiosis Isosporiasis Strongyloidiasis Cytomegalovirus Progressive multifocal leukoencephalopathy Kaposi's sarcoma Lymphoma PLH/LIP complex	Microscopy (histologic or cytologic)
Candidiasis	Microscopy (histologic or cytologic) on a specimen obtained directly from the affected tissues (including scrapings from the mucosal surface) or gross inspection by endoscopy or autopsy
Cryptococcosis Histoplasmosis Coccidioidomycosis Herpes simplex virus	Microscopy (histologic or cytologic), *or* culture, *or* antigen detection in a specimen obtained directly from the affected tissue or a fluid from those tissues
Tuberculosis Other mycobacteriosis Other bacterial infections	Culture

REFERENCES

1. Barre-Sinoussi, F., Chermann, J. C., Rey, F. et al. (1983). Isolation of a T-lymphotropic retrovirus from a patient at risk for acquired immune deficiency syndrome (AIDS). *Science 220*:868-871.
2. Levy, J. A., Hoffman, A. D., Kramer, S. M. et al. (1984). Isolation of lymphocytopathic retroviruses from San Francisco patients with AIDS. *Science 25*:840-842.
3. Gallo, R. C., Salahuddin, S. Z., Popovic, M. et al. (1984). Frequent detection and isolation of cytopathic retroviruses (HTLV-III) from patients with AIDS and at risk for AIDS. *Science 224*:500-502.
4. Clavel, F., Mansinho, K., Chamaret, S. et al. (1987). Human immunodeficiency virus type 2 infection associated with AIDS in West Africa. *N. Engl. J. Med. 316*: 1180-1185.
5. Haase, A. T. (1986). Pathogenesis of lentivirus infections. *Nature 322*:130-136.
6. Sonigo, P., Alizon, M., Staskus, K. et al. (1985). Nucleotide sequence of the visna lentivirus: Relationship to the AIDS virus. *Cell 42*:369-382.

7. Maddon, P. J., Dalgleish, A. G., McDougal, J. S., Clapham, P. R., Weiss, R. A., and Axel, R. (1986). The T4 gene encodes the AIDS virus receptor and is expressed in the immune system and the brain. *Cell 47*:333-348.

8. Gyorkey, F., Melnick, J. L., and Gyorkey, P. (1987). Human immunodeficiency virus in brain biopsies of patients with AIDS and progressive encephalopathy. *J. Infect. Dis. 155*:870-876.

9. Resnick, L., DiMarzo-Veronese, F., Schupbach, J. et al. (1985). Intra-blood-brain-barrier synthesis of HTLV-III-specific IgG in patients with neurologic symptoms associated with AIDS or AIDS-related complex. *N. Engl. J. Med. 313*:1498-1504.

10. Ho, D. D., Rota, T. R., Schooley, R. T. et al. (1985). Isolation of HTLV-III from cerebrospinal fluid and neural tissues of patients with neurologic syndromes related to the acquired immunodeficiency syndrome. *N. Engl. J. Med. 313*: 1493-1497.

11. Wiley, C. A., Schrier, R. D., Nelson, J. A., Lampert, P. W., and Oldstone, M. B. A. (1986). Cellular localization of human immunodeficiency virus infection within the brains of acquired immune deficiency syndrome patients. *Proc. Natl. Acad. Sci. USA 83*:7089-7093.

12. Levy, J. A., Shimabukuro, J., McHugh, T., Casavant, C., Stites, D., and Oshiro, L. (1985). AIDS-associated retroviruses (ARV) can productively infect other cells besides human T helper cells. *Virology 147*:441-448.

13. Gartner, S., Markovits, P., Markovitz, D. M., Kaplan, M. H., Gallo, R. C., and Popovic, M. (1986). The role of mononuclear phagocytes in HTLV-III/LAV infection. *Science 233*:215-219.

14. Morgan, D. A., Ruscetti, F. W., and Gallo, R. C. (1976). Selective in vitro growth of T-lymphocytes from normal human bone marrow. *Science 193*:1007-1008.

15. Barre-Sinoussi, F., Montagnier, L., Lidereau, R., Sisman, J., Wood, J., and Chermann, J. C. (1979). Enhancement of retrovirus production by anti-interferon serum. *Ann. Microbiol. (Paris) 130B*:349-362.

16. Lifson, J. D., Reyes, G. R., McGrath, M. S., Stein, B. S., and Engleman, E. G. (1986). AIDS retrovirus induced cytopathology: Giant cell formation and involvement of CD4 antigen. *Science 232*:1123-1127.

17. Wittek, A. E., Phelan, M. A., Wells, M. A. et al. (1987). Detection of human immunodeficiency virus core protein in plasma by enzyme immunoassay. *Ann. Intern. Med. 107*:286-292.

18. Wofsy, C. B., Cohen, J. B., Hauer, L. B. et al. (1986). Isolation of AIDS-associated retrovirus from genital secretions of women with antibodies to the virus. *Lancet 1*:527-529.

19. Vogt, M. W., Witt, D. J., Craven, D. E. et al. (1986). Isolation of HTLV-III/LAV from cervical secretions of women at risk for AIDS. *Lancet 1*:525-527.

20. Archibald, D. W., Zon, L., Groopman, J. E. et al. (1986). Antibodies to human T-lymphotropic virus type III (HTLV-III) in saliva of acquired immunodeficiency syndrome (AIDS) patients and in persons at risk for AIDS. *Blood 67*:831-834.

21. Archibald, D. W., Witt, D. J., Craven, D. E. et al. (1987). Antibodies to human immunodeficiency virus in cervical secretions from women at risk for AIDS. *J. Infect. Dis. 156*:240-241.

22. Gallo, D., Kimpton, J. S., and Dailey, P. J. (1987). Comparative studies on use of fresh and frozen peripheral blood lymphocyte specimens for isolation of human immunodeficiency virus and effects of cell lysis on isolation efficiency. *J. Clin. Microbiol. 25*:1291-1294.

23. Lee, M. H., Sano, K., Morales, F. E., and Imagawa, D. T. (1987). Sensitive reverse transcriptase assay to detect and quantitate human immunodeficiency virus. *J. Clin. Microbiol. 25*:1717-1721.

24. Gupta, P., Balachandran, K., Grovit, K., Webster, D., Rinaldi, C., Jr. (1987). Detection of human immunodeficiency virus by reverse transcriptase assay, antigen capture assay, and radioimmunoassay. *J. Clin. Microbiol. 25*:1122-1125.

25. Higgins, J. R., Pedersen, N. C., and Carlson, J. R. (1986). Detection and differentiation by sandwich enzyme-linked immunosorbent assay of human T-cell lymphotropic virus type III/lymphadenopathy-associated virus and acquired immunodeficiency syndrome-associated retroviruslike clinical isolates. *J. Clin. Microbiol. 24*:424-430.

26. Resnick, L. and Novatt, G. (1986). Human T-cell lymphotropic viruses: syncytia formation. *JAMA 255*:3421.

27. Mitsuya, H., Popovic, M., Yarchoan, R., Matsushita, S., Gallo, R. C., and Broder, S. (1984). Suramin protection of T cells in vitro against infectivity and cytopathic effect of HTLV-III. *Science 226*:172-174.

28. Cooper, D. A., Gold, J., Maclean, P. et al. (1985). Acute AIDS retrovirus infection. *Lancet 1*:537-540.

29. Cooper, D. A., Imrie, A. A., and Penny, R. (1987). Antibody response to human immunodeficiency virus after primary infection. *J. Infect. Dis. 155*:1113-1118.

30. CDC (1987). Update: Human immunodeficiency virus infections in health-care workers exposed to blood of infected patients. *MMWR 36*:285-289.

31. *Lancet* (1984). Needlestick transmission of HTLV-III from a patient infected in Africa. *2*:1376-1377.

32. Esteban, J. I., Shih, J. W.-K., Tai, C. C., Bodner, A. J., Kay, J. W. D., and Alter, H. J. (1985). Importance of Western blot analysis in predicting infectivity of HTLV-III/LAV positive blood. *Lancet 2*:1083-1086.

33. Schupbach, J., Haller, O., Vogt, M. et al. (1985). Antibodies to HTLV-III in Swiss patients with AIDS and pre-AIDS and in groups at risk for AIDS. *N. Engl. J. Med. 312*:265-270.

34. Goudsmit, J., Lange, J. M. A., Paul, D. A., and Dawson, G. J. (1987). Antigenemia and antibody titers to core and envelope antigens in AIDS, AIDS-related complex, and subclinical human immunodeficiency virus infection. *J. Infect. Dis. 155*:558-560.

35. Burke, D. S., Redfield, R. R., Putman, P., and Alexander, S. S. (1987). Variations in Western blot banding patterns of human T-cell lymphotropic virus type III/lymphadenopathy-associated virus. *J. Clin. Microbiol. 25*:81-84.

36. Weiss, S. H., Goedert, J. J., Sargadharan, M. G. et al. (1985). Screening test for HTLV-III (AIDS agent) antibodies. *JAMA 253*:221-225.

37. Carlson, J. R., Hinrichs, S. H., Yee, J., Gardner, M. B., and Pedersen, J. C. (1986). Evaluation of three commercial screening tests for AIDS virus antibodies. *Am. J. Clin. Pathol. 86*:357-359.

38. Handsfield, H. H., Wandell, M., Goldstein, L. et al. (1987). Screening and diagnostic performance of enzyme immunoassay for antibody to lymphadenopathy-associated virus. *J. Clin. Microbiol. 25*:879-884.

39. Barrett, J. E., Dawson, G., Heller, J. et al. (1986). Performance evaluation of the Abbott HTLV-III EIA, a test for antibody to HTLV-III in donor blood. *Am. J. Clin. Pathol. 86*:180-185.

40. Martin, P. W., Burger, D. R., Caouette, S., Goldstein, A. S., and Peetoom, F. (1986). Importance of confirmatory tests after strongly positive HTLV-III screening tests. *N. Engl. J. Med. 314*:1577.

41. Thorn, R. M., Beltz, G. A., Hung, C.-H. et al. (1987). Enzyme immunoassay using a novel recombinant polypeptide to detect human immunodeficiency virus env antibody. *J. Clin. Microbiol. 25*:1207-1212.

42. Wang, J. J. G., Steel, S., Wisniewolski, R., and Wang, C. Y. (1986). Detection of antibodies to human T-lymphotropic virus type III by using a synthetic peptide of 21 amino acid residues corresponding to a highly antigenic segment of gp42 envelope protein. *Proc. Natl. Acad. Sci. USA 83*:6159-6163.

43. Bayes, T. (1763). An essay toward solving a problem in the doctrine of chance. *Philos. Trans. R. Soc. Lond. 53*:370.

44. CDC (1985). Results of human T-lymphotropic virus type III test kits reported from blood collection centers—United States, April 22-May 19, 1985. *MMWR 34*:375-376.

45. Kuhnl, P., Seidl, S., Kurth, R. et al. (1985). Human T-cell lymphotropic virus antibody screening: Data survey on 33,603 German blood donors correlated to confirmatory tests. *Vox Sang. 49*:327-330.

46. Heneson, N. (1986). AIDS and the blood testing program. *ASM News 52*:458-459.

47. Mendenhall, C. L., Roselle, G. A., Grossman, C. J., Rouster, S. D., Weesner, R. E., and Dumaswala, U. (1986). False-positive tests for HTLV-III antibodies in alcoholic patients with hepatitis. *N. Engl. J. Med. 314*:921-922.

48. Moore, J. D., Cone, E. F., and Alexander, S. S., Jr. (1986). HTLV-III seropositivity in 1971-1972 parenteral drug abusers—a case of false positives or evidence of viral exposure? *N. Engl. J. Med. 314*:1387-1388.

49. Neale, T. J., Dagger, J., Fong, R. et al. (1985). False positive anti-HTLV-III serology. *N. Z. Med. J. 98*:914.

50. Sayers, M. H., Beatty, P. G., and Hansen, J. A. (1986). HLA antibodies as a cause of false-positive reactions in screening enzyme immunoassays for antibodies to human T-lymphotropic virus type III. *Transfusion 26*:113-115.

51. Saag, M. S. and Britz, J. (1986). Asymptomatic blood donor with a false positive HTLV-III Western blot. *N. Engl. J. Med. 314*:118.

52. Zarling, J. M., Eichberg, J. W., Moran, P. A. et al. (1987). Proliferative and cytotoxic T cells to AIDS virus glycoproteins in chimpanzees immunized with a recombinant vaccinia virus expressing AIDS virus envelope glycoproteins. *J. Immunol. 139*:988-990.

53. Sivak, S. L. and Wormser, G. P. (1986). Predictive value of a screening test for antibodies to HTLV-III. *Am. J. Clin. Pathol. 85*:700-703.

54. Petricciani, J. C. (1985). Licensed tests for antibody to human T-lymphotropic virus type III. Sensitivity and specificity. *Ann. Intern. Med. 103*:726-729.

55. Yomtovian, R. (1986). HTLV-III antibody testing: The false-negative rate. *JAMA* 255:609.

56. *JAMA* (1986). Transfusion-associated human T-lymphotropic virus type III/ lymphadenopathy-associated virus infection from a seronegative donor—Colorado. *256*:574-575.

57. Fox, J. L. (1987). AIDS: The public health-public policy crisis. *ASM News 53*: 428-430.

58. Towbin, H., Staehelin, T., and Gordon, J. (1979). Electrophoretic transfer of proteins from polyacrylamide gels to nitrocellulose sheets: Procedure and some applications. *Proc. Natl. Acad. Sci. USA 76*:4350-4354.

59. Tsang, V. C. W., Hancock, K., Wilson, M., Palmer, D. F., Whaley, S., McDougal, J. S., and Kennedy, S. (1986). *Enzyme-Linked Immunoelectrotransfer blot technique (EITB) (Western blot) for HTLV-III/LAV Antibodies. Developmental Guidelines, December 1986*. U.S. Department of Health and Human Services, Public Health Service, Centers for Disease Control, Atlanta, Ga.

60. Martin, K., Katz, B. Z., and Miller, G. (1987). AIDS and antibodies to human immunodeficiency virus (HIV) in children and their families. *J. Infect. Dis. 155*: 54-63.

61. Berstein, J. M., Stokes, C. E., and Fernie, B. (1987). Comparative sensitivity of ^{125}I-protein A and enzyme-conjugated antibodies for detection of immunoblotted proteins. *J. Clin. Microbiol. 25*:72-75.

62. Burke, D. and Wilber, J. (1987). Work Group IV—Supplemental tests for antibody detection. In *Second Consensus Conference on HIV Testing. Report and Recommendations*. Committee on HIV, Association of State and Territorial Public Health Laboratory Directors, March 16-18, 1987, Atlanta, Ga, pp. 12-14.

63. Package insert for the Human Immunodeficiency Virus (HIV) Biotech/Dupont HIV Western Blot Kit for Detection of Antibodies to HIV. E.I. du Pont de Nemours & Company (Inc.), Medical Products Department, Wilmington, Del.

64. Carlson, J. C., Yee, J., Hinrichs, S. H., Bryant, M. L., Gardner, M. B., and Pedersen, N. C. (1987). Comparison of indirect immunofluorescence and Western blot for detection of anti-human immunodeficiency virus antibodies. *J. Clin. Microbiol. 25*:494-497.

65. Gallo, D., Diggs, J. L., Shell, G. R., Dailey, P. J., Hoffman, M. J., and Riggs, J. L. (1986). Comparison of detection of antibody to the acquired immune deficiency syndrome virus by enzyme immunoassay, immunofluorescence, and Western blot methods. *J. Clin. Microbiol. 23*:1049-1051.

66. Lennette, E. T., Karpatkin, S., and Levy, J. A. (1987). Indirect immunofluorescence assay for antibodies to human immunodeficiency virus. *J. Clin. Microbiol. 25*:199-202.

67. Essex, M., McLane, M. F., Lee, T. H. et al. (1983). Antibodies to cell membrane antigens associated with human T-cell leukemia virus in patients with AIDS. *Science 220*:859-862.

68. Saah, A. J., Farzadegan, H., Fox, R. et al. (1987). Detection of early antibodies in human immunodeficiency virus infection by enzyme-linked immunosorbent assay, Western blot, and radioimmunoprecipitation. *J. Clin. Microbiol. 25*: 1605-1610.

69. Chaisson, R. E., Allain, J.-P., Leuther, M., and Volberding, P. A. (1986). Significant changes in HIV antigen level in the serum of patients treated with azidothymidine. *N. Engl. J. Med. 315*:1610-1611.

70. Gaub, J., Lindhardt, B. O., Poulsen, A. G., Pedersen, C., Nielsen, C. M., Faber, V. et al. (1987). Anti-CMV treatment with DHPG does not affect HIV antigen levels in AIDS patients. *Abstr. III Int. Conf. AIDS.* Washington, D.C., p. 47, Abstr. MP224.

71. Vernon, A., Schulof, R. S. for the Ribavirin ARC Study Group (1987). Serum HIV core antigen in symptomatic ARC patients taking oral ribavirin or placebo. *Abstr. III Int. Conf. AIDS.* Washington, D.C., p. 58, Abstr. T8.6.

72. Tregellas, W. M. and Olive, J. A. (1986). Positive HTLV-III antibody tests due to apparent cross-reactivity with p24 region of HTLV-III [Abstr. S129]. *Transfusion 26*:577.

73. Mintz, L., Drew, W. L., Miner, R. C., and Braff, E. H. (1983). Cytomegalovirus infections in homosexual men. An epidemiological study. *Ann. Intern. Med. 99*:326-329.

74. Schmidt, N. J., Dennis, J., Devlin, V., Gallo, D., and Mills, J. (1983). Comparison of direct immunofluorescence and direct immunoperoxidase procedures for detection of herpes simplex virus antigen in lesion specimens. *J. Clin. Microbiol. 18*:445-448.

75. Salahuddin, S. Z., Ablashi, D. V., Markham, P. D. et al. (1986). Isolation of a new virus, HBLV, in patients with lymphoproliferative disorders. *Science 234*: 596-603.

76. Whimbey, E., Gold, J. W. M., Polsky, B. et al. (1986). Bacteremia and fungemia in patients with the acquired immunodeficiency syndrome. *Ann. Intern. Med. 104*:511-514.

77. Eng, R. H. K., Bishburg, E., Smith, S. M., Geller, H., and Kapila, R. (1986). Bacteremia and fungemia in patients with acquired immune deficiency syndrome. *Am. J. Clin. Pathol. 86*:105-107.

78. Celum, C. L., Chaisson, R. E., Rutherford, G. W., Barnhart, J. L., and Echenberg, D. F. (1987). Incidence of salmonellosis in patients with acquired immunodeficiency syndrome. *J. Infect. Dis. 156*:998-1002.

79. Gerberding, J. L., Krieger, K., and Sande, M. A. (1986). Recurrent bactermic infection with *S. pneumoniae* in patients with AIDS virus (AV) infection. *Abstr. 26th Intersci. Conf. Antimicrob. Agents Chemother.* New Orleans, La, p. 177; Abstr. 443.

80. Feeley, J. C., Gorman, G. W., Weaver, R. E. et al. (1978). Primary isolation media for Legionnaires' disease bacterium. *J. Clin. Microbiol. 8*:320-325.

81. England, A. C., Fraser, D. W., Plikaytis, B. D., Tsai, T. F., Storch, G., and Broome, C. v. (1981). Sporadic legionellosis in the United States: The first thousand cases. *Ann. Intern. Med. 94*:164-170.

82. Zuravleff, J. J., Yu, V. L., Shonnard, J. W., Davis, B. K., and Rihs, J. D. (1983). Diagnosis of Legionnaires' disease. An update of laboratory methods with new emphasis on isolation by culture. *JAMA 250*:1981-1985.

83. Meyer, R. D. (1983). Legionella infections: A review of five years of research. *Rev. Infect. Dis. 5*:258-278.

84. Edelstein, P. H. and Finegold, S. J. (1979). Use of a semi-selective medium to culture *Legionella pneumophila* from contaminated lung specimens. *J. Clin. Microbiol. 10*:141-143.

85. Moncada, J. V., Schachter, J., and Wofsy, C. (1986). Prevalence of *Chlamydia trachomatis* lung infection in patients with acquired immune deficiency syndrome. *J. Clin. Microbiol. 23*:986.

86. Kuo, C. C., Chen, H. H., Wang, S. P., and Grayston, J. T. (1986). Identification of a new group of *Chlamydia psittaci* strains called TWAR. *J. Clin. Microbiol. 24*:1034-1037.

87. Regan, J. and Lowe, F. (1977). Enrichment medium for the isolation of *Bordetella*. *J. Clin. Microbiol. 6*:303-309.

88. Totten, P. A., Fennell, C. L., Tenover, F. C. et al. (1985). *Campylobacter cinaedi* (sp. nov.) and *Campylobacter fennelliae* (sp. nov.): Two new *Campylobacter* species associated with enteric disease in homosexual men. *J. Infect. Dis. 151*:131-139.

89. Pasternak, C., Bolivar, R., Hopfer, R. L. et al. (1984). Bacteremia caused by *Campylobacter*-like organisms in two male homosexuals. *Ann. Intern. Med. 101*:339-341.

90. Cimolai, N., Gill, M. J., Jones, A. et al. (1987). *Campylobacter cinaedi* bacteremia: Case report and laboratory findings. *J. Clin. Microbiol. 25*:942-943.

91. Ng, V. L., Hadley, W. K., Fennell, C. L., Flores, B. M., and Stamm, W. E. (1987). Successive bacteremias with *Campylobacter cinaedi* and *Campylobacter fennelliae* in a bisexual male. *J. Clin. Microbiol. 25*:2008-2009.

92. Flores, B. M., Fennell, C. L., Holmes, K. K., and Stamm, W. E. (1985). In vitro susceptibilities of *Campylobacter*-like organisms to twenty antimicrobial agents. *Antimicrob. Agents Chemother. 28*:188-191.

93. Greene, J. B., Sidhu, G. S., Lewis, S. et al. (1982). *Mycobacterium avium-intracellulare*: A cause of disseminated life-threatening infection in homosexuals and drug abusers. *Ann. Intern. Med. 97*:539-546.

94. Macher, A. M., Kovacs, J. A., Gill, V. et al. (1983). Bacteremia due to *Mycobacterium avium-intracellulare* in the acquired immunodeficiency syndrome. *Ann. Intern. Med. 99*:782-785.

95. Zakowski, P., Fligiel, S., Berlin, O. G. W., and Johnson, B. L., Jr. (1982). Disseminated *Mycobacterium avium-intracellulare* infection in homosexual men dying of acquired immunodeficiency. *JAMA 248*:2980-2982.

96. Wong, B., Edwards, F. F., Kiehn, T. E. et al. (1985). Continuous high-grade *Mycobacterium avium-intracellulare* bacteremia in patients with the acquired immune deficiency syndrome. *Am. J. Med. 78*:35-40.

97. Poropatich, C. O., Labriola, A. M., and Tuazon, C. U. (1987). Acid-fast smear and culture of respiratory secretions, bone marrows, and stools as predictors of disseminated *Mycobacterium avium* complex infection. *J. Clin. Microbiol. 25*: 929-930.

98. Kiehn, T. E., Edwards, F. F., Brannon, P. et al. (1985). Infections caused by *Mycobacterium avium* complex in immunocompromised patients: Diagnosis by blood culture and fecal examination, antimicrobial susceptibility tests, and morphological and seroagglutination characteristics. *J. Clin. Microbiol. 21*:168-173.

99. Yajko, D. M., Nassos, P. S., and Hadley, W. K. (1987). Broth microdilution testing of susceptibilities to 30 antimicrobial agents of *Mycobacterium avium* strains from patients with acquired immune deficiency syndrome. *Antimicrob. Agents Chemother. 31*:1579-1584.

100. Yajko, D. M., Nassos, P. S., and Hadley, W. K. (1987). Therapeutic implications of inhibition versus killing of *Mycobacterium avium* complex by antimicrobial agents. *Antimicrob. Agents Chemother. 31*:117-120.

101. Masur, H., Tuazon, C., Gill, V. et al. (1987). Effect of combined clofazimine and ansamycin therapy on *Mycobacterium avium-Mycobacterium intracellulare* bacteremia in patients with AIDS. *J. Infect. Dis. 155*:127-129.

102. Kirihara, J. M., Hillier, S. L., and Coyle, M. B. (1985). Improved detection times for *Mycobacterium avium* complex and *Mycobacterium tuberculosis* with the BACTEC radiometric system. *J. Clin. Microbiol. 22*:841-845.

103. Kiehn, T. E., Gold, J. E., Brannon, P., Timberger, R. J., and Armstrong, D. (1985). *Mycobacterium tuberculosis* bacteremia detected by the isolator lysis-centrifugation blood culture system. *J. Clin. Microbiol. 21*:647-648.

104. Roberts, M. C., McMillan, C., and Coyle, M. B. (1987). Whole chromosomal DNA probes for rapid identification of *Mycobacterium tuberculosis* and *Mycobacterium avium* complex. *J. Clin. Microbiol. 25*:1239-1243.

105. Drake, T. A., Hindler, J. A., Berlin, O. G. W., and Bruckner, D. A. (1987). Rapid identification of *Mycobacterium avium* complex in culture using DNA probes. *J. Clin. Microbiol. 25*:1442-1445.

106. Kiehn, T. E. and Edwards, F. F. (1987). Rapid identification using a specific DNA probe of *Mycobacterium avium* complex from patients with acquired immunodeficiency syndrome. *J. Clin. Microbiol. 25*:1551-1552.

107. Gordon, M. A. and Lapa, E. W. (1974). Elimination of rheumatoid factor in the latex test for cryptococcosis. *Am. J. Clin. Pathol. 61*:488-494.

108. Stamm, A. M. and Polt, S. S. (1980). False-negative cryptococcal antigen test. *JAMA 244*:1359.

109. Kaufman, L. and Reiss, E. (1985). Serodiagnosis of fungal diseases. In *Manual of Clinical Microbiology*, 4th ed. (Lennette, E. H., Balows, A., Hausler, W. J., Jr., and Shadomy, H. J., eds.). Washington, D.C., American Society for Microbiology, pp. 937-939.

110. Mandell, W., Goldberg, D. M., and Neu, H. C. (1986). Histoplasmosis in patients with the acquired immune deficiency syndrome. *Am. J. Med. 81*:974-978.

111. McNabb, S. J. N., Hensel, D. M., Welch, D. F., Heijbel, H., McKee, G. L., and Istre, G. R. (1985). Comparison of sedimentation and flotation techniques for identification of *Cryptosporidium* sp. oocysts in a large outbreak of human diarrhea. *J. Clin. Microbiol. 22*:587-589.

112. Garcia, L., Bruckner, D. A., Brewer, T. C., and Shimizu, R. Y. (1983). Techniques for the recovery and identification of *Cryptosporidium* oocysts from stool specimens. *J. Clin. Microbiol. 18*:185-190.

113. Package insert for the Merifluor-Cryptosporidium Indirect Immunofluorescent Detection Procedure. Meridian Diagnostics, Inc., Cincinnati, Ohio.

114. Ma, P., Villanueva, T. G., Kaufman, D., and Gillooley, J. F. (1984). Respiratory cryptosporidiosis in the acquired immunodeficiency syndrome. *JAMA* *252*:1298-1301.

115. Restrepo, C., Macher, A. M., and Radany, E. H. (1987). Disseminated extraintestinal isosporiasis in a patient with acquired immune deficiency syndrome. *Am. J. Clin. Pathol. 87*:536-542.

116. DeHovitz, J. A., Pape, J. W., Boncy, M., and Johnson, W. D., Jr. (1986). Clinical manifestations and therapy of *Isospora belli* infection in patients with the acquired immunodeficiency syndrome. *N. Engl. J. Med. 315*:87-90.

117. Luft, B. J., Brooks, R. G., Conley, F. K., McCabe, R. E., and Remington, J. S. (1984). Toxoplasmic encephalitis in patients with acquired immune deficiency syndrome. *JAMA 252*:913-917.

118. Ruskin, J. and Remington, J. S. (1976). Toxoplasmosis in the compromised host. *Ann. Intern. Med. 84*:193-199.

119. Snider, W. K., Simpson, D. M., Nielsen, S. et al. (1983). Neurological complications of acquired immune deficiency syndrome: Analysis of 50 patients. *Ann. Neurol. 14*:403-418.

120. Levy, R. M., Bredesen, D. E., and Rosenblum, M. L. (1985). Neurological manifestations of the acquired immunodeficiency syndrome (AIDS): Experience at UCSF and review of the literature. *J. Neurosurg. 62*:475-495.

121. Hauser, W. E., Luft, B. J., Conley, F. K., and Remington, J. S. (1982). Central nervous system toxoplasmosis in homosexual and heterosexual adults. *N. Engl. J. Med. 307*:498-499.

122. Conley, F. K., Jenkins, K. A., and Remington, J. S. (1981). *Toxoplasma gondii* infection of the central nervous system. *Hum. Pathol. 12*:690-698.

123. Broaddus, C., Dake, M. D., Stulbarg, M. S. et al. (1985). Bronchoalveolar lavage and transbronchial biopsy for the diagnosis of pulmonary infections in the acquired immunodeficiency syndrome. *Ann. Intern. Med. 102*:747-752.

124. Bigby, T. D., Margolskee, D., Curtis, J. L. et al. (1986). The usefulness of induced sputum in the diagnosis of *Pneumocystis carinii* pneumonia in patients with the acquired immunodeficiency syndrome. *Am. Rev. Resp. Dis. 133*:515-518.

125. Ng, V. L., Gartner, I., Weymouth, L. A., Goodman, C. D., Hopewell, P. C., and Hadley, W. K. (1989). The use of mucolysed induced sputum for the identification of pulmonary pathogens associated with human immunodeficiency virus infection. Submitted.

126. Blumenfeld, W., Wagar, E., and Hadley, W. K. (1984). Use of the transbronchial biopsy for diagnosis of opportunistic pulmonary infections in acquired immunodeficiency syndrome (AIDS). *Am. J. Clin. Pathol. 81*:1-5.

127. Pitchenik, A. E., Ganjei, P., Torres, A. et al. (1986). Sputum examination for the diagnosis of *Pneumocystis carinii* pneumonia in the acquired immunodeficiency syndrome. *Am. Rev. Resp. Dis. 133*:226-229.

128. Gosbey, L. L., Howard, R. M., Witebsky, F. G. et al. (1985). Advantages of a modified toluidine blue O stain and bronchoalveolar lavage for the diagnosis of *Pneumocystis carinii* pneumonia. *J. Clin. Microbiol. 22*:803-807.

129. Kovacs, J. A., Ng, V. L., Masur, H. et al. (1988). Diagnosis of *Pneumocystis carinii* pneumonia: Improved detection in sputum with use of monoclonal antibodies. *New. Engl. J. Med. 318*:589-593.

130. Medina, I., Mills, J., and Wofsy, C. (1987). Serum lactate dehydrogenase (LDH) in *Pneumocystis carinii* pneumonia (PCP) in AIDS: Possible indicator and predictor of disease activity. *Abstr. III Int. Conf. AIDS.* Washington, D.C., p. 109, Abstr. W5.5.

131. Zimmerman, H. J. and Henry, J. B. (1984). Clinical enzymology. In *Clinical Diagnosis and management by Laboratory Methods*, 17th ed. (Henry, J. B., ed.). Philadelphia, W.B. Saunders, pp. 259-269.

132. Schneiderman, D. J., Cello, J. P., and Laing, F. C. (1987). Papillary stenosis and sclerosing cholangitis in the acquired immunodeficiency syndrome. *Ann. Intern. Med. 106*:546-549.

133. Nath, N., Wunderlich, C., Darr, F. W. II, Douglas, D. K., and Dodd, R. Y. (1987). Immunoglobulin level in donor blood reactive for antibodies to human immunodeficiency virus. *J. Clin. Microbiol. 25*:364-369.

134. Heriot, K., Hallquist, A. E., and Tomar, R. H. (1985). Paraproteinemia in patients with acquired immunodeficiency syndrome (AIDS) or lymphadeno- pathy syndrome (LAS). *Clin. Chem. 31*:1224-1226.

135. Deutsch, M., Brown, M. A., and Repetti, C. F. (1987). The frequency and characterization of oligoclonal protein (OCP) bands in individuals with HIV antibodies. *Abstr. III Int. Conf. AIDS.* Washington, D.C., p. 29, Abstr. MP114.

136. Bratt, G., Waldenlind, L., von Krogh, G., Karlsson, A., Moberg, L., and Sandstrom, E. (1987). Oligoclonal IgG bands on serum-electrophoresis in a cohort of homosexual men in Stockholm, Sweden. *Abstr. III Int. Conf. AIDS.* Washington, D.C., p. 185, Abstr. THP130.

137. Ng, V. L., Hwang, K. M., Reyes, G. R., Kaplan, L. D., Khayam-Bashi, H., Hadley, W. K., and McGrath, M. S. (1988). High titer anti-HIV antibody re- activity associated with a paraprotein spike in a homosexual male with AIDS related complex. *Blood 71*:1397-1401.

138. Klatzmann, D., Champagne, E., Chamaret, S., Gruest, J., Guetard, D., Her- cend, T., Gluckman, J. C., and Montagnier, L. (1984). T-lymphocyte T4 mole- cule behaves as the receptor for human retrovirus LAV. *Nature 312*:767-768.

139. Sattentau, Q. J., Dalgleish, A. G., Weiss, R. A., and Beverley, P. C. L. (1986). Epitopes of the CD4 antigen and HIV infection. *Science 234*:1120-1123.

140. Stites, D. P. (1987). Clinical laboratory methods for detection of cellular im- mune function. In *Basic and Clinical Immunology*, 6th ed. (Stites, D. P., Stobo, J. D., and Wells, J. V., eds.). Norwalk, Conn., Appleton & Lange, p. 289.

141. CDC (1987). Revision of the CDC surveillance case definition for acquired im- munodeficiency syndrome. *MMWR 36*(suppl.):1S.

142. Polk, B. F., Fox, R., Brookmeyer, R. et al. (1987). Predictors of the acquired immunodeficiency syndrome developing in a cohort of seropositive homo- sexual men. *N. Engl. J. Med. 316*:61-66.

143. Reddy, M. M., Englard, A., Brown, D., Buimovici-Klien, E., and Grieco, M. H. (1987). Lymphoproliferative responses to human immunodeficiency virus antigen in asymptomatic intravenous drug abusers and in patients with lym- phadenopathy or AIDS. *J. Infect. Dis. 156*:374-376.

Index

About the Editors

GIFFORD S. LEOUNG is Assistant Clinical Professor of Medicine, Department of Medicine, University of California, San Francisco. He is also affiliated with the Division of AIDS Activities and has appointments in the Division of Infectious Diseases and the Chest Service at San Francisco General Hospital, California. An invited speaker or panel member at many conferences, Dr. Leoung has published some 20 research articles, abstracts, and book chapters. He is also an investigator in the National Institutes of Health AIDS Clinical Trials Group. Among the professional organizations he belongs to are the American College of Chest Physicians, American Thoracic Society, American Society of Microbiology, California Medical Association, and American College of Physicians. He received the B.S. degree (1975) in chemical engineering from Columbia University, New York, New York, and M.D. degree (1979) from Cornell University, New York, New York.

JOHN MILLS is Professor of Medicine, Department of Medicine, University of California, San Francisco, as well as Chief, Division of Infectious Diseases, San Francisco General Hospital, California. Dr. Mills has published over 250 research articles, book chapters, books, and abstracts. A principal investigator of the University of California, San Francisco AIDS Clinical Trials Unit, Dr. Mills is also the Chairman of the Opportunistic Infection Committee of the national AIDS Clinical Trials Group effort. He is a Fellow of the American College of Physicians and Infectious Diseases Society of America, and a member of the American Society of Microbiology, American Thoracic Society, American Federation for Clinical Research, and several others. Dr. Mills received the B.S. degree (1961) in medicine from the University of Chicago, Illinois, and M.D. degree (1966) from Harvard University Medical School, Boston, Massachusetts.

T - #1055 - 101024 - C4 - 229/152/22 [24] - CB - 9780824780807 - Gloss Lamination